MIND AND BRAIN

JOURNEY THROUGH THE MIND AND BODY

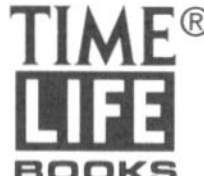

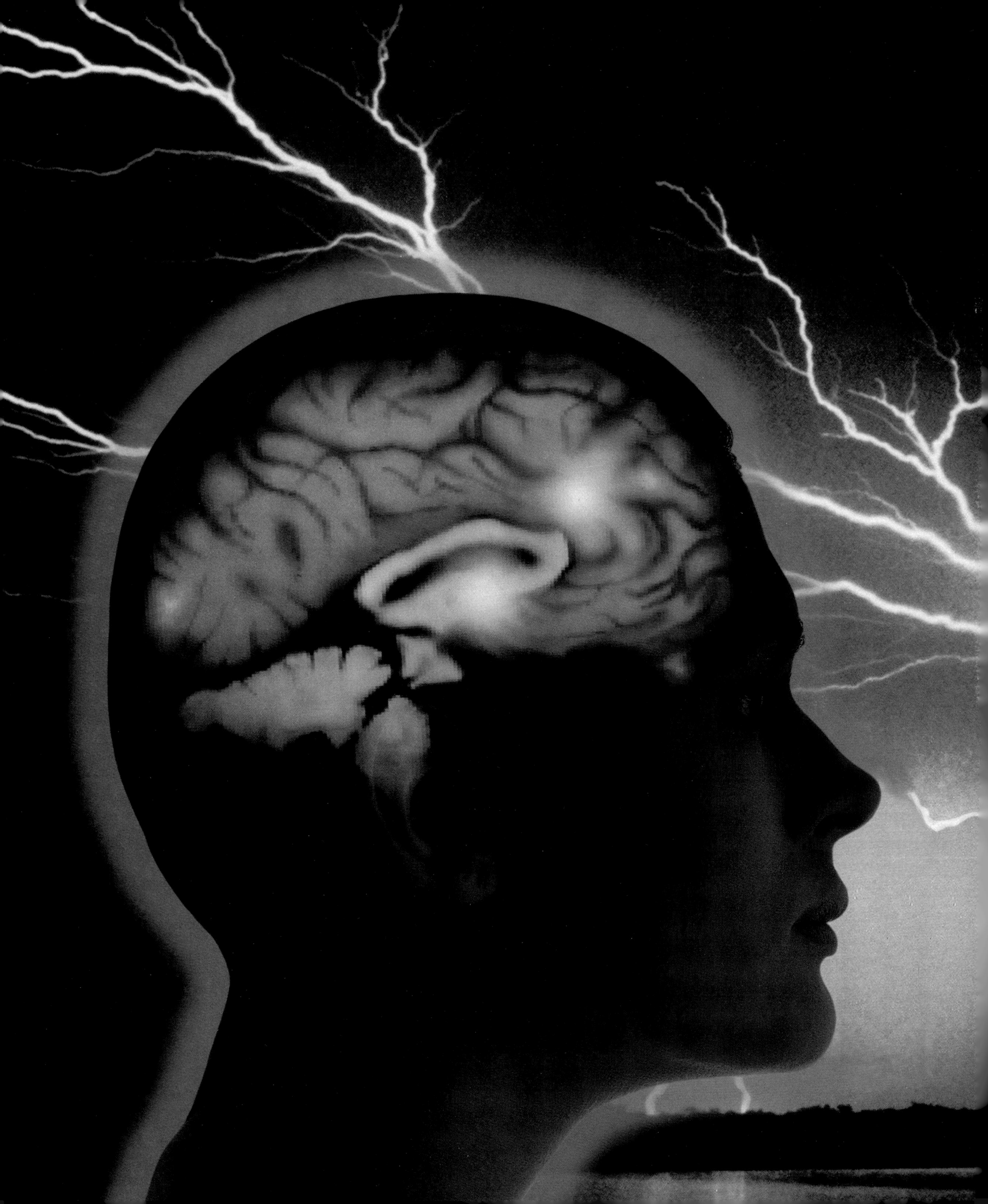

CONTENTS

JOURNEY THROUGH THE MIND AND BODY

SERIES EDITOR: Roberta Conlan
Administrative Editor: Judith W. Shanks

Editorial Staff for *Mind and Brain*
Deputy Editors: Tina S. McDowell (pictures); Robert Somerville (text)
Art Directors: Barbara Sheppard, Fatima Taylor
Text Editors: Lee Hassig, Jim Hicks, Jim Watson
Associate Editors/Research: Mark H. Rogers (principal), Karen Monks, Barbara Sause
Assistant Editors/Research: Ruth Goldberg, Jennifer Mendelsohn, Narisara Murray
Writer: Mark Galan
Assistant Art Director: Sue Pratt
Senior Copyeditor: Juli Duncan
Copyeditor: Donna D. Carey
Editorial Assistant: Julia Kendrick
Picture Coordinator: Mark C. Burnett

Special Contributors:
Joseph Alper, Sharon Begley, George Constable, Tucker Coombe, Elizabeth Corcoran, Margery A. duMond, Elaine Friebele, Stephen Hart, Gina Maranto, Dave Thomson, Mitch Waldrop (text); Jocelyn Lindsay, Maureen McHugh (research); Barbara L. Klein (index); John Drummond, Cynthia T. Richardson (design).

Correspondents:
Elisabeth Kraemer-Singh (Bonn); Christine Hinze (London); Christina Lieberman (New York); Dag Christensen (Oslo); Maria Vincenza Aloisi (Paris); Ann Natanson (Rome); Mary Johnson (Stockholm). Valuable assistance was also provided by Elizabeth Brown, Katheryn White (New York).

Library of Congress Cataloging in Publication Data

Mind and brain / by the editors of Time-Life Books.
p. cm. — (Journey through the mind and body)
Includes bibliographical references and index.
ISBN 0-7835-1000-4 (Trade) —
ISBN 0-7835-1001-2 (Library)
1. Cognitive neuroscience—Popular works.
I. Time-Life Books. II. Series.
QP360.5.M545 1993
612.8'2—dc20 93-1152

First printing. Printed in U.S.A. Published simultaneously in Canada. School and library distribution by Simon & Schuster, New York, New York 10020.

This volume is one of a series that explores the fascinating inner universe of the human mind and body.

CONSULTANTS

ALBERT J. BERGER teaches physiology and biophysics at the School of Medicine of the University of Washington. His research focuses on the neurons responsible for generating respiratory rhythms.

ALAN GEVINS is director of the EEG Systems Laboratory and president of SAM Technology in San Francisco.

JOHN HART, JR., who teaches neurology at the Johns Hopkins School of Medicine in Baltimore, is also an associate member of the Zanvyl Krieger Mind/Brain Institute of the Johns Hopkins University with a special interest in how objects are represented visually and verbally in the brain.

RONALD LESSER teaches neurology at the Johns Hopkins University in Baltimore; his special interests include epilepsy, higher cortical function, and electrophysiology.

ARTHUR D. LOEWY teaches at Washington University School of Medicine in St. Louis. His research is to understand the basic brain circuits and mechanisms that control vital life functions.

JOHN R. MOFFETT teaches at Georgetown University, where he does research on neurotransmitters in the visual system.

DEEPAK N. PANDYA's research specialty is the architecture of the cerebral cortex. He is a neurologist at the Bedford Veterans Administration Hospital and teaches at the Boston University School of Medicine and the Harvard Medical School.

RICHARD M. RESTAK, who has a private practice in neurology in Washington, D.C., also teaches at Georgetown University and consults for numerous scientific and lay organizations.

MICHAEL E. SMITH is employed at EEG Systems Laboratory and SAM Technology in San Francisco, where he works on advanced technologies for measuring human neurocognitive functions.

LARRY R. SQUIRE works at the Veterans Affairs Medical Center in San Diego, teaches in the Department of Psychiatry at the University of California, and specializes in memory and learning.

MIND AND BRAIN

JOURNEY THROUGH THE MIND AND BODY

BY THE EDITORS OF TIME-LIFE BOOKS
ALEXANDRIA, VIRGINIA

1

The Search for the Mind's "I"

"He keeps asking for the time or date again and again all day," George's wife told his doctor several months after the 52-year-old engineer's heart bypass surgery. "He's even eaten breakfast two or three times in a morning, each time as if it's the first."

This disturbing memory problem had become evident shortly after the operation, a serious procedure made riskier because of a severely clogged artery that reduced blood flow to George's brain. At the end of the operation, his heart had unexpectedly refused to beat on its own. Sustained by life-support systems, he had lain in a coma for nearly two days before his heart had miraculously started pumping again.

At first doctors thought that George—and more specifically, his brain—had come through unharmed. When he woke up, his perceptual skills and native intellect were intact, and he could vividly recall events and people from his life before surgery. Within hours, however, the hospital staff recognized that George could remember nothing that had happened since the operation. Every minute or so, the blackboard of recent events was simply wiped clean.

A brain scan confirmed what the doctors had feared. George had suffered a stroke that damaged each of his two hippocampi—tiny, whorled structures in the brain that direct the formation of long-term memory. Although he eventually managed to understand that his memory was impaired, George's condition did not improve. As he told his neurologist many months later, "I'm aware of today and so forth, but tomorrow I'll forget it." Trying to follow a conversation gave George a headache. "They don't finish their sentences," he said of other people. "I feel like I'm in a box, hearing little bits and pieces." Trapped in an eternal present, unable to learn or to forge new memories, George sensed that the thread of his life was broken. Turning to his wife, he asked a question no one could answer with certainty: "When is my mind coming back?"

George's rare and nightmarish condition demonstrates the intimate connection between one's sense of self, or any of the various things we mean by "mind," and the wrinkled, three-pound mass of fatty tissue encased in the skull. As scientists have come to realize with increasing certitude, everything that makes up the self-aware "I" who experiences and interacts with the world "out there" arises somehow from the activity of the brain's intricate network of somewhere between 10 billion and 100 billion nerve cells, or neurons. Although these specialized cells never touch one another, they communicate electrochemically across minuscule gaps called synapses. Numbering perhaps as many as 20 quadrillion (2 followed by 16 zeros), the synapses form a web of connections whose complexity far surpasses that of the most sophisticated supercomputers.

In ways that researchers have barely begun to fathom, this incessant neuronal activity regulates every bodily function. It enables us to walk and talk; to ride a bike, flip a pancake, play the guitar; to recognize the face of a friend in a crowd of strangers. And it generates our every thought, dream, and desire.

Astonishingly, humans are born with all or close to all of the neurons they will ever possess. Unlike most other cells in the body, neurons typically do not replicate, and early in life they begin to die off. The rate is by no means constant and seems to be more pronounced before adulthood. Studies suggest that these early losses may be a normal part of brain development—a kind of natural selection at the neuronal level that preserves the most efficient connections. According to this view, mental capacity is not a matter of strength in numbers but of effective networking of neurons.

The brain has been the subject of sustained scientific inquiry for some two centuries, as researchers have attempted to map its principal structures and divisions and identify their functions. Most of the early insights into brain function resulted from studies of patients who, like George, had suffered brain injury through accident or illness. Other work was done on cadavers, and much of what was learned about basic brain function came from animal studies—still a major source of information.

New horizons opened in the 1930s with the advent of fine-gauge electric probes, used to stimulate the brain during surgery. The still-common practice—during which patients are conscious so they can describe sensations caused by the stimulation—is primarily intended to help surgeons

AN INTRICATE WEB. Tinted green in this false-color image, individual neurons—in reality fractions of a millimeter across—display the spidery structure that enables them to form elaborate networks of interconnections throughout the brain. Electrochemical signals flow between neurons through the branching fibers extending from each cell body.

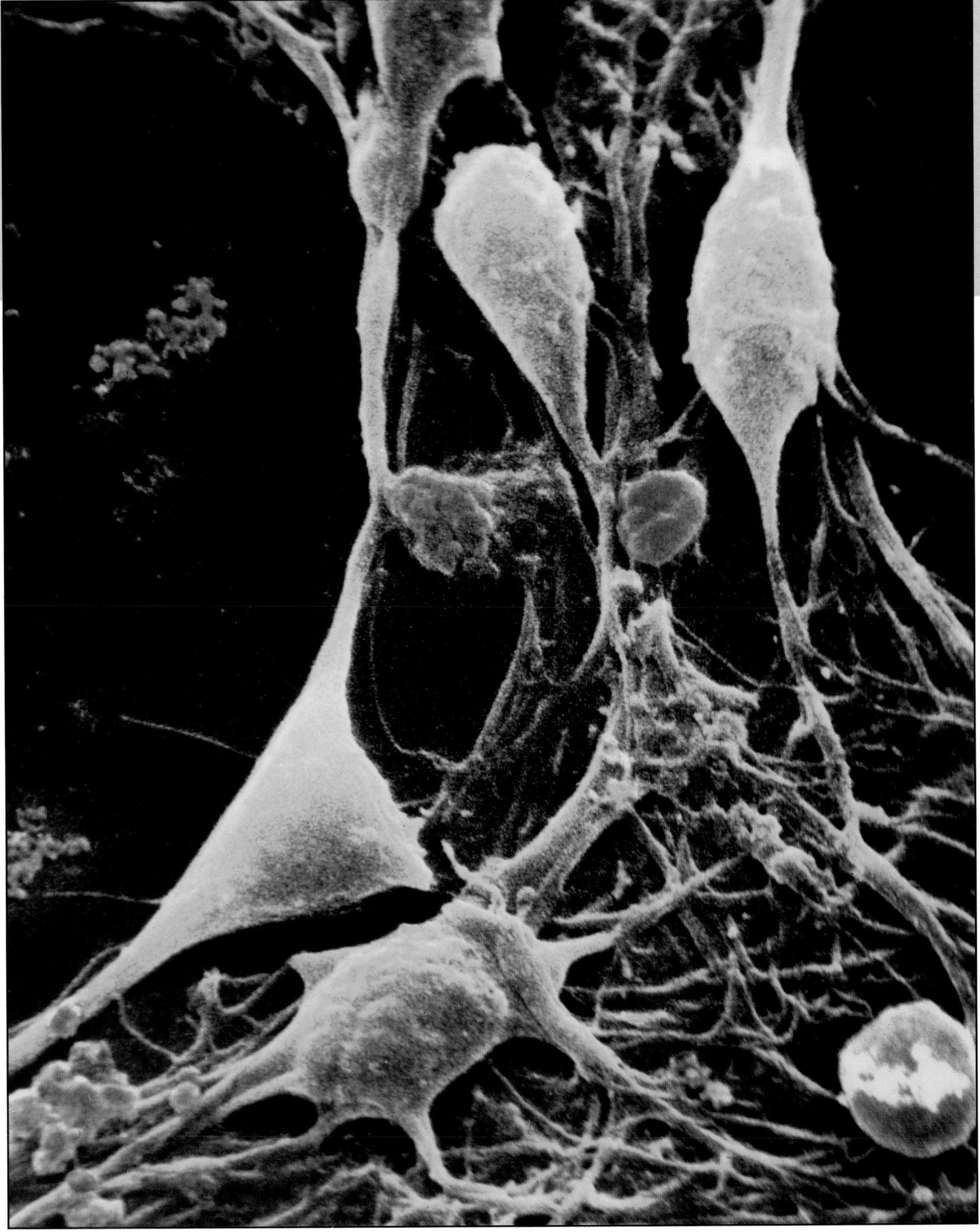

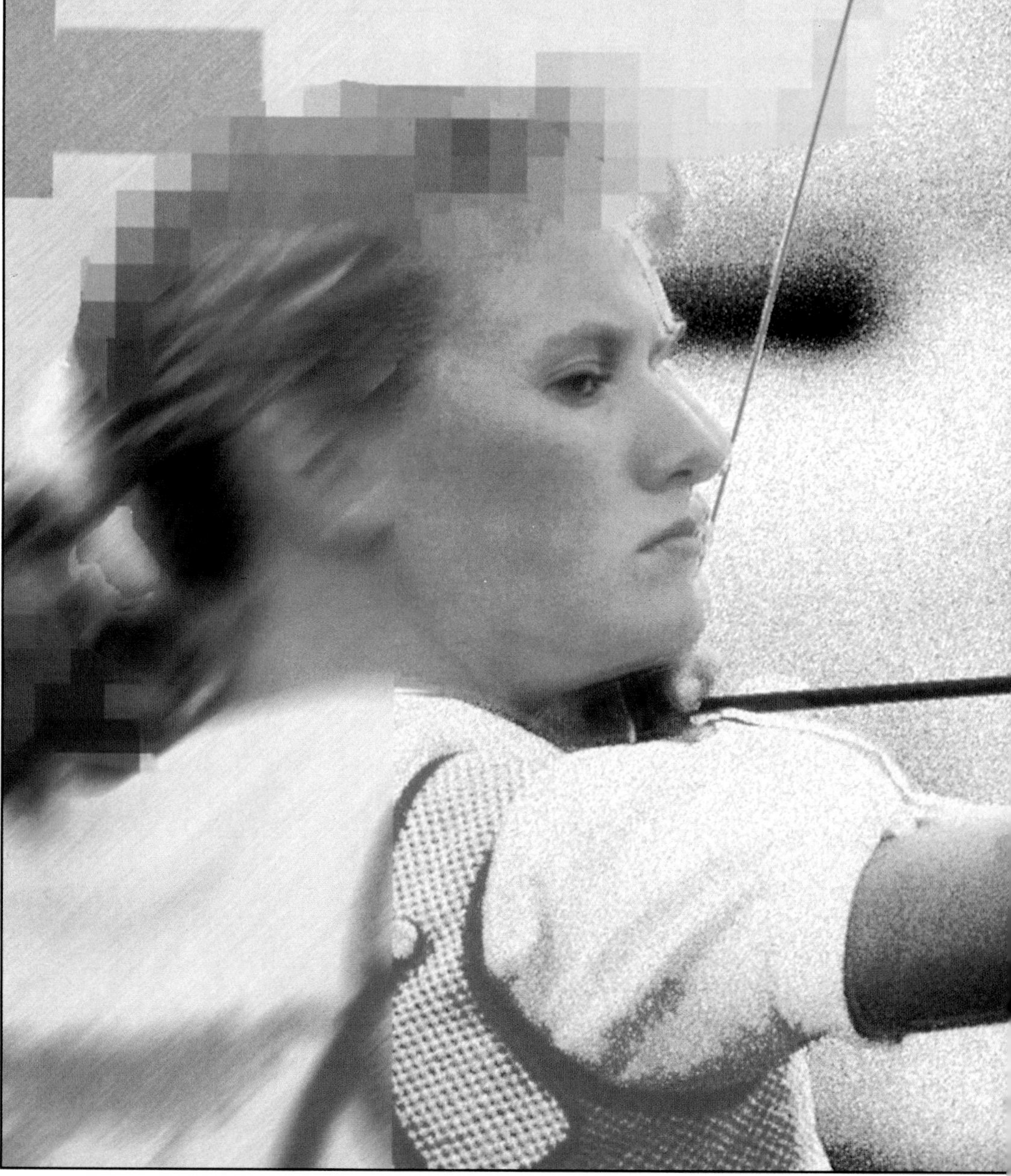

identify crucial areas to avoid, for example, in the course of removing a tumor. The side benefit has been an increasingly detailed portrait of the brain's functional organization.

The last two decades or so have brought about even more dramatic progress. Noninvasive brain scanning procedures—with handy acronyms such as PET, CT, and MRI (*pages 16-19*)—have enabled researchers to examine the structure of living brains and watch them in action over much wider territory than just a few electrode sites. For example, while scientists have known since the 1860s that certain parts of the brain are involved with language, PET scans show that brain activity shifts from one localized area to another depending on whether the subject is reading words or hearing or speaking them.

The rich and varied landscape of the brain that such investigations have revealed can be viewed from several different perspectives. Much has been gleaned, for example, from a fine focus on the electrochemical flow of information between neurons and throughout the brain's myriad networks. At another level, an apparent hierarchy in the brain's architecture—ranging from its most primitive to its most highly evolved features—has served as a particularly effective guide to the full gamut of the brain's activities. Almost every approach, however, ultimately confronts the most intriguing question of all: What, precisely, is the relationship between the brain and the mind?

Over the last several decades, the search for answers has been drawing together two disciplines that were once widely separated—cognitive psychology, the science of the mind, and neurobiology, the science of the brain and the nervous system. The dichotomy dates back to the fourth century BC, when Plato declared that human beings were inhabited by a nonphysical entity called the soul. Ever since, Western philosophers have struggled to resolve this split between substance and psyche—the so-called mind-body problem.

The debate was cast in its most enduring form in the mid-17th century by French mathematician René Des-

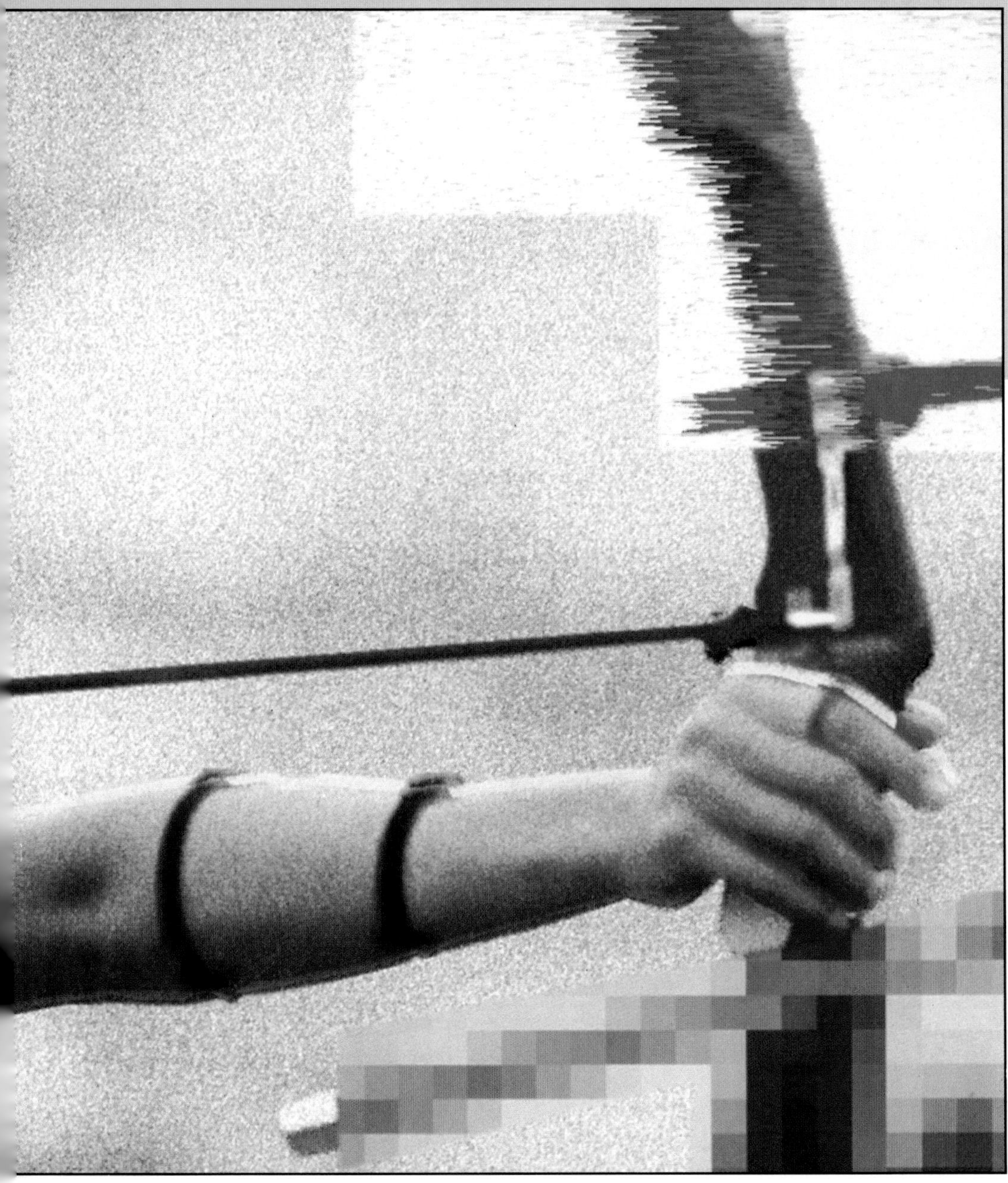

BODY, BRAIN, AND MIND AT WORK. Her attention riveted on the target, an archer takes aim—a process that involves her brain at both conscious and unconscious levels. Without her awareness, her brain fine-tunes such physical details as her body's position, the tension in her muscles, and her eyes' focus. But it also creates the state of mental concentration that helps her block out distractions—and decide the perfect moment to let the arrow fly.

cartes, who formulated the approach known as dualism. Central to his concept was the notion that the mind (what he called *res cogitans*, or "the thinking thing") was distinct from the physical body, including the brain. As he laid out the argument, because the brain was physical, it had to obey physical laws and, like a machine, was capable of performing only a set program of actions from which it could not deviate. The apparently free-ranging nature of human thought, however, clearly had to stem from a separate phenomenon that was unrestricted by physical laws. Such, Descartes asserted, was the mind.

Although dualism long held sway and still has proponents, it has remained an essentially unsatisfying philosophy for most scientists. According to Daniel Dennett, a professor at Tufts University and director of its Center for Cognitive Studies, the dualist position sidesteps the problem of understanding the mind. "What the dualist does is invent a magical space and inhabit it with some new substance, the mind," Dennett says. "But that couldn't solve the problem—that is just giving up. It leaves all the truly interesting questions of how the mind works not only unanswered but unanswerable."

In the face of such shortcomings—and because of increasingly sophisticated knowledge of how the brain itself works—dualism has for the most part given way to its opposite, the philosophy known as materialism, which holds that mind and body are one and that the brain and the mind are therefore inseparable. Although many fundamental questions remain unanswered, the basis for most investigations into the nature of the mind has become the relatively simple notion that, as neurologist and noted author Richard Restak has put it, "Mind is what the brain does."

While not all materialists are students of the nervous system or even of biology, the research that supports their position derives largely from those

1 **THE SPINAL CORD** conveys impulses from the brain to other parts of the body, and relays messages from them back to various brain structures.

2 **THE MEDULLA** helps regulate breathing, swallowing, blood pressure, such responses as sneezing, and more complex functions like sleep.

3 **THE PONS** serves to link the cortex with the cerebellum. Neurons within the pons are associated with facial expression and eye movements.

4 **THE MIDBRAIN** forwards sensory impulses from the spinal cord to other parts of the brain and controls reflex responses to certain stimuli.

5 **THE CEREBELLUM** is responsible for balance and posture, incorporating the sense of the body's position in space and coordinating all of its motions.

6 **THE HIPPOCAMPUS** is involved in emotional reactions and also apparently in learning, helping to process information and to store it in memory.

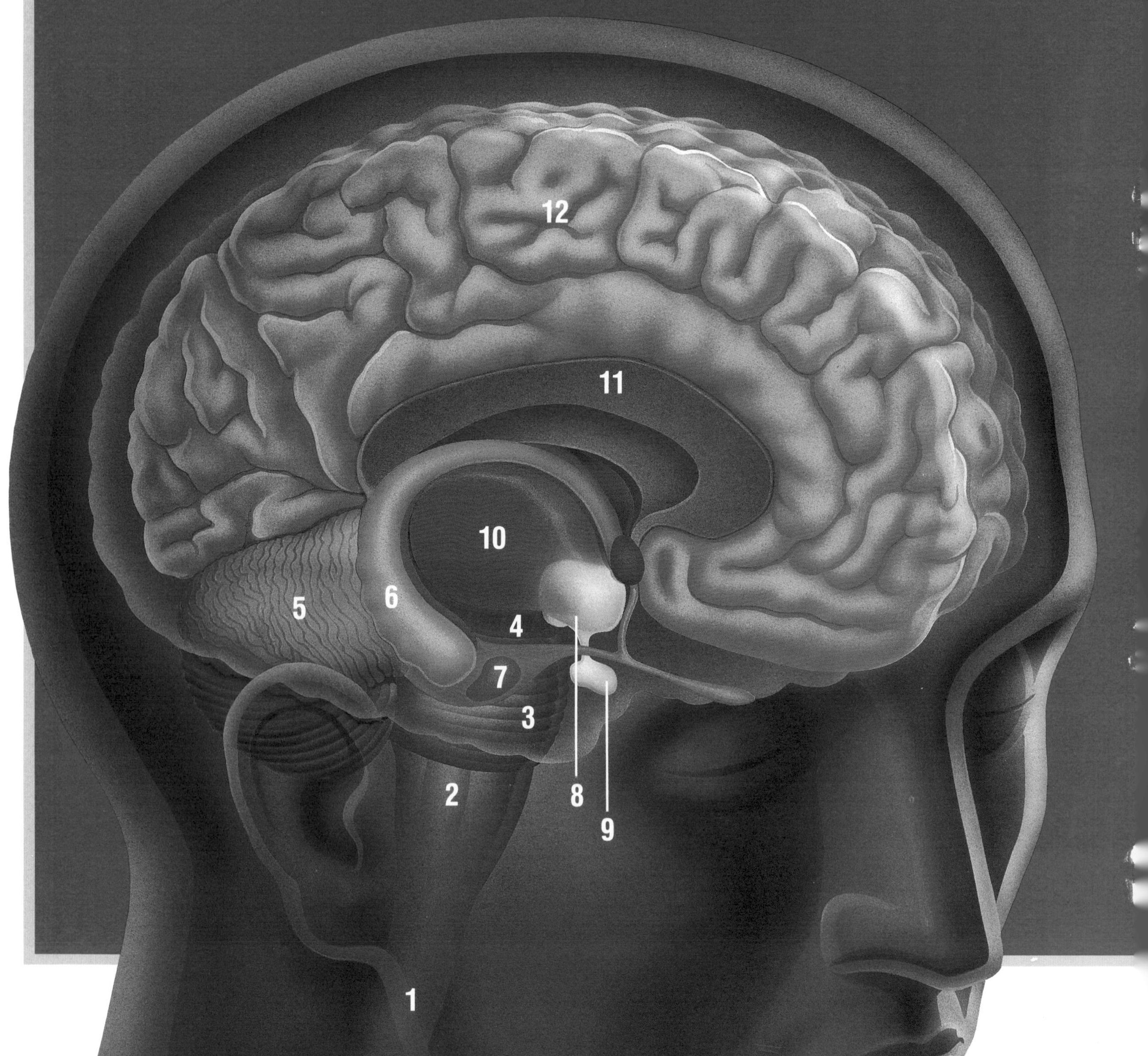

7 THE AMYGDALA, working with the hippocampus, generates emotions from perceptions and thoughts; it also plays a role in the sense of smell.

8 THE HYPOTHALAMUS controls adjustments in such processes as heart rate and body temperature, and regulates sleep cycles and hormone levels.

9 THE PITUITARY GLAND, under the direction of the hypothalamus, secretes hormones that circulate through the body and control other glands.

10 THE THALAMUS deals with all senses except smell. Many types of information destined for the cerebral cortex are routed through this structure.

11 THE CORPUS CALLOSUM is a band of fibers that connects the two hemispheres of the cerebral cortex, allowing them to exchange information.

12 THE CEREBRAL CORTEX, the surface of the cerebrum, is only an eighth-inch thick. It carries out sophisticated processes like thought and language.

The Master of Life

From such basics as breathing to the profound mysteries of emotion and personality, every aspect of human life is governed by the grapefruit-size organ housed within the skull. The key to the brain's awesome power and versatility is both division of labor and communal action: Each of the brain's many components performs its own special tasks, but most also take part in joint efforts.

The vital life-support duties are handled by the medulla, pons, and midbrain, which together constitute the brainstem. A tapered, three-inch-long segment situated where the brain meets the spinal cord, the brainstem regulates heartbeat and breathing, and also governs many other body functions that proceed without conscious effort. Above the brainstem lie the various components of the limbic system—the thalamus, hypothalamus, hippocampus, and amygdala, as well as several other elements. Their tasks include a host of basic brain activities, from the processing of sensory information to the physical expression of emotions.

These structures are almost completely enveloped by the two hemispheres of the cerebrum, the largest part of the brain, whose most significant feature is its thin outer layer, the cerebral cortex. Consisting of four lobes in each hemisphere (*below*), the cortex is so deeply fissured and folded that if it were spread out flat, its surface area would be three times greater. Among its myriad functions—many of which involve interactions with the brain's other components—this distinctively human part of the brain produces thoughts, governs language, and stores memories.

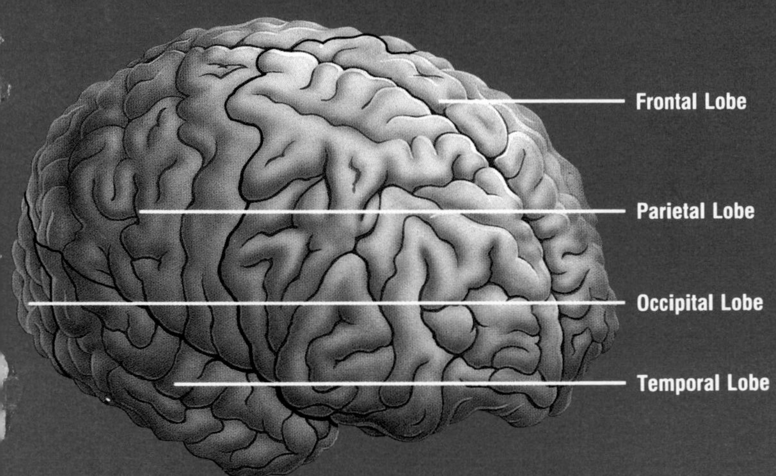

THE FOUR LOBES in each hemisphere of the cerebral cortex handle the brain's most impressive workings. The frontal lobes oversee such complex mental activities as decision making. Behind them lie the parietal lobes, primarily responsible for sensory perception. The occipital lobes, at the rear of the brain, are devoted mainly to vision, while the temporal lobes are involved in hearing, expression, and memory.

Yielding Secrets to Technology

Within the past few decades, a handful of sophisticated imaging techniques have emerged that allow doctors and researchers to peer, without exploratory surgery, into the brains of healthy human beings, shedding new light on the brain's closely held secrets. Perhaps the most widely known of these techniques is called computed tomography (CT). Like its predecessor the x-ray, CT translates relative tissue densities into a structural portrait. Unlike conventional x-rays, however, CT scans can provide a three-dimensional representation of a region of the brain. Each picture is actually a composite image, crafted from thousands of x-rays taken by a scanner that revolves around the skull.

Methods for mapping brain activity rather than structure take a more roundabout approach. Positron emission tomography (PET), for example, draws on the principle that blood rushes to the busiest areas of the brain to deliver oxygen and nutrients to active neurons. By injecting a subject with radioactive glucose, then scanning the brain for the gamma rays emitted as the solution metabolizes, researchers can pinpoint active neuronal sites.

For mapping both structure and activity of the brain, scientists often rely on magnetic resonance imaging, or MRI, which extracts clues from hydrogen atoms that are associated with water molecules in the blood. In structural MRI, a subject's head is immersed in a strong magnetic field and then subjected to several pulses of radio waves. The hydrogen atoms' nuclei respond by emitting signals that can be translated into an exceptionally precise three-dimensional representation of the scanned region. To map brain activity, researchers use a process called functional MRI, which detects variations in the response of hydrogen nuclei when oxygen is present in the blood. By deducing which parts of the brain are being replenished by oxygen, scientists can target and then scan specific sites of neuronal activity.

One drawback of functional MRI is its relative sluggishness: Anywhere from one to four seconds may elapse between the firing of neurons and the arrival of oxygen—an eternity in a realm where impulses can travel at 200 feet per second. To capture brain activity more quickly, researchers often turn to electroencephalography, or EEG, which can identify sparking neurons within one-thousandth of a second. Superimposing EEG data over an MRI-generated blueprint of a subject's brain yields a map that combines blinding speed with a high degree of spatial precision.

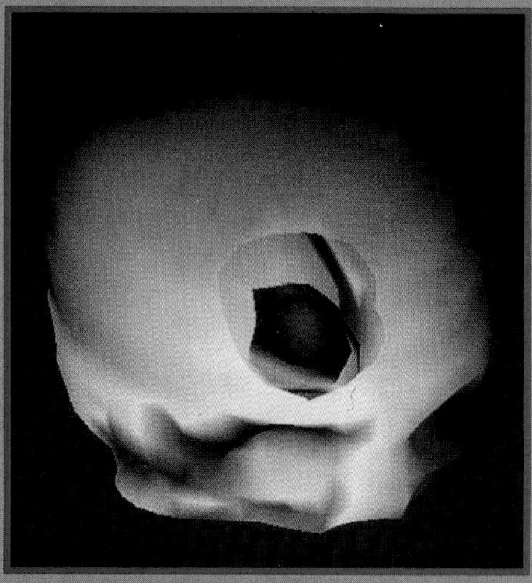

Betrayed by its greater density, a deeply embedded brain tumor *(red, above)* shows through a "window" opened by computed tomography (CT) in a living subject's forehead. Doctors used the computer-generated image, produced by piecing together thousands of x-rays, as a guide during surgery to remove the tumor.

disciplines. As early as the second century AD, the Greek physician Galen of Pergamum performed dissections on such animals as an African monkey sometimes called the Barbary ape. Galen's descriptions of the nervous system, tracing fibers now known to carry sensations from the body to the brain and to relay messages back to the muscles and sense organs, were prized by medieval Arab scholars. They were, however, all but lost to Europeans through the Dark Ages, and not until much later did researchers begin to build on the foundations Galen had laid.

A signal event came in the middle

PET images depict levels of activity in the brains of two people playing a computer game. With red and yellow indicating high levels of activity, the scans reveal that an experienced player *(below, right)* burns significantly less energy than a novice *(below, left)*. Learning, then, seems to be a function not of greater effort but of increased neuronal efficiency. Indeed, players who score high on standard IQ tests show the most precipitous drop in mental exertion while learning the game.

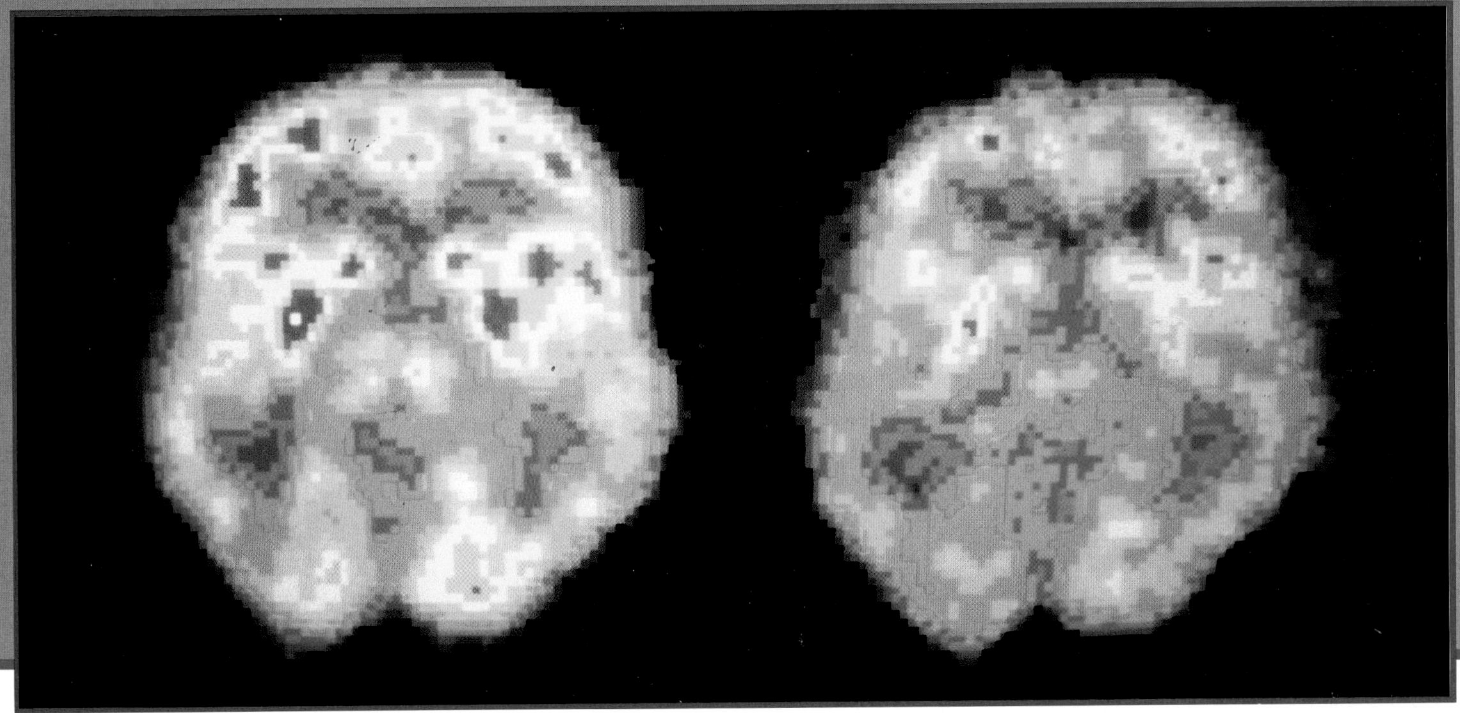

of the 18th century, when the French physician François Gigot de La Peyronie stumbled upon an important connection. While treating a patient felled by a deep gash in the head that penetrated the skull, La Peyronie bathed the wound in water, whereupon the man promptly fainted; when the doctor drew off the pool of water in the wound, the patient came to. The surprising result of La Peyronie's ministrations, which he described to colleagues in a 1741 paper, provided an unassailable, albeit general, observation: Somehow, basic consciousness and the physical stuff of the brain were linked. The more specific idea that certain mental processes could be located in, or associated with, discrete parts of the brain came several decades later.

Functional localization, as this notion is called, gained attention just after the turn of the 19th century with the work of Franz Joseph Gall, a doctor with a special interest in physiology who worked in both Vienna and Paris between 1785 and his death in 1828. Gall has come down to the modern age as something of a quack, a proponent of the pseudoscientific practice of phrenology, or the study of bumps on the skull. The large-scale anatomy of the human brain was known by this time, but Gall claimed in 1810 to have pinpointed areas of the brain responsible for such faculties and traits as memory, musical talent, cautiousness, faithfulness, acquisitiveness, and dozens of others. He based his findings on extensive comparisons of people's behavior and abilities and the contours of their skulls. A bump directly over the right ear, for example, was supposed to reveal a person's destructive tendencies; one in front of the ear was proof of extraordinary attentiveness. At the height of its popularity during the Victorian era, phrenology became a parlor game favored by the well-to-do in England and on the Continent.

Though Gall's investigations were founded on several mistaken assumptions—among them that brain contours rise or fall depending on the prominence of a faculty or trait—his concept of localization turned out to be a worthy contribution to brain sci-

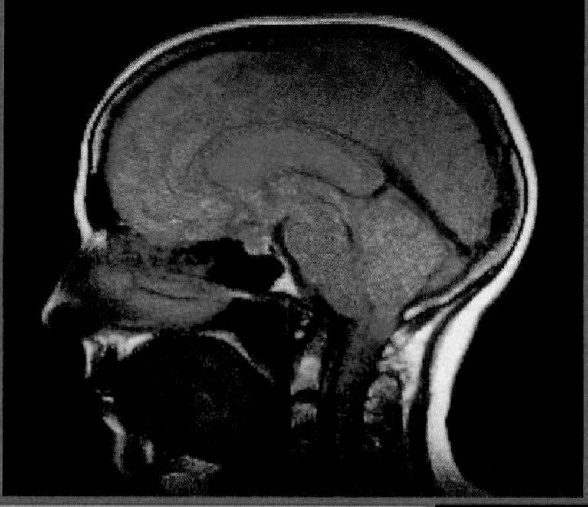

Red and yellow displays on a functional MRI scan taken over a period of 45 milliseconds *(below)* identify a region in a subject's motor cortex activated by the rapid tapping together of the thumb and fingers of the right hand. Small yellow dots represent neuronal "noise."

In the structural MRI scan of a human brain shown above, fluid-filled components such as blood vessels appear dark, while fat and other relatively fluid-free tissues show up in lighter hues. Accurate to within one millimeter, the technique has been used successfully to chart the progression of diseases such as multiple sclerosis, which destroys patches of the fatty myelin sheath encasing an axon.

ence. Over the next half-century, it played a significant role in the research of many investigators, including French surgeon Paul Broca. In 1861 Broca performed an autopsy on a man who had received the nickname "Tan-Tan" because those were the only sounds he had been able to utter. Broca noted that Tan-Tan had suffered damage to a certain area of the left frontal lobe between the eyebrow and the temple. After finding damage in the same region in the autopsy of a similarly impaired patient, Broca concluded that this area of the brain is responsible for the ability to put sounds together to form syllables, words, and phrases.

Broca also found that this mechanism is confined to the brain's left hemisphere; injury to an equivalent area on the right side of the brain seemed to have no effect. Patients who suffer damage to what is now called Broca's area can understand what is said to them, and they can still make sounds, but they are usually able to say only very simple words such as yes and no, or put together rudimentary phrases.

Because of Broca's work and his reputation as a pathologist, the idea that different areas of the brain control various bodily responses and senses soon gained wide acceptance in the scientific community. In 1874, just 13 years after Broca's autopsy of Tan-Tan, the German neurologist Carl Wernicke pinpointed another region, later called Wernicke's area, where damage caused a different sort of language problem, seemingly interfering with the ability to grasp meaning. For example, a patient with damage in Broca's area might reply, if asked about the weather, "Sunny" or, if pushed, "Sunny day." But a patient injured in Wernicke's area would spout nonsense—a string of words bearing no relation to the question.

Clearly there was much more to be learned about where and how the brain processes and produces the highly prized human capacity for language, and the investigation today has drawn researchers from such diverse fields as psychobiology, linguistics, and artificial intelligence. Meanwhile, neuroanatomists—who

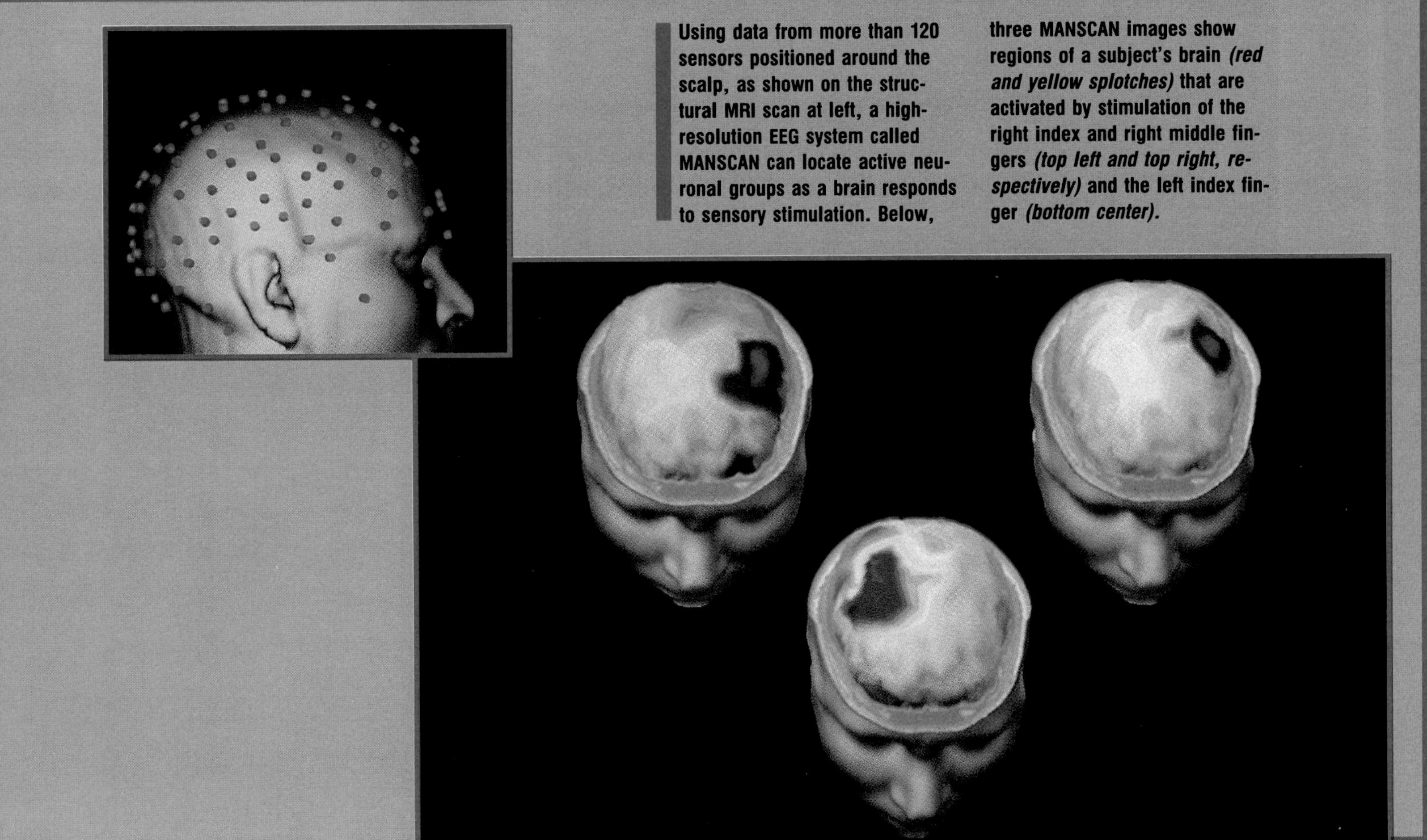

Using data from more than 120 sensors positioned around the scalp, as shown on the structural MRI scan at left, a high-resolution EEG system called MANSCAN can locate active neuronal groups as a brain responds to sensory stimulation. Below, three MANSCAN images show regions of a subject's brain *(red and yellow splotches)* that are activated by stimulation of the right index and right middle fingers *(top left and top right, respectively)* and the left index finger *(bottom center).*

specialize in the brain's physical structure—began to develop a hierarchical model of the brain and all its functions. Starting at the literal and conceptual bottom with the brainstem and cerebellum (*pages* 14-15), which regulate autonomic functions like breathing and heartbeat and coordinate muscular activity, researchers went on to identify areas responsible for basic drives like hunger and thirst (the hypothalamus), sexual development (the pituitary gland), and cognition, memory, and awareness (the cortex). In the course of this work, one important figure, British physiologist Sir Charles Sherrington, demonstrated the close interaction of different parts of the brain in controlling reflexes—an interaction far more extensive than had been previously realized.

In his 1906 classic, *The Integrative Action of the Nervous System*, Sherrington argued that the brain and body constitute an elaborate mechanism regulated by feedback loops, a kind of process control in which information on the effects of a particular action is continuously returned to the source of that action. Feedback, said Sherrington, enables the brain to evaluate a range of stimuli and produce appropriate levels of response. This scheme accounts for certain instinctive, automatic reactions—jerking one's hand away from a flame, for instance—which might be owed to simple feedback loops involving relatively few nerve pathways, as well as for other activities far more complex. In the ongoing balancing act of maintaining the body's posture, for example, whole arrays of nerves come into play, including those that respond to external stimuli (heat, noise, light, touch, and smells) and others that check the status of internal systems like the muscles. Both types of nerves interact not in strictly predetermined ways but in shifting patterns, depending on circumstances.

Around the time that Sherrington was carrying out the investigations that led to his book (he would win a Nobel Prize in 1932, shared with colleague Edgar Adrian), a Spanish physician and professor of physiology named Santiago Ramón y Cajal was furthering knowledge of the brain's cellular structure. Using an adapted version of a silver stain invented in 1873 by Italian physician Camillo Golgi—himself a noted theorist on brain physiology—Ramón y Cajal brought nerve cells into sharp focus for the first time. Peering through a microscope at thin slices from the brains of cadavers, he discerned in the densely tangled world of brain tissue the distinctive features of the brain's specialized cells—the compact nucleus; the long, whiplike axon; the spiky halo of dendrites. He also noted that the neurons were embedded in a sponge of supporting cells called glial (glue) cells.

Ultimately more significant, however, was Ramón y Cajal's landmark observation in 1901 that neurons pass impulses to one another without touching. This finding was hotly contested by, among others, Golgi, who firmly subscribed to the concept of an interconnected web of cells. The debate was still unresolved in 1906, when the Nobel Prize committee chose to make that year's award to both Golgi and Ramón y Cajal, acknowledging that each had contributed mightily but that neither had yet won the day.

(Several decades later, in the 1950s, scientists equipped with powerful biochemical tools would reveal that the Spanish professor had been right. Impulses travel from one neuron to another across narrow gaps, or synapses, by means of special-purpose chemicals called neurotransmitters that neurons produce.)

Brain science was now poised to make large strides through the middle decades of the 20th century. Teams of investigators around the world carried out painstaking experiments designed to translate neuronal activity into an integrated portrait of the brain going about its multifaceted business. Adding to earlier findings on localization, for example, research showed that incoming signals register not indiscriminately across the whole cortex but only among certain neurons, depending on the origin of the stimulus. Impulses from the optic nerve, for instance, are received in the so-called visual cortex, while sound, taste, touch, and painful pressure are each received in other discrete cortical regions.

While physiologists gathered ever more data on the brain itself, inquiries into the nature of the mind set off in a different direction entirely. Indeed, until sometime around 1900 psychology was considered a branch of philosophy, and in that realm there were few who challenged Descartes's dualist argument. Even as investigators of the brain followed a strategy of discovering ever-smaller constituent parts of the brain, the mind remained whole and indivisible.

Then Sigmund Freud, the giant of modern psychology, overthrew this Cartesian dogma. Practicing in Vienna between 1882 and 1938, the year he fled the Nazi regime for London, Freud used his own grounding in neurology as a springboard for his exploration of the mind. Where others had seen unity, Freud discerned partitions, most notably a cleaving of the conscious from the unconscious. In his scheme, one's mental outlook, which develops as an individual matures, bears the stamp of both heredity and the influences of family and society. As a consequence, why individuals behave as they do is far from obvious. Freud postulated that much of the time—and especially for patients with psychological problems—true motives lie swamped in the unconscious, emerging only in the perplexing imagery of dreams and in everyday slips of the tongue. Freud's solution, which profoundly influenced the treatment of mental illness in Europe and the United States, was for patients to practice a regimen of retrieving and confronting unconscious conflicts. Since the 1960s, however, Freudian psychoanalysis, as this practice is known, has been increasingly superseded—if not in the clinical, then in the experimental, domain—by theories of the mind and consciousness that more closely parallel advances in neuroscience.

It is now amply evident, for example, that mental states, emotions, and behavior, whether conscious or unconscious, can often be linked to levels of neurotransmitters in the synaptic gaps between neurons in the brain. When brain chemistry goes awry, for reasons and in ways that are not always apparent, mood swings and even full-blown mental illnesses result. For instance, excessive levels of the neurotransmitter dopamine have been tied to the delusionary state that constitutes schizophrenia. Elsewhere in the brain, an imbalance of serotonin, a potent sleep-causing neurotransmitter, and norepinephrine, a chemical related to adrenaline, may yield the torpor, bleak outlook, and dismay of chronic depression. In light of such discoveries, treatment of mental illness has increasingly turned toward drugs that help regulate the chemistry of the nervous system.

Although many of the factors that influence mental states and govern behavior now appear to have a basis in brain chemistry, not all human behavior can be explained in this way. One way to complete the picture is to take into account the brain's evolutionary history. In the 1970s, Paul MacLean, a scientist in the Laboratory of Neurophysiology at the National Institute of Mental Health, near Washington, D.C., offered an evolutionary theory that has since stimulated considerable controversy and research. MacLean suggested that the brain of *Homo sapiens* is actually, in effect, a three-level archaeological site, with old, intermediate, and new layers added sequentially in the course of animal evolution.

At the bottom of this hierarchy, MacLean said, lies an ancient reptilian core, the brainstem, which was responsible for behavior that might well be termed irrational in that it happens without the benefit of logic or reason. The R-complex, as MacLean named this region, was deemed to run a fixed set of programs that regulate basic life-sustaining functions such as breathing. MacLean also suggested that the R-complex plays a role in other responses that are virtually instinctive, such as the almost unconscious bow of greeting when people meet, or the hard-to-suppress body language of two people who react strongly to each other—either positively or negatively.

In MacLean's scheme, the limbic system, which includes the hippocampus, the thalamus, the amygdala, and several other structures, overlies the R-complex and is in control of the ebb and flow of emotions, as well as the rhythms of reproduction and of hunger. Somewhat similar in structure to the brain of a mouse, this paleomammalian ("old mammalian") brain, as MacLean called it, also does not operate on logic. Love—or hate—at first sight and all the nuances of feeling and emotion are the province of the limbic system.

The final stage of evolution, in the triune hypothesis, is the wrinkled, multilobed cap of the cerebral cortex, sometimes called the neocortex—"new covering"—a reference to its relative youth in evolutionary terms. This most sophisticated component of the human brain generates language and abstractions, anticipates and plans for the future, reasons and calculates, deliberates, fantasizes.

According to MacLean's theory, these three parts of the brain are separated evolutionarily by eons. Indeed, as he put it, each has "its own special intelligence, its own subjectiv-

Explorers of the Brain and Mind

Throughout much of the history of investigations into the workings of the human brain, many scholars found it implausible that something as ethereal as the mind could arise from something as tangible as the brain. In fact, the accepted wisdom—at least in the Western world—was that the mind and the body were distinctly different entities, a concept that was first articulated in systematic detail by the French mathematician René Descartes in the 1600s. A fundamental divide thus existed between those trying to understand the physical processes of the brain and those focusing on such philosophical and psychological matters as the nature of thought and the constitution of personality.

But Descartes himself had acknowledged some kind of link between the mind and the brain, and as studies continued—and scientists attempted to define the parameters of that link more precisely—evidence began to mount that the brain might indeed be responsible for even the most profound mysteries of the mind. The investigators at right represent some of the key theories and discoveries that have shaped today's efforts to see mind and brain with the same eye.

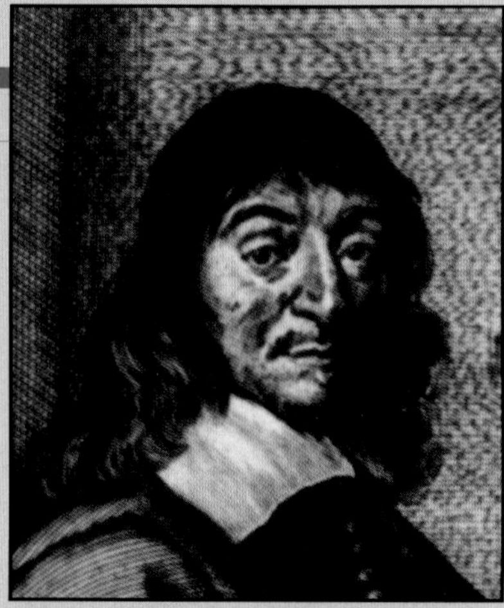

RENÉ DESCARTES formalized the concept of dualism in 1641, arguing that mind and body are separate.

SIGMUND FREUD, schooled in neurology, turned the study of the mind into a science early in the 20th century.

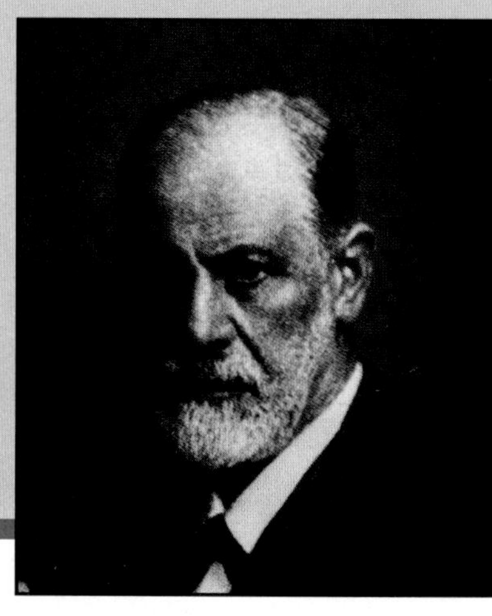

ity, its own sense of time and space and its own memory." Perhaps the most salient issue, however—for some the most controversial part of his proposal—is the notion that after tens of thousands of years as a distinct species, *Homo sapiens* operates with a brain that is two-thirds animal, equipment that is governed by instinct and knows nothing of reason. Indeed, MacLean asserted, much of what we do intellectually is rationalize decisions and actions—from voting for the "candidate of our choice" to choosing a spouse—made by the unreasoning parts of the brain.

If nothing else, MacLean's triune hypothesis spurred many researchers toward a more systematic analysis of the anatomy, physiology, and function of the human brain as compared with its animal counterparts. And many scientists will admit a certain utility in discussing the interactions of three hypothetical divisions of the brain—the neocortex, the limbic system, and the brainstem—as a way to grapple with the brain's enormous complexity. But most would balk at any implication that the divisions operate independently or that the brain is anything but a single organ. Rather, as research increasingly shows, the various parts of the brain are in constant communication. For example, it is possible, at least some of the time, to bring the reasoning cortex into play to control an emotional response.

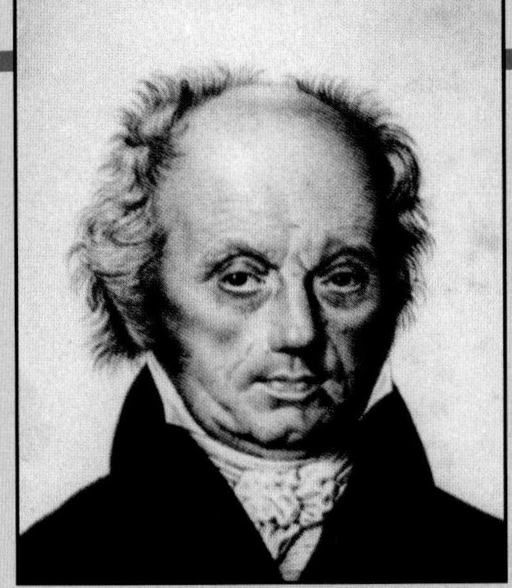

FRANZ JOSEPH GALL linked anatomy to mental traits with his 1810 claim that he "read" bumps on people's skulls.

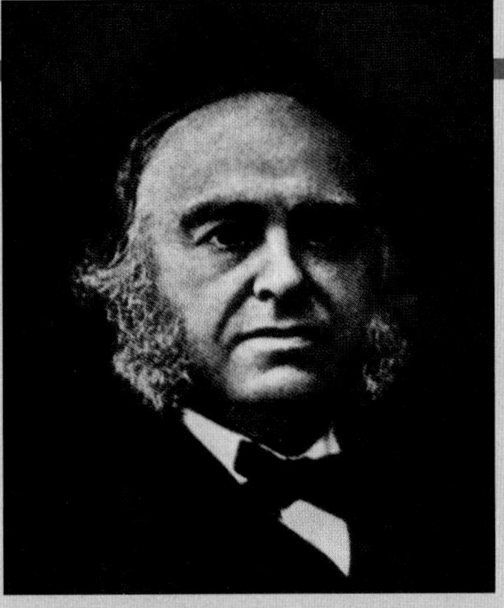

PAUL BROCA identified a speech center in the brain in 1861, helping to establish the principle of localization.

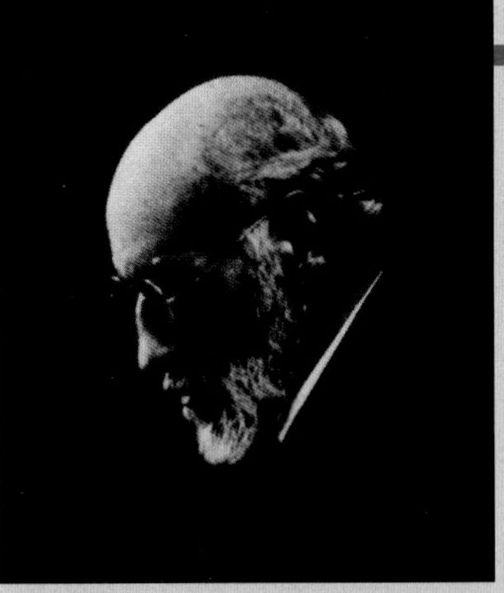

SANTIAGO RAMON Y CAJAL discovered the synapse in 1901, paving the way for studies of how neurons communicate.

JOHN ECCLES, who started analyzing the chemistry of nerve impulses in the 1920s, never abandoned dualism.

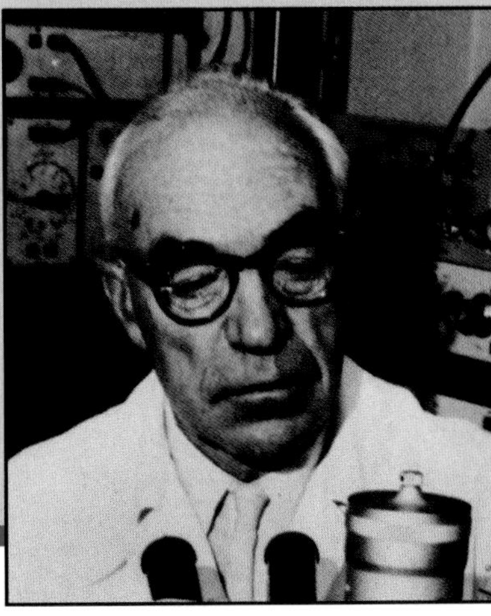

PAUL MACLEAN named the limbic system in 1952 and later developed the concept of the triune brain.

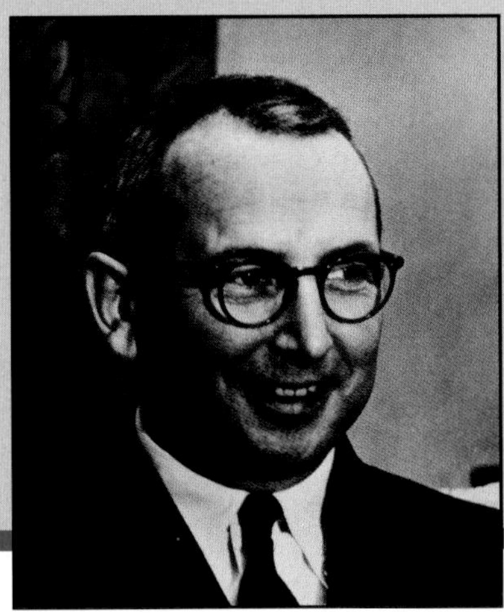

ERIC KANDEL began research in the 1960s that has shown how learning causes physical changes in the brain.

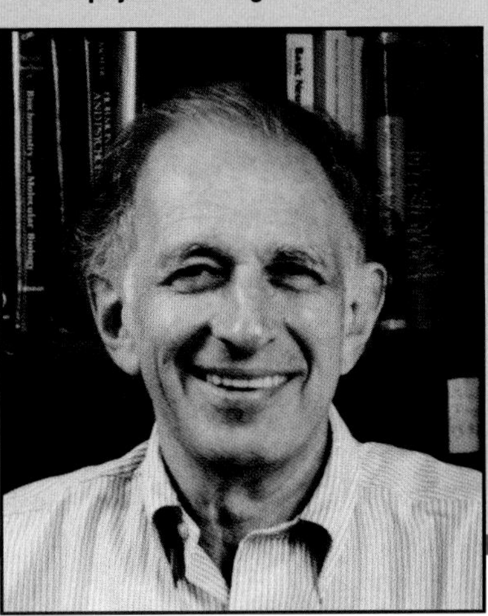

Furthermore, the workings of the brain, although constrained in part by heredity, are also influenced by individual experience. According to Michael Merzenich, a brain researcher at the University of California, "Anatomy lays down a crude topographic map of the body on the surface of the cortex, which is fixed and immutable in early life. But the fine-grained map is not fixed. Experience sketches in all the details, altering the map continually throughout life."

The principal instrument of this alteration process is learning. To understand how learning causes physical changes in the brain, scientists have turned to an organism with a relatively simple nervous system, a giant marine snail whose nerve cells number only about 20,000. Since 1963 Eric Kandel at Columbia University in New York City has been among the leading researchers in this area. Kandel has found that training the snail to shrink from a mild touch by associating it with a strong shock produces distinct changes in the animal's synapses. Neurotransmitter release between nerve cells goes up, and eventually additional dendrites grow, multiplying contacts with neighboring cells.

The conclusion that brain activity can alter connections among neurons in the brains of Kandel's snails probably applies to at least some forms of learning in humans, including both rote memorization and the mastery of simple motor skills. However, to discover the mechanics of recall, attention, imagination, and other more complex mental processes, neuroscientists still face the challenge of understanding the intricacies of memory and learning that involve the cortex and other parts of the brain. How the brain redirects its own activities, or analyzes its own analyses—how the thinking cortex can overcome some of the unyielding programs of the brain's nonreasoning components—are other mysteries yet to be fathomed.

Not everyone in the field believes such puzzles can be unraveled by scientific investigation. One such skeptic is Sir John Eccles, a respected physiologist who studied under Sherrington at Oxford University in the 1920s and shared a Nobel Prize in medicine in 1963 for his work on the chemistry of nerve impulses. Eccles and others have remarked that however much they poke and prod the brain, the mind remains elusive. As far as anyone knows, even the jagged trace of an electroencephalogram, which records patterns of electrical activity among neurons, reveals nothing about the thought or feeling that produced the pattern. Eccles simply considers insupportable the assertion that cells entirely lacking in self-awareness can somehow unite to produce consciousness. Rather, he concludes that some nonmaterial force flows into the brain and animates the body. Dualism is not yet dead.

Eccles and other skeptics may have deserted the materialist camp too soon. Perhaps what they perceive as a chasm between science and the nature of the mind is simply a gap in knowledge that will eventually be closed by research. Certainly modern mind-brain studies are undergoing a major expansion, drawing recruits from many other avenues of science.

But there is a sense in which those who see shortcomings in the materialist approach may be right. For example, most researchers nowadays doubt that behaviorism—an extreme form of materialism that attempts to describe all aspects of the mind in purely objective terms, as predictable behavioral responses to various stimuli—is an accurate reflection of how the brain works. Indeed, when it comes to the relationship between the mind and the brain, the whole is so clearly greater than the sum of its parts that brain science may always have to leave room for a touch of magic. The most appropriate metaphor may be that of Sherrington, who described the intricate networks of the brain as an "enchanted loom."

According to Richard Restak, among others, the fact that materialism may never supply all the answers is hardly surprising. As he has put it, "Our search for everything there is to know about the human brain would have to include the operation of that very brain that asks, impishly, 'Will scientists ever discover everything there is to know about the human brain?' "

Yet Restak himself would be the first to acknowledge that much more than was ever thought possible has already been learned about how the brain works and what those workings reveal about the mind. Even if a complete picture never emerges, the details already gleaned remain boundlessly fascinating.

INTO THE NEURONAL UNIVERSE

The incomparable power of the human brain is generated by the actions and interactions of its many billions of neurons, specialized cells that transmit information in the form of electrochemical impulses. Neuronal impulses convey messages that result in everything from bodily sensations of thirst or hunger to the shape and meaning of words on a page.

The impulses travel along neuron fibers called axons, which link regions of the central nervous system (the brain and spinal cord). Outside the central nervous system, axons are bundled together into the nerves that make up the peripheral nervous system, relaying messages between the central nervous system and every organ and muscle in the body (*right*).

In the brain itself, as shown on the following pages, neurons are joined by a supporting cast of cells that help in signal transmission and also assist in protecting the brain from certain blood-borne substances. Thus aided, neurons go about the work of transforming electrochemical signals into the act of throwing a ball or pounding a nail, laughing at a joke or falling in love—in short, into everything that makes us human.

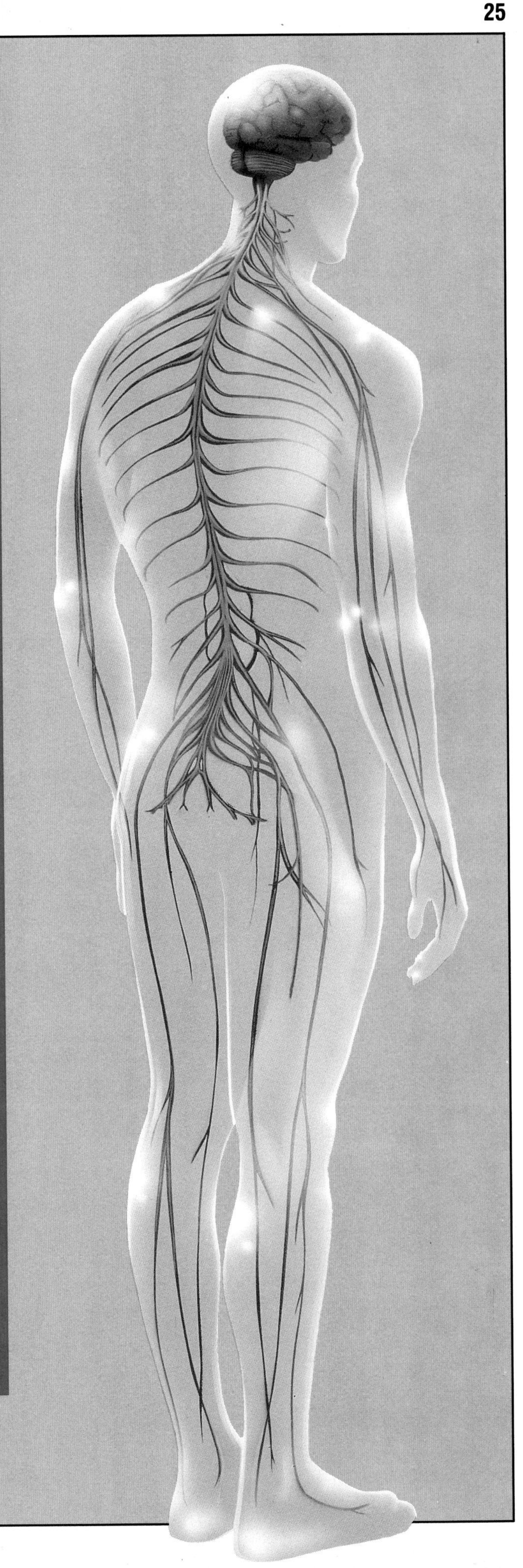

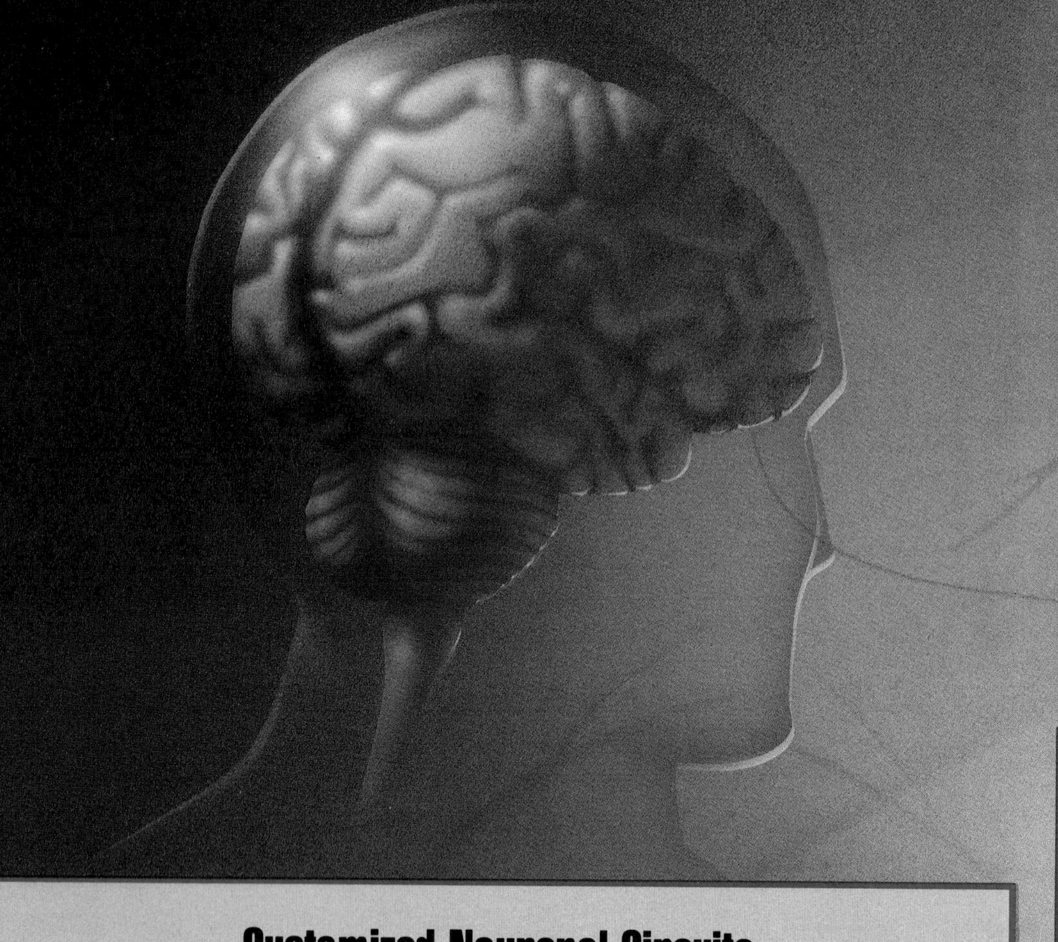

NEURON ANATOMY. The cell body of a neuron contains a nucleus, which holds the cell's DNA, and life-support structures including energy-producing mitochondria; the endoplasmic reticulum, a network that makes proteins and chemicals called neurotransmitters; and membrane-lined canals called Golgi bodies, involved in the transport of nutrients. Unique to the neuron are the long axon fiber for sending electrochemical signals, the many-branched dendrites for receiving them, and the narrow gaps, or synapses, the signals must cross *(pages 28-29)*.

Customized Neuronal Circuits

While animals share the mechanism for neuronal action, the numbers of nerve cells in the human brain and their patterns of connection are several orders of magnitude greater and more complex than those of almost all other creatures. Some relatively simple wiring schemes are shown here, from the linear action of parallel circuits, useful for basic relaying of signals, to the feedback loops of reverberating circuits, which can keep a signal going for as long as several hours. (Such circuits may be related to short-term memory; abnormal versions may cause epileptic seizures.) Divergent circuits are at work in, for example, muscle movement, when a signal from a single motor neuron in the brain ultimately stimulates a number of skeletal muscles. And convergent circuits can produce one strong reaction to different stimuli. The sight, smell, and taste of blood, for example, might induce nausea.

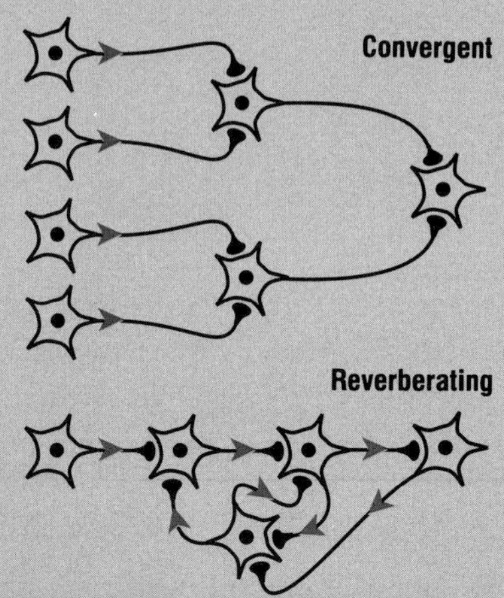

BUILDING BLOCKS OF THE BRAIN

Nothing in the known universe can match the complexity of the human brain, each of whose billions of neurons can communicate with anywhere from 2,000 to 200,000 others. The connecting circuits themselves may be relatively simple in design (*box, opposite*), but, somehow, out of their interactions arises the ineffable phenomenon of human consciousness.

The three types of neurons—sensory, motor, and so-called interneurons, which communicate within the central nervous system—resemble other cells in the organization of their cell bodies (*below*). However, they have evolved specialized structures for transmitting and receiving information. The transmitting structure is the axon, a single long fiber that extends from the cell body, in some cases for as much as three feet (akin to a kite three feet across with a tail 40 miles long). The axon splits at its end into terminals, ranging in number from a few to several hundred, each of which conveys the signal across a tiny gap called the synapse. Sometimes a muscle or gland is on the receiving end, but more often the signal arrives at the cell bodies of other neurons or at one of their dendrites (from the Greek for "tree"). Anywhere from a few micrometers to several millimeters in length, the dendritic fibers form a spiky fringe around the cell body, allowing each cell to receive signals from more than 100,000 others. As shown on the next few pages, the method of moving information from neuron to neuron is partly electrical, partly chemical—a system we human beings share with all other animals from jellyfish on up.

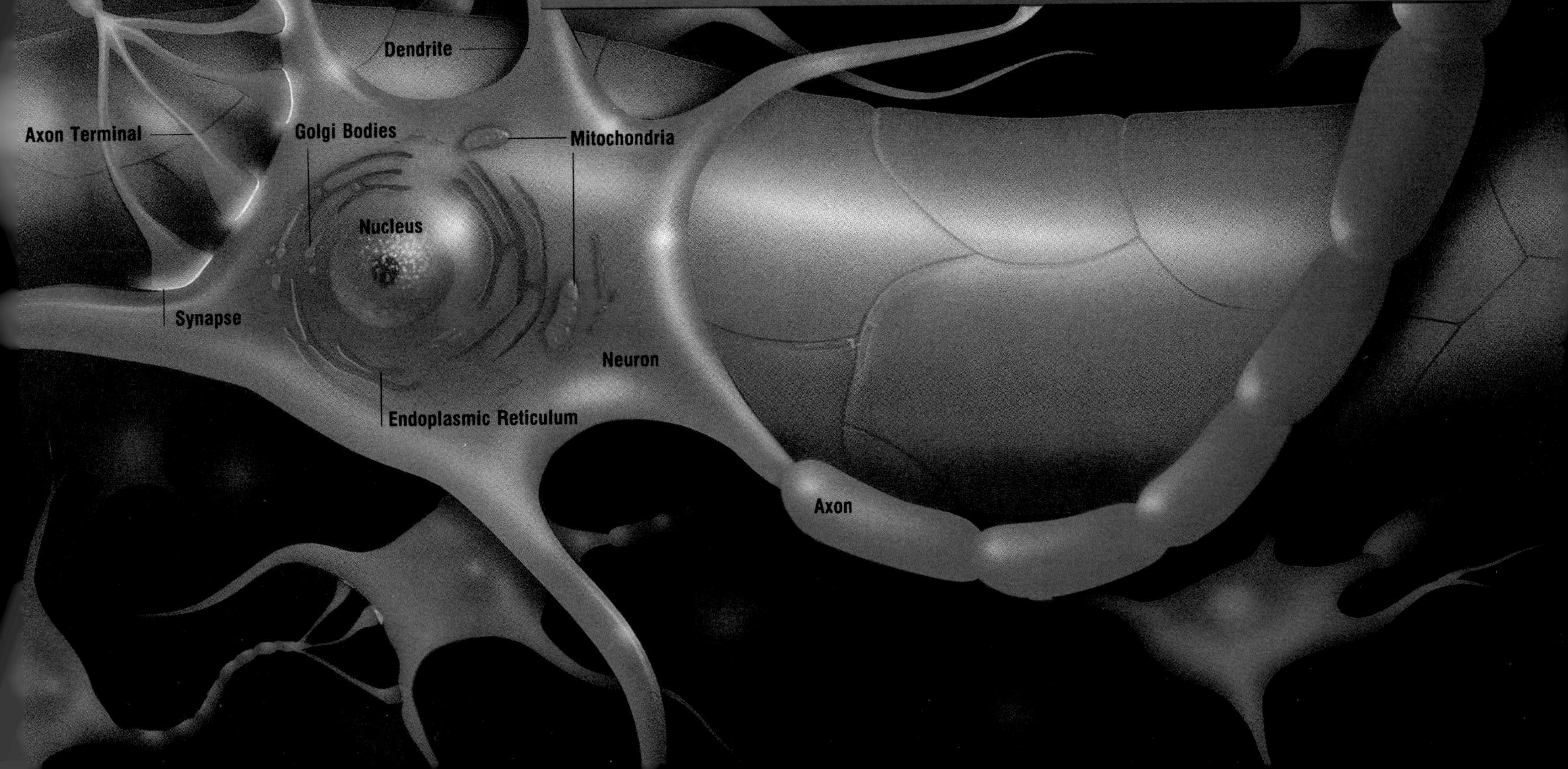

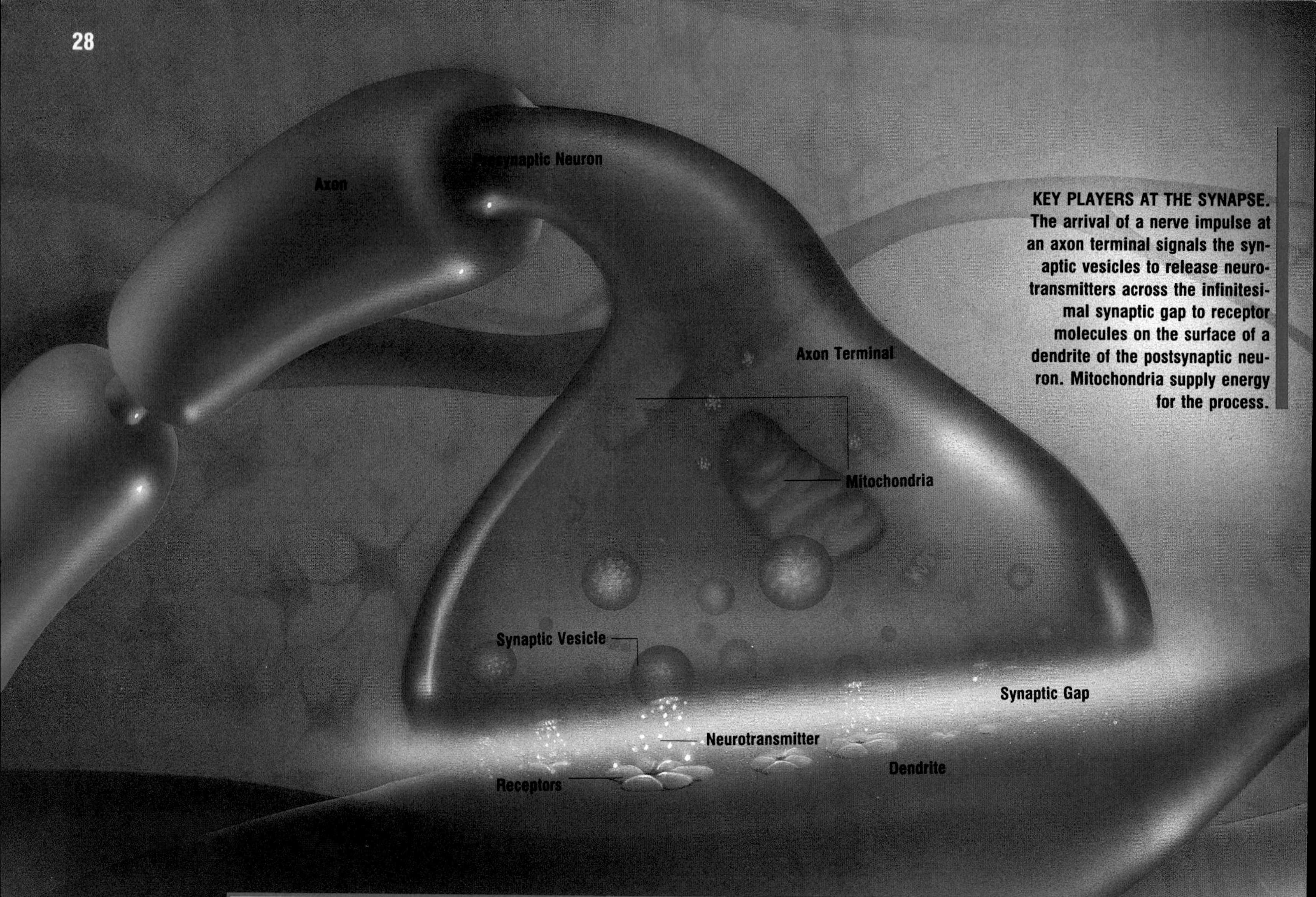

KEY PLAYERS AT THE SYNAPSE. The arrival of a nerve impulse at an axon terminal signals the synaptic vesicles to release neurotransmitters across the infinitesimal synaptic gap to receptor molecules on the surface of a dendrite of the postsynaptic neuron. Mitochondria supply energy for the process.

Nerve Impulses and Synaptic Transmission

As seen here, the basic mechanism of a nerve impulse is the inflow of sodium ions and the outflow of potassium ions through the nodes of Ranvier, in such a way as to render the electrical potential, or polarity, of the axon membrane slightly positive relative to the outside. Molecular ion pumps quickly restore the negative resting potential by pumping sodium back out and potassium back in, but already a similar change has occurred in the next node. When the impulse reaches an axon terminal, neurotransmitters are released that excite the target neuron to fire or prevent it from generating its own nerve impulse.

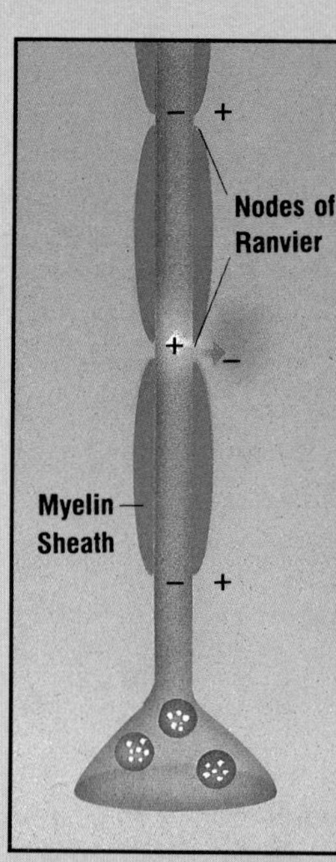

The resting potential at one node of Ranvier *(top)* is restored as an impulse moves to the next node.

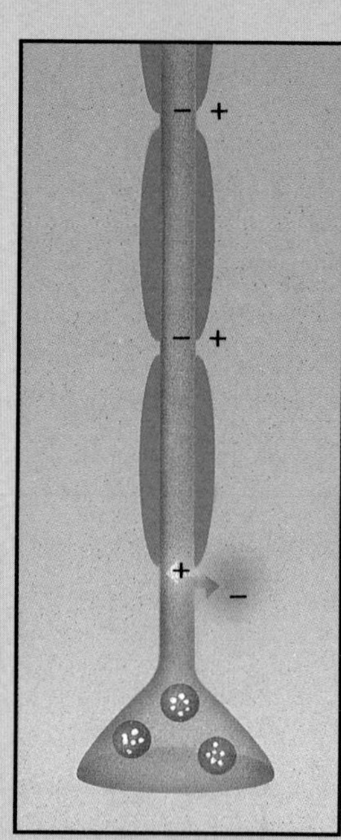

The middle node resumes its resting state; sodium and potassium rush into and out of the last node.

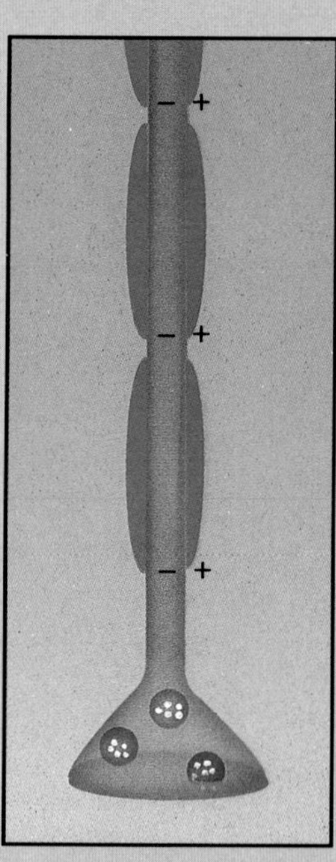

The impulse reaches the axon terminal, where vesicles prepare to release neurotransmitters.

Postsynaptic Neuron

THE DUAL LANGUAGES OF CELL COMMUNICATION

Like a soldier stationed at a critical post, each neuron in the brain and nervous system is subject to continuous bombardment by hundreds or thousands of relayed signals, each of which is saying, in effect, "Fire!" or "Don't fire!" But unlike a soldier who acts at one commander's order, a neuron fires or not according to a kind of majority rule.

To carry out this democratic action, nerve cells communicate in two different languages. One is the electrical nerve impulse, or action potential, which develops at the point where the axon leaves the cell body. In axons that are covered with a fatty sheath of insulating myelin, the wavelike impulse occurs in gaps in the myelin called nodes of Ranvier, as depicted in the sequence below, left. Depending on factors such as the axon's size and the intensity of the stimulation, the impulse moves at a rate ranging from about nine to 400 feet per second. (In nonmyelinated axons, the lack of insulation slows the speed of the action potential to less than six feet per second.)

With the arrival of the impulse at the axon terminals of the sending, or presynaptic, neuron, the language of synaptic transmission takes over. Structures called synaptic vesicles release molecules of neurotransmitters, which diffuse across the synaptic gap to receptor sites on the target, or postsynaptic, neuron. A given neurotransmitter sends a message that is either excitatory ("Fire!") or inhibiting ("Don't fire!"). Only if the excitatory messages exceed a threshold does the target neuron fire—starting a nerve impulse of its own.

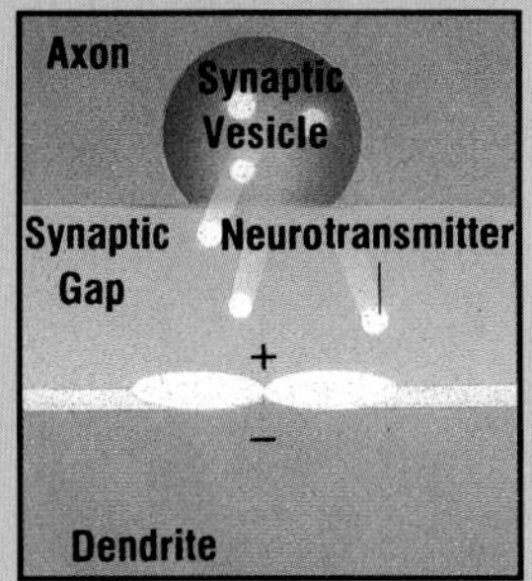

Neurotransmitters *(white balls)* diffuse across the synaptic gap toward the postsynaptic neuron.

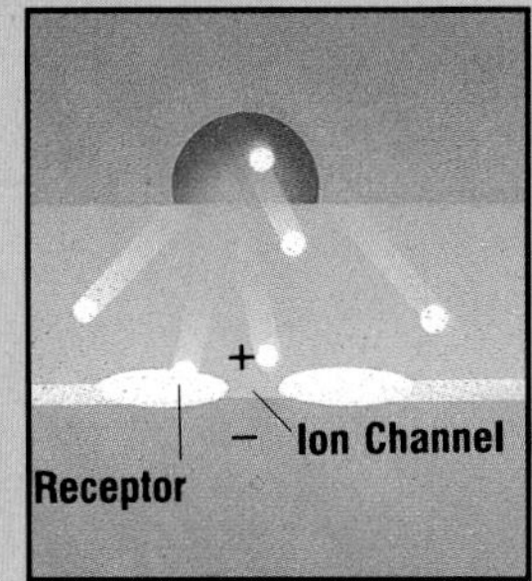

Neurotransmitters bind to receptor molecules on the target neuron, causing ion channels to open.

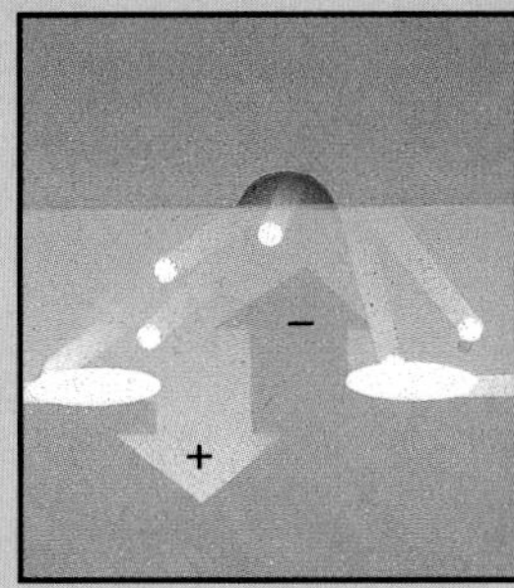

As sodium flows in and potassium out, the neuron's polarity grows positive relative to outside.

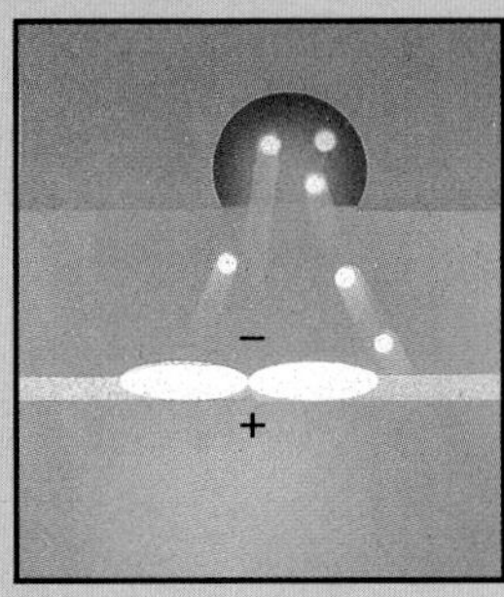

Released by the receptors, neurotransmitters are reabsorbed by the sending neuron or destroyed.

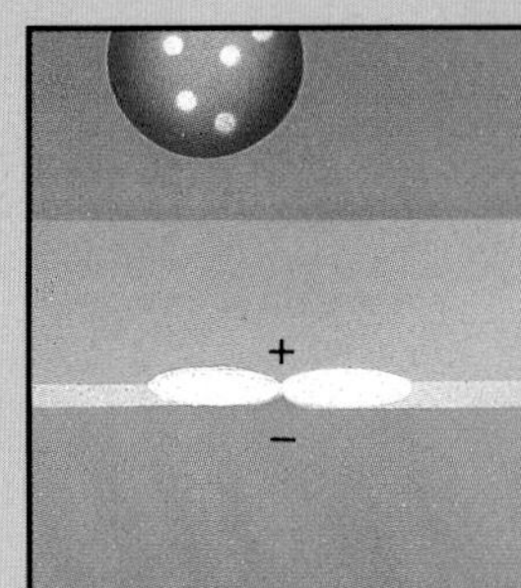

The resting state in this region of the neuron is restored by ion pumps as the impulse moves on.

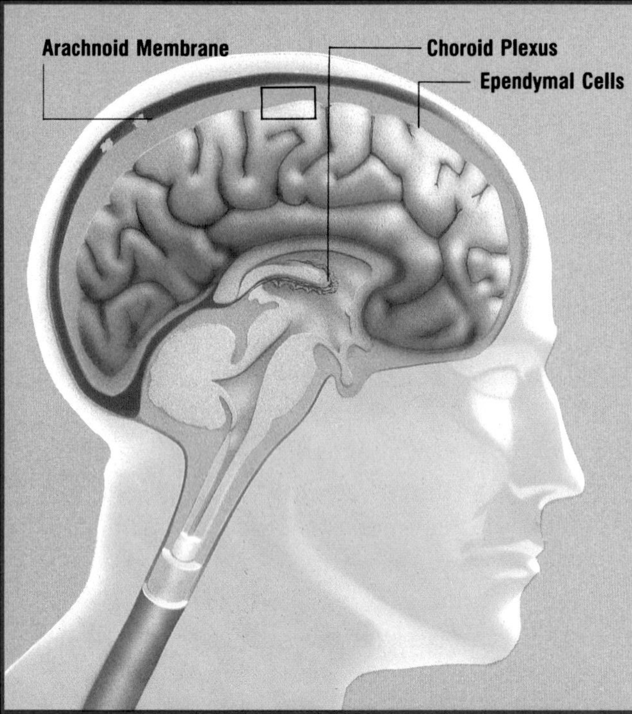

Arachnoid Membrane
Choroid Plexus
Ependymal Cells

A CRANIAL CUSHION. Flowing through the narrow spaces between the brain and skull, as well as in the spinal cord, is a watery broth called cerebrospinal fluid (*blue, left*). Secreted primarily by a structure in the brain called the choroid plexus, the fluid carries nutrients to brain tissue and cushions that organ against impacts. (Indeed, the cushion effectively reduces the weight of the brain from three pounds to less than two ounces.) Although the brain requires only about half a cup of fluid at a time, the choroid plexus produces about a quart per day, for reasons unknown. Much of the spent fluid is absorbed by ependymal cells, and a weblike structure called the arachnoid membrane pumps the rest into the bloodstream.

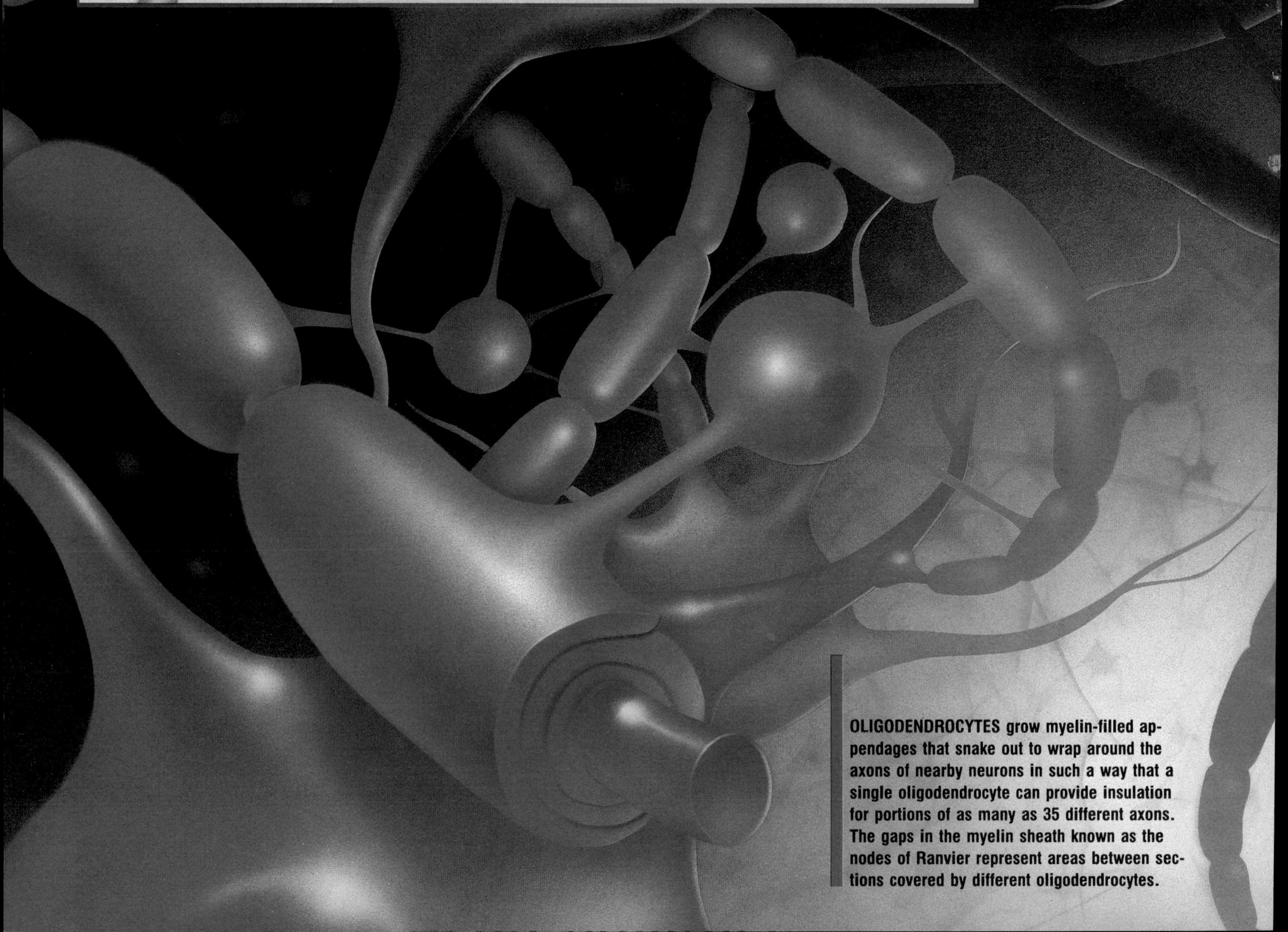

OLIGODENDROCYTES grow myelin-filled appendages that snake out to wrap around the axons of nearby neurons in such a way that a single oligodendrocyte can provide insulation for portions of as many as 35 different axons. The gaps in the myelin sheath known as the nodes of Ranvier represent areas between sections covered by different oligodendrocytes.

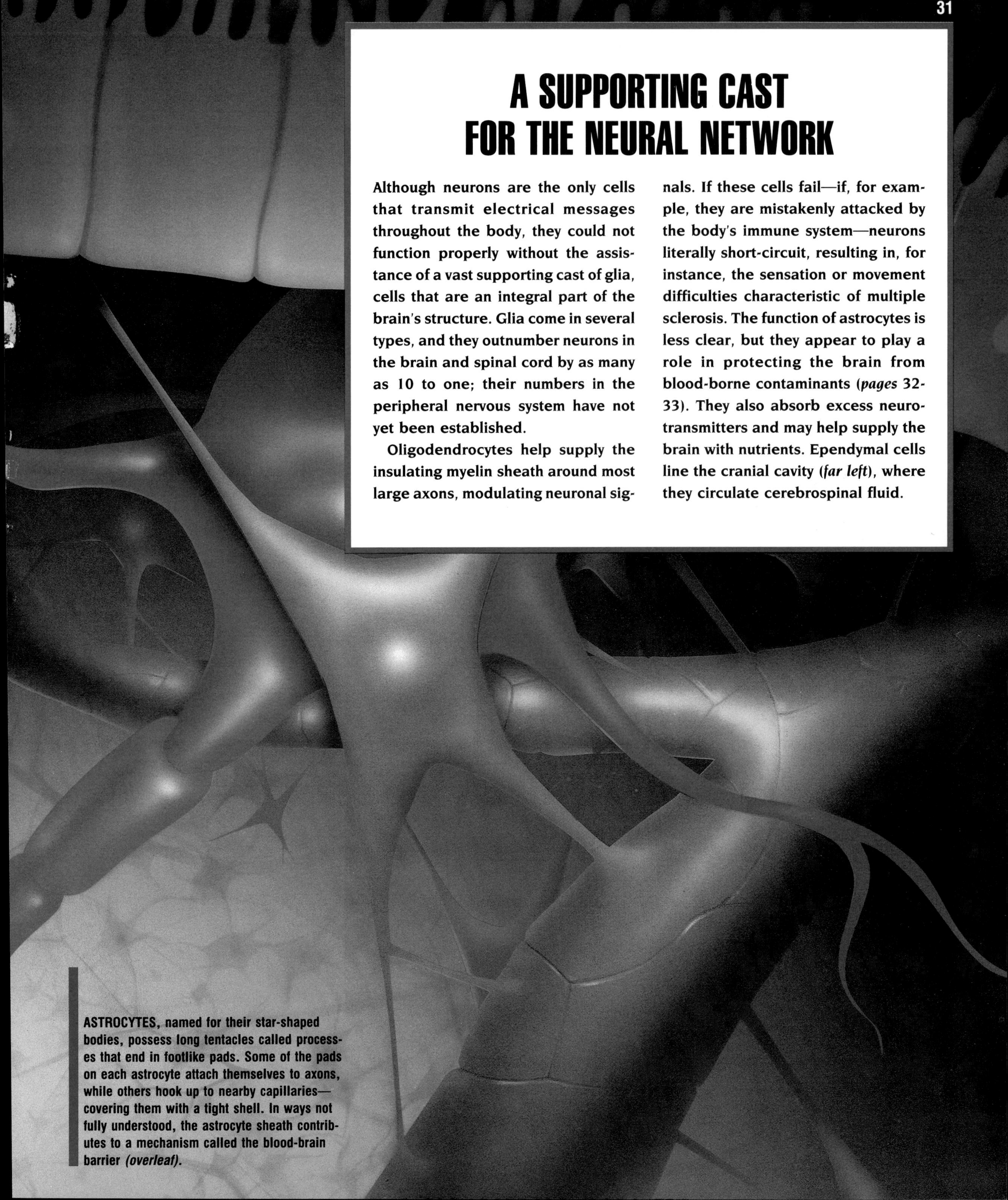

A SUPPORTING CAST FOR THE NEURAL NETWORK

Although neurons are the only cells that transmit electrical messages throughout the body, they could not function properly without the assistance of a vast supporting cast of glia, cells that are an integral part of the brain's structure. Glia come in several types, and they outnumber neurons in the brain and spinal cord by as many as 10 to one; their numbers in the peripheral nervous system have not yet been established.

Oligodendrocytes help supply the insulating myelin sheath around most large axons, modulating neuronal signals. If these cells fail—if, for example, they are mistakenly attacked by the body's immune system—neurons literally short-circuit, resulting in, for instance, the sensation or movement difficulties characteristic of multiple sclerosis. The function of astrocytes is less clear, but they appear to play a role in protecting the brain from blood-borne contaminants (*pages* 32-33). They also absorb excess neurotransmitters and may help supply the brain with nutrients. Ependymal cells line the cranial cavity (*far left*), where they circulate cerebrospinal fluid.

ASTROCYTES, named for their star-shaped bodies, possess long tentacles called processes that end in footlike pads. Some of the pads on each astrocyte attach themselves to axons, while others hook up to nearby capillaries—covering them with a tight shell. In ways not fully understood, the astrocyte sheath contributes to a mechanism called the blood-brain barrier *(overleaf).*

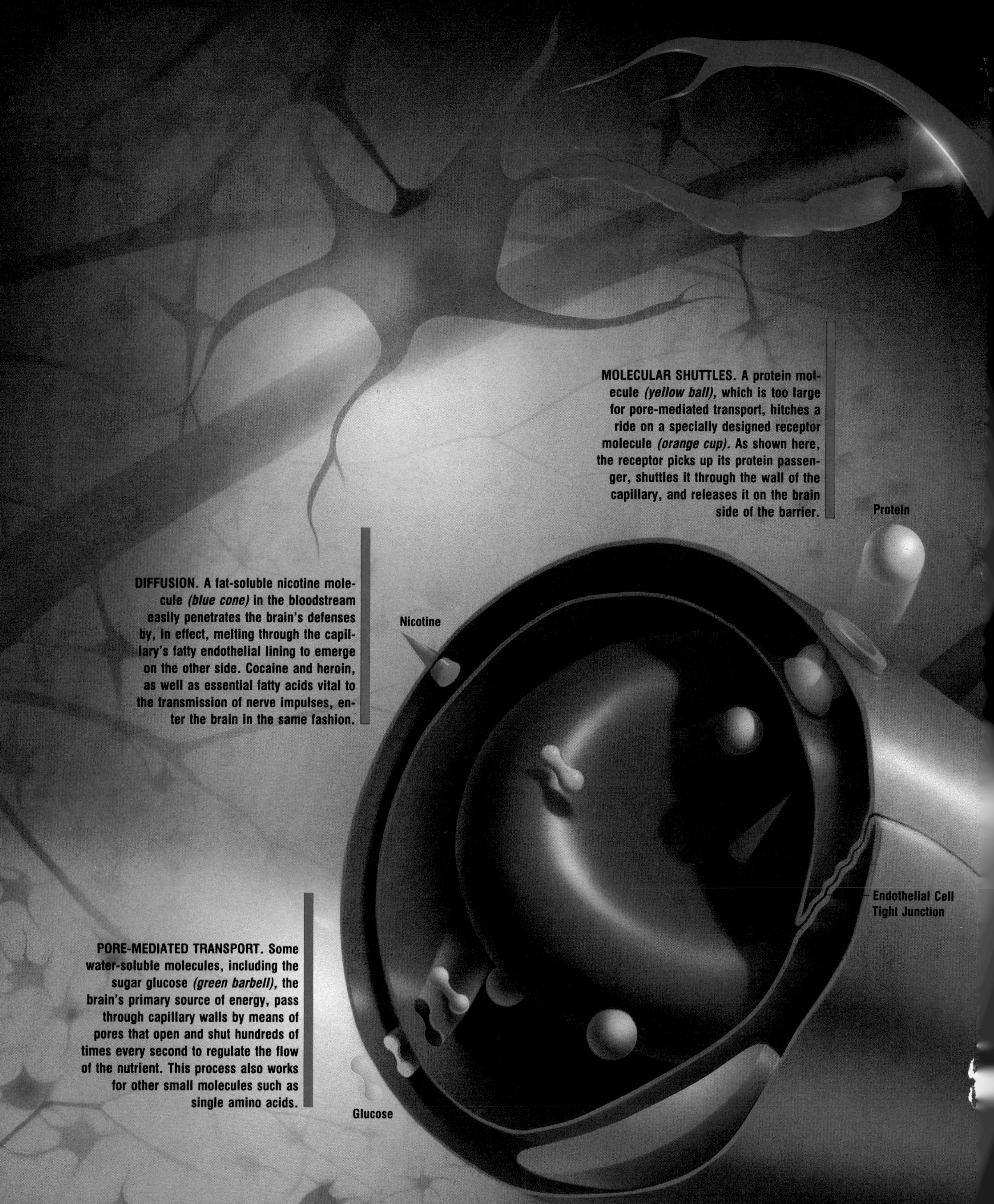
MOLECULAR SHUTTLES. A protein molecule (yellow ball), which is too large for pore-mediated transport, hitches a ride on a specially designed receptor molecule (orange cup). As shown here, the receptor picks up its protein passenger, shuttles it through the wall of the capillary, and releases it on the brain side of the barrier.
Protein
DIFFUSION. A fat-soluble nicotine molecule (blue cone) in the bloodstream easily penetrates the brain's defenses by, in effect, melting through the capillary's fatty endothelial lining to emerge on the other side. Cocaine and heroin, as well as essential fatty acids vital to the transmission of nerve impulses, enter the brain in the same fashion.
Nicotine
Endothelial Cell Tight Junction
PORE-MEDIATED TRANSPORT. Some water-soluble molecules, including the sugar glucose (green barbell), the brain's primary source of energy, pass through capillary walls by means of pores that open and shut hundreds of times every second to regulate the flow of the nutrient. This process also works for other small molecules such as single amino acids.
Glucose

KEYS TO THE BRAIN'S GUARDED SANCTUM

In the packed confines of the brain are capillaries so fine that red blood cells must pass single file. Not only do they supply nutrients to the brain's billions of neurons, they also keep brain tissue isolated from the effects of most harmful blood-borne agents. The protective mechanism—an ancient defense shared by all vertebrates—is known as the blood-brain barrier. Elsewhere in the body, crescent-shaped endothelial cells that form capillaries are separated by minuscule gaps that allow most nutrients and chemicals to pass freely from blood to nearby tissues. In the brain, however, not only do endothelial cells overlap, they are further sealed by their jigsawlike tight junctions and encased by foot processes of nearby astrocytes. Without this protection, the surge of neurotransmitters and hormones stimulated by the mere act of eating, for example, would upset the delicate chemical balance in the brain, triggering potentially fatal seizures or other difficulties.

The barrier shields the brain from bacteria and viruses, as well as from most toxic chemicals. Oddly, however, it also blocks the body's own disease-fighting white blood cells, and it allows substances like nicotine, alcohol, and cocaine to pass, while denying entry to many medicines. Scientists have thus begun to focus on the mechanisms by which chemicals cross the barrier. By creating drugs that take advantage of these methods, three of which are shown here, researchers hope to trick the brain's defenses into letting lifesaving medications reach the organ that above all others is responsible for making us who we are.

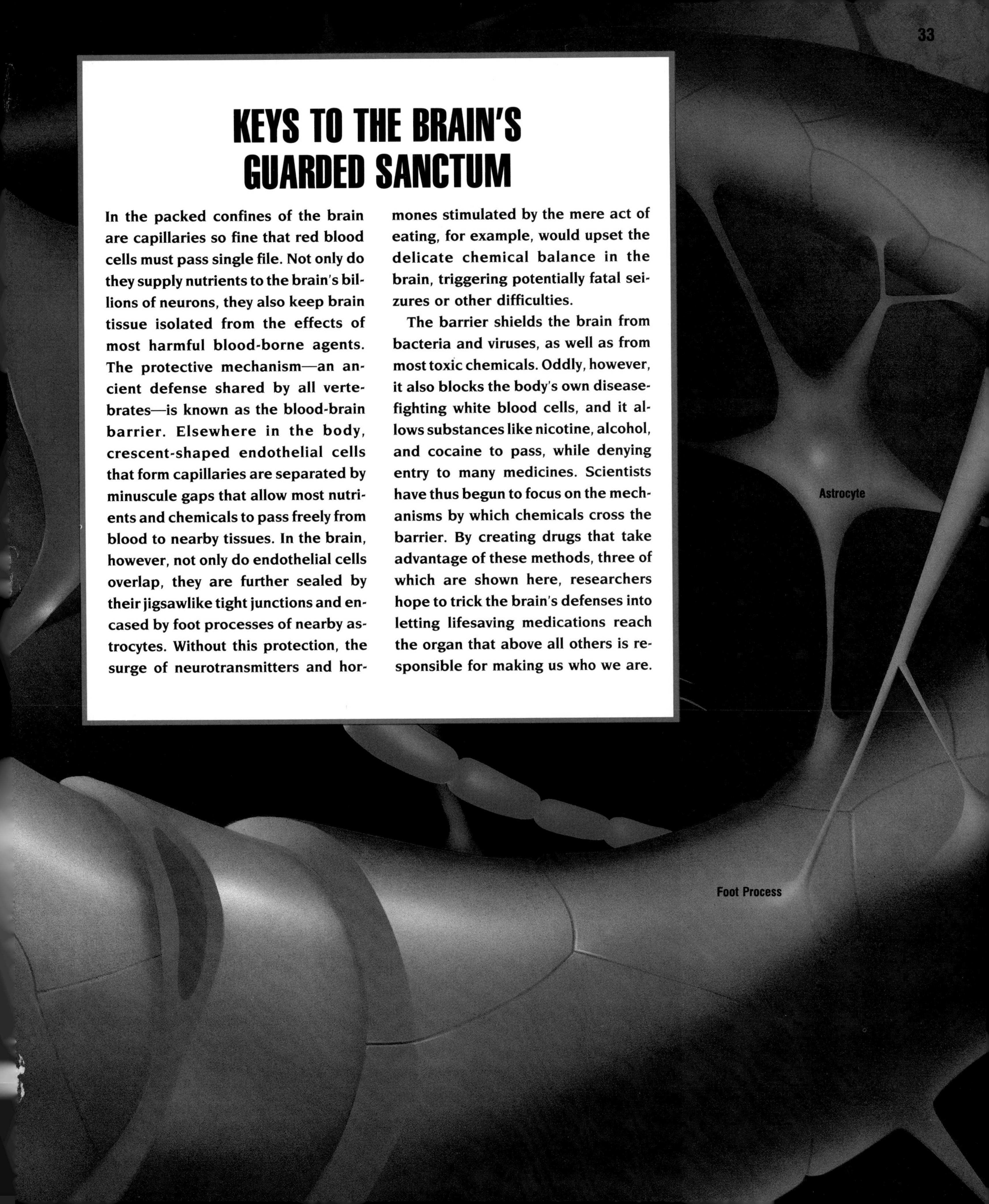

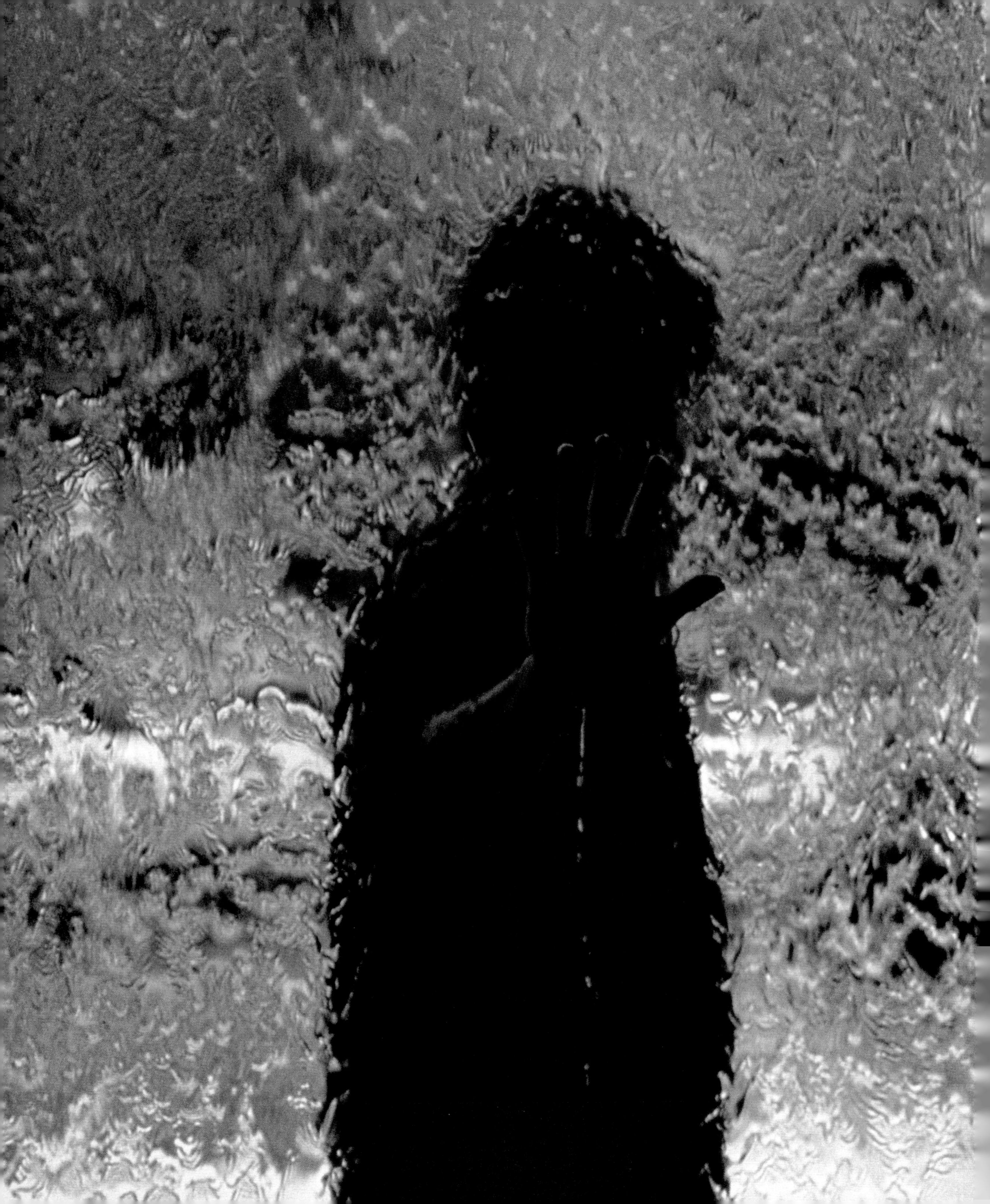

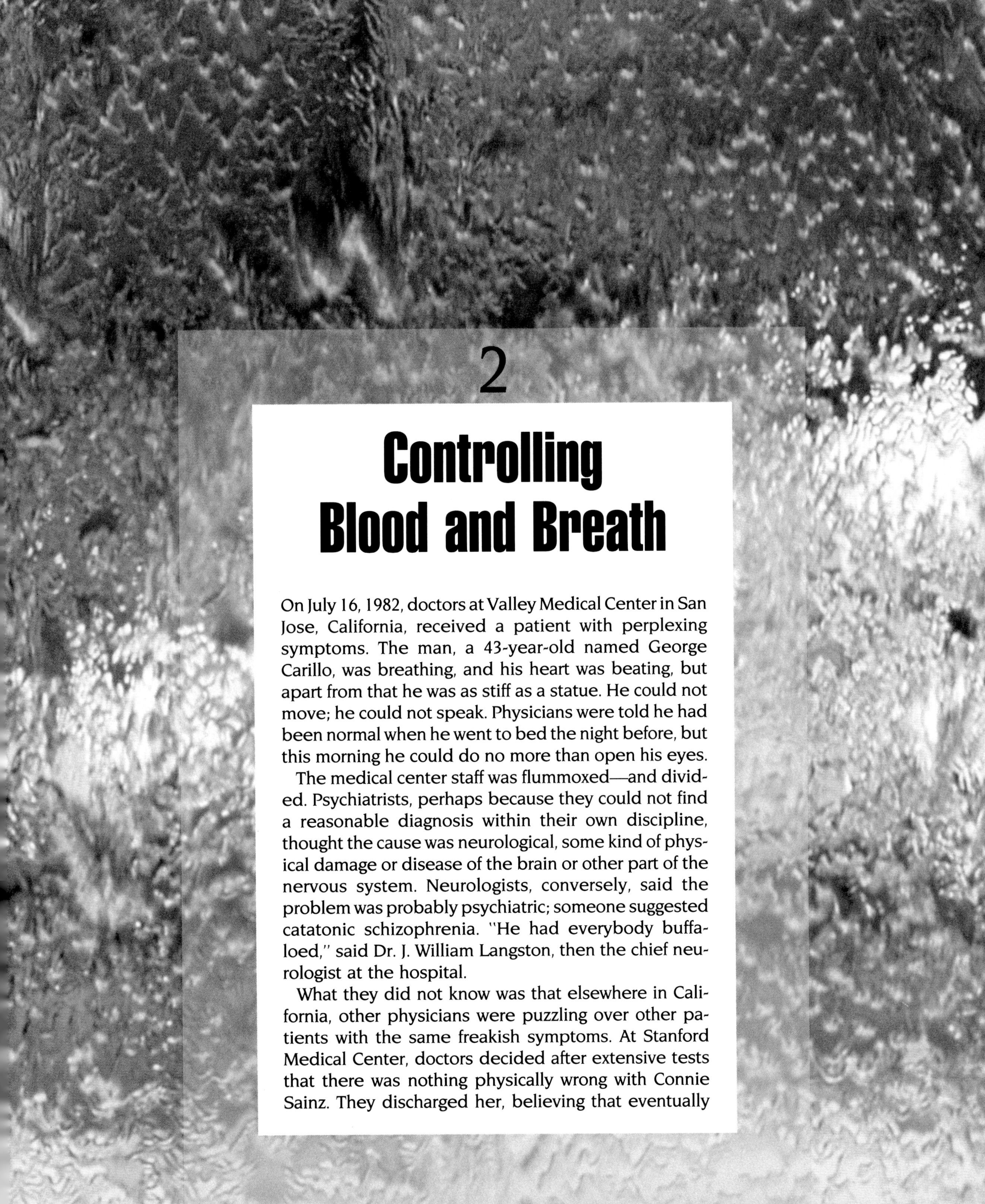

2

Controlling Blood and Breath

On July 16, 1982, doctors at Valley Medical Center in San Jose, California, received a patient with perplexing symptoms. The man, a 43-year-old named George Carillo, was breathing, and his heart was beating, but apart from that he was as stiff as a statue. He could not move; he could not speak. Physicians were told he had been normal when he went to bed the night before, but this morning he could do no more than open his eyes.

The medical center staff was flummoxed—and divided. Psychiatrists, perhaps because they could not find a reasonable diagnosis within their own discipline, thought the cause was neurological, some kind of physical damage or disease of the brain or other part of the nervous system. Neurologists, conversely, said the problem was probably psychiatric; someone suggested catatonic schizophrenia. "He had everybody buffaloed," said Dr. J. William Langston, then the chief neurologist at the hospital.

What they did not know was that elsewhere in California, other physicians were puzzling over other patients with the same freakish symptoms. At Stanford Medical Center, doctors decided after extensive tests that there was nothing physically wrong with Connie Sainz. They discharged her, believing that eventually

Muhammad Ali, shown at right fending off a flurry of blows during his 1980 loss to Larry Holmes, is one of millions worldwide diagnosed with the nervous disorder known as parkinsonism. Attributed to a shortage of the neurotransmitter dopamine in motor areas of the brain, parkinsonism brings movement problems, including tremors and slurred speech. The disorder has a number of causes, but it is most commonly associated with Parkinson's disease, a degenerative illness that destroys a key dopamine production site in the midbrain. Doctors suspect that in Ali's brain, dopamine depletion resulted from the repeated blows to the head sustained during his long boxing career.

she would get over what appeared to be a psychological problem and recover her ability to move and talk. In Watsonville, California, the mother of David and Bill Silvey was shocked to find her two sons, both in their 20s, lying mute and immobilized in the apartment they shared. Doctors at the Watsonville Community Hospital were mystified. In all, at least six "frozen" individuals sought medical attention within a few days, but in each instance the physicians involved thought they were dealing with isolated, unique cases.

Questions about these patients abounded. Was this frozen state tantamount or akin to a coma? Could the victims understand what was going on around them? Could they think? Or were their minds completely blank, zapped clean by some unknown calamity? Desperate for any clues, William Langston and his colleagues noticed one day that George Carillo seemed able to move one of his hands, although extremely slowly. They wrapped his fingers around a pencil and asked if he could hear them and tell them what was wrong.

"I can't move right," he scrawled painstakingly in a shaky script. "I know what I want to do, it just won't come out right."

As slowly as he scratched it out, Carillo's answer nonetheless struck like a thunderbolt. Trapped within his statuelike body, his mind still operated. For a neurologist such as Langston, who knows the geography of the brain and the functions of its parts, this revelation was a clue to the mystery of the puzzling patient.

The portion of George Carillo's brain that observed, interpreted, reasoned, and gave expression to thought—the outer layer called the cerebral cortex—was apparently unharmed by whatever had happened to him. If the problem was within his brain, it lay somewhere in deeper sections that transmit and coordinate messages telling muscles when and how to contract or relax in order to effect movements, perhaps in the basal ganglia—large masses of neurons beneath the cerebral cortex that are involved in motor control (*pages* 62-63)—or even deeper, in the brainstem and cerebellum, lower-brain structures that also have roles in movement.

Indeed, scientists have come to appreciate that no part of the brain operates in total isolation from all the other parts. Virtually every experiment seems to reveal interconnections that cast new doubts on long-held, simplistic views of the brain that assigned particular responsibilities exclusively to clearly defined areas.

The brainstem and cerebellum (or "little brain") are no exception. Although these two structures are still believed to manage all kinds of muscle activity, from breathing and heartbeat to the coordinated movements required of a prima ballerina or a skilled neurosurgeon (*pages* 49-57), they are also influenced by the cerebral cortex and the complex of brain centers, known as the limbic system, involved with emotions. Moreover, the influence probably goes both ways, though only controversial evidence has surfaced so far.

Part of the evidence for the scope of communications within the brain comes from research into neurotransmitters, highly specialized chemicals that carry nerve impulses across the tiny synaptic gaps between neurons (*pages* 28-29). Of the 50 or so known chemicals in this family (and scientists suspect that neurotransmitters may come in more than 200 varieties), most are produced in several parts of the central nervous system, and each one is implicated in multiple activities.

A well-studied neurotransmitter called dopamine, for example, is manufactured at three different sites in the brain. Supplies originating in neurons of the hypothalamus ultimately affect the production of various hormones from glands located

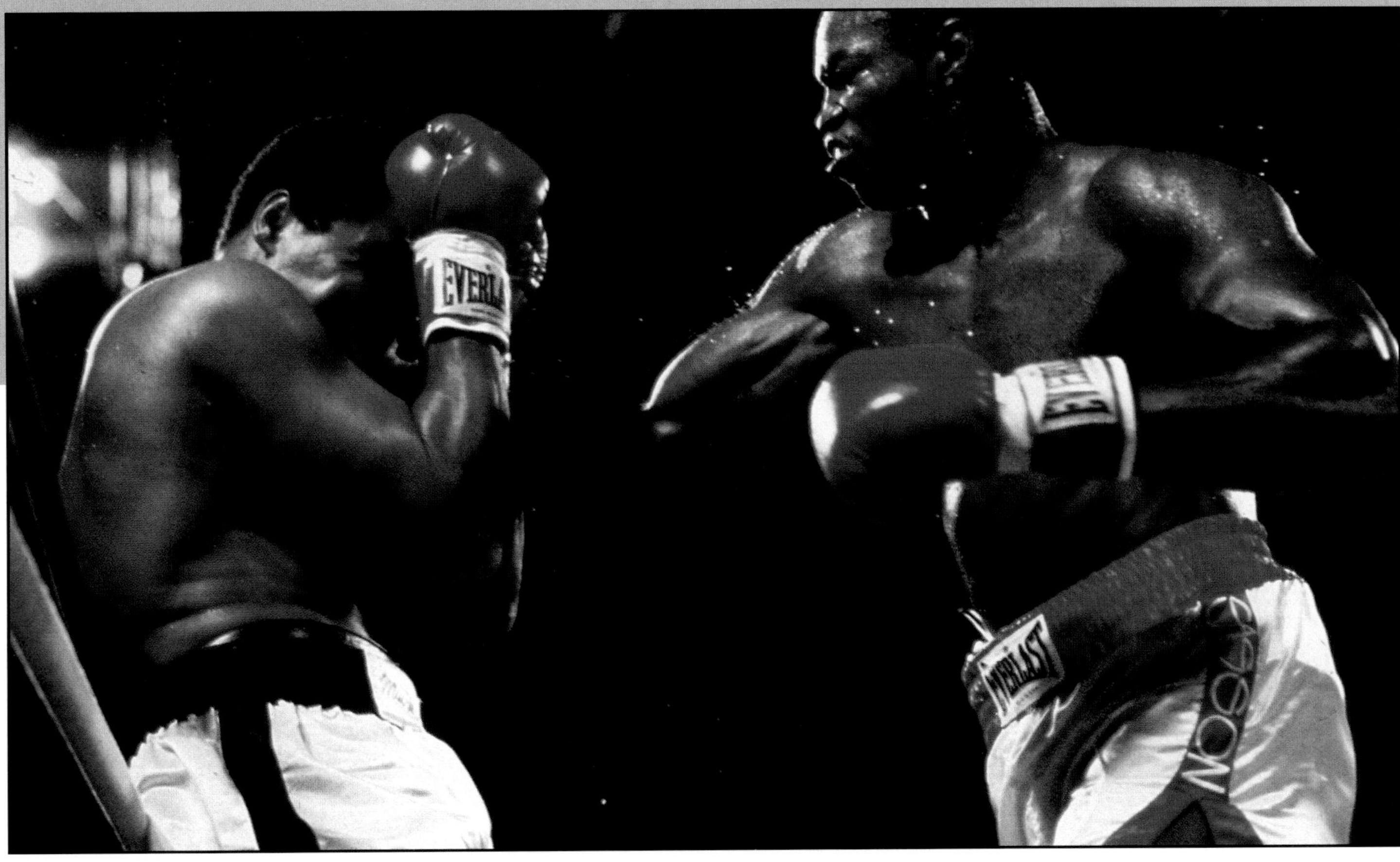

throughout the body. Dopamine from one part of the midbrain is associated with neurons that extend into the limbic system and thus influence emotional behavior. The major source of dopamine, however, is a structure found in the midbrain called (because of its normally dark hue) the substantia nigra, or "black substance." Dopamine from the substantia nigra helps the brainstem, cerebellum, and basal ganglia perform their muscle-control functions.

When the substantia nigra fails to supply sufficient amounts of dopamine, those nerve cells are short-circuited. This disorder, called Parkinson's disease, is characterized by rhythmic tremors of the extremities, rigidity of the arms and legs, unblinking eyes fixed in a zombielike stare, an unchanging facial expression, and glacial slowness of movement.

George Carillo wanted to move, but the action would not "come out right." Soon Dr. Langston learned that other people shared the symptoms and that all of them were heroin abusers. (In Carillo's case the information came as a written response to a query about what medicine he had taken lately.) Langston doubted that heroin had caused the victims' difficulties, though the drug affects the brainstem. "These addicts exhibited virtually every one of the signs that we see in Parkinson's disease," he said.

A standard treatment for Parkinson's disease is a drug called levodopa, or L-dopa, which the brain converts into dopamine. Even though Parkinson's usually attacks much older people, takes years to develop, and rarely if ever reaches the severity that had all but paralyzed the young addicts literally overnight, Langston tried L-dopa on Carillo—with dramatic results. Like a statue come to life, he was soon able to move his arms, to walk, to speak. The other addicts responded similarly to the treatment.

Analysis of the heroin recently purchased by some of the victims revealed that the substance was not heroin at all, but a so-called designer drug called MPPP, a chemical that simulates heroin's effects. The illegal laboratory that manufactured this batch had somehow fouled up the process, tainting the drug with a by-product compound identified as 1-methyl-4-phenyl-1,2,3,6-tetrahydropyridine, or MPTP. Tests on animals showed that MPTP killed dopamine-producing cells of the substantia nigra, just as Parkinson's disease does. The victims were unlikely to recover fully, but the physicians and researchers trying to help them now at least understood what was wrong.

Parkinson's disease was named for London physician James Parkinson, who first described its characteristic "involuntary tremulous motion" in 1817. For well over a century after its discovery, the disease was considered an ailment of the spinal cord, the muscles, and even the motor regions of the cerebral cortex, which was thought to be totally responsible for control of movement.

In 1915, however, a Parisian neuroanatomist named Tretiakoff offered a different theory. Upon examining the brains of people who had died after suffering Parkinson's, he and other researchers in several countries discovered that the normally black cells of the substantia nigra had undergone a transformation, paling significantly or turning virtually white. Tretiakoff suggested the damage indicated by the loss of pigment could be at the root of Parkinson's disease. He even proposed that the problem was a chemical deficiency and that Parkinson's might be alleviated by replacing the hypothetical missing chemical—this insight before chemical neurotransmitters were even known to exist.

In the 1930s, animal studies conducted by three Soviet brain researchers indirectly bolstered the notion that Parkinson's was not a disease of the cerebrum. Employing procedures typical of the period, the scientists worked with cats trained to run on a treadmill, cutting all nerve connections between each animal's brainstem and its motor cortex. Unable to walk or even to stand on its own, the cat was then suspended above the treadmill in a harness, and the researchers hooked up an electrical stimulator to the midbrain, the upper part of the brainstem. When this area, which came to be called the midbrain locomotor region, was rhythmically stimulated, the cat walked—then trotted, then galloped as the frequency of stimulations was increased.

By demonstrating that motion was possible without input from the motor cortex, the experiments suggested that Parkinson's disease, with its profound effects on movement, could originate elsewhere in the brain. Moreover, they showed that the brainstem is involved in transmitting the message that begins motion, a finding confirmed by more recent studies of nerve fibers running through the brainstem. These fibers, often called the reticular formation (from a Latin word meaning "small net"), are essential both for delivering the brain's motor commands to appropriate muscles and for receiving the feedback information the brain needs about whether the movements are taking place as intended.

All animals—from snakes slithering along the ground and porpoises undulating through the sea to two- and four-legged creatures walking and running on land—have wired in their brains from birth a basic repertoire of locomotive motions. But other kinds of movement come much less naturally. While all humans may be preprogrammed to walk, for example, there is much evidence that we are not all born dancers or hockey players or violinists. Somehow, though, we learn how to do all manner of things, from tying a shoe to driving a car, which then become second nature.

Mastery of these skills, sometimes called "muscle memory," seems to be held in the cerebellum, located behind the brainstem. This control center, which also deals with the subtleties of posture and muscle tone, receives nerve signals from nearly every part of the brain, every muscle in the body, and all the sensory organs, and processes such information to ensure that the muscles are doing exactly what was intended.

The cerebellum's role in movement is apparent in nearly every motion a person makes. Shaking hands with a friend, for example, requires the cerebellum to compute—from visual as well as muscular cues—the relative positions of the two hands and to automatically adjust speed and direction for smooth contact. Damage to the cerebellum can cause the hand to swing about wildly, unable to connect with its target.

For a time, scientists were reasonably certain that both the cerebellum and the brainstem acted only as accomplices to the cerebrum's motor cortex when it calls for movement. But then experimental evidence began to mount that the source of the impulse or decision to take action does not rest in the cerebrum alone.

In 1972 Edward Evarts of the National Institutes of Health restrained a monkey in a chair placed within reach of a fruit-juice dispenser with a push-pull handle. The monkey learned to pull the handle for a fruit-juice reward when a red light came on and to push it when a green light appeared. An extremely thin electrode inserted through a hole in the animal's skull and into a single cell of its motor cortex measured electrical activity there.

Evarts found that the cell's rate of firing rose above normal when the monkey received a "pull" command and fell below normal when the display signaled "push." Moreover, the change in firing rate always preceded the monkey's actual movement. So far, the evidence indicated that the command to push or pull definitely originated in the motor cortex.

But Evarts wanted to discover more about how the brain's activity is coordinated. He added microelectrodes to record what happened in the monkey's cerebellum and basal ganglia. Much to Evarts's surprise, cells in those sections of the lower brain fired simultaneously with the cell in the motor cortex—and all before the monkey moved a muscle to push or pull. The monkey's decision to move the handle came from all three areas, not just from the higher brain.

These experiments and others strongly suggest that the mind does not occupy a single location in the brain. Instead, it seems more likely that "mind" is the name we give to the result of all the brain's parts cooperating in ways that scientists are just beginning to understand. Future brain-mapping research will no doubt identify more control centers in the brain and further expose the influences that different parts of the brain exert on each other. A large portion of that influence arises in the chemical universe of neurotransmitters, the medium for the messages of the central nervous system; pinning down their identities and roles is an ongoing challenge for neuroscientists.

The first neurotransmitter was discovered in 1921 by German pharmacologist Otto Loewi with an experiment involving the still-beating heart excised from a living frog. Still attached to the heart was the vagus nerve, which carries signals to the heart muscle from the frog's medulla. Loewi knew from earlier work that stimulating the vagus nerve with an electrical current would dramatically slow the heartbeat.

Loewi immersed the frog heart in a saline solution similar to a natural fluid found in living tissue, then he applied electrical stimulation to the vagus nerve until the heart slowed. Next, he used the fluid to bathe the beating heart of another frog. The second heart, too, slowed, even though it had not been subjected to an electrical stimulus.

The dendrite filigree of a Purkinje cell *(right, top)* echoes the intricacy in the cortex of the cerebellum *(cross section, bottom)*, where these neurons reside. Receiving input from as many as 150,000 other neurons, these cells enable the cortex to process a stream of information from all over the body. To accommodate the huge numbers of neurons needed for this task, the cortex folds deeply in on itself, following a convoluted coastline of supporting structure in a continuous layer about a millimeter thick.

This proved to Loewi that the neurons of the vagus nerve had sent the cease-beating signal to the first heart not through direct electrical contact but by the release of a chemical agent that acted on the heart muscle's nerves. He reasoned that some of that chemical agent, having mixed with the saline solution, must have caused the second heart to stop beating as well. After some five more years of research, Loewi isolated the chemical involved. The agent was acetylcholine, named for two ingredients: choline, which helps convert fat to energy; and a form of acetic acid, the component of vinegar that makes it sour. Later, lower than normal levels of acetylcholine would be found during postmortem examination of people who had been victims of Alzheimer's disease and its attendant memory loss. However, no one has yet discovered the equivalent of an L-dopa to treat this disorder.

In the 1930s the neurotransmitter norepinephrine, important to the fight-or-flight response, was identified. Norepinephrine production was found to be concentrated in a tiny oval structure called the locus ceruleus—"blue place"—for its color. The locus ceruleus lies within the pons, a bulge in the brainstem between the medulla and midbrain, and contains the cell bodies of only about 3,000 neurons, an infinitesimal fraction of the brain's many billions of such cells. But these are most remarkable neurons indeed. Not only do they constitute the brain's biggest production center for any known neurotransmitter, their influence extends throughout the brain.

Few scientists believed this astounding news when Sweden's Kjell Fuxe and Annica Dahlström announced it in the early 1960s, but their research could not be faulted. In the course of investigating the bright green fluorescence that norepinephrine and some other brain chemicals emit after exposure to formaldehyde vapor, the two researchers placed thin slices of rat brain in a box containing the vapor. Examined under the microscope, the brain samples displayed a glowing tracery showing clearly that norepinephrine-dispensing axons of nerve cells originating in the locus ceruleus reach out to amazing distances in every direction, sprouting branches on branches on branches in such multiplicity that they defy counting.

In a remarkable demonstration of how the brainstem converses with every other part of the brain, axons from the blue place stretch backward to the cerebellum, forward into the prefrontal cortex, down into the spinal cord, up into the whole of the cerebral cortex and outward through the limbic system surrounding the top end of the brainstem. Experiments have shown that these cells release norepinephrine when they fire.

Some scientists theorize that the norepinephrine alerts neurons of the cerebral cortex that something out of the ordinary has happened and that the "thinking" part of the brain should pay attention, perhaps to prepare for danger. And because most of the locus ceruleus's neurons also reach into various parts of the limbic system, implicated in the welling up of emotions, norepinephrine may take part in triggering feelings associated with love or fear or anger. It is also fairly certain that the axons descending into the spinal cord increase muscle tension, possibly as a prelude to action. Researchers are still trying to puzzle out all the ramifications of this network—whether the fight-or-flight response, which is known to involve norepinephrine, is enough by itself to demand such complexity or whether this neurotransmitter plays other roles as well.

Similar uncertainties are associated with dopamine. Scientists discovered dopamine's presence in the brain during the mid-1950s, but they thought at first that it was merely a chemical steppingstone in the manufacture of a handful of neurotransmit-

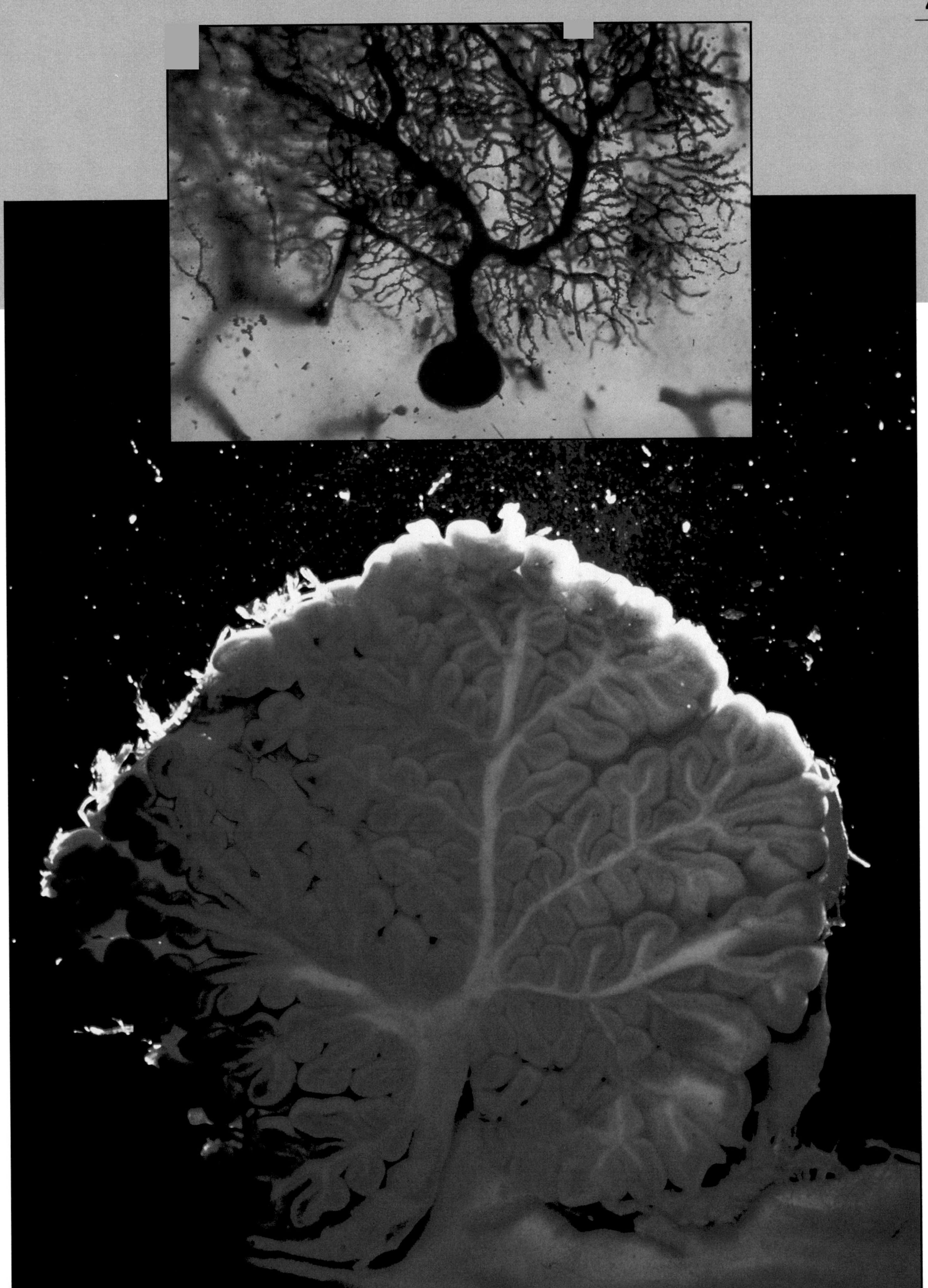

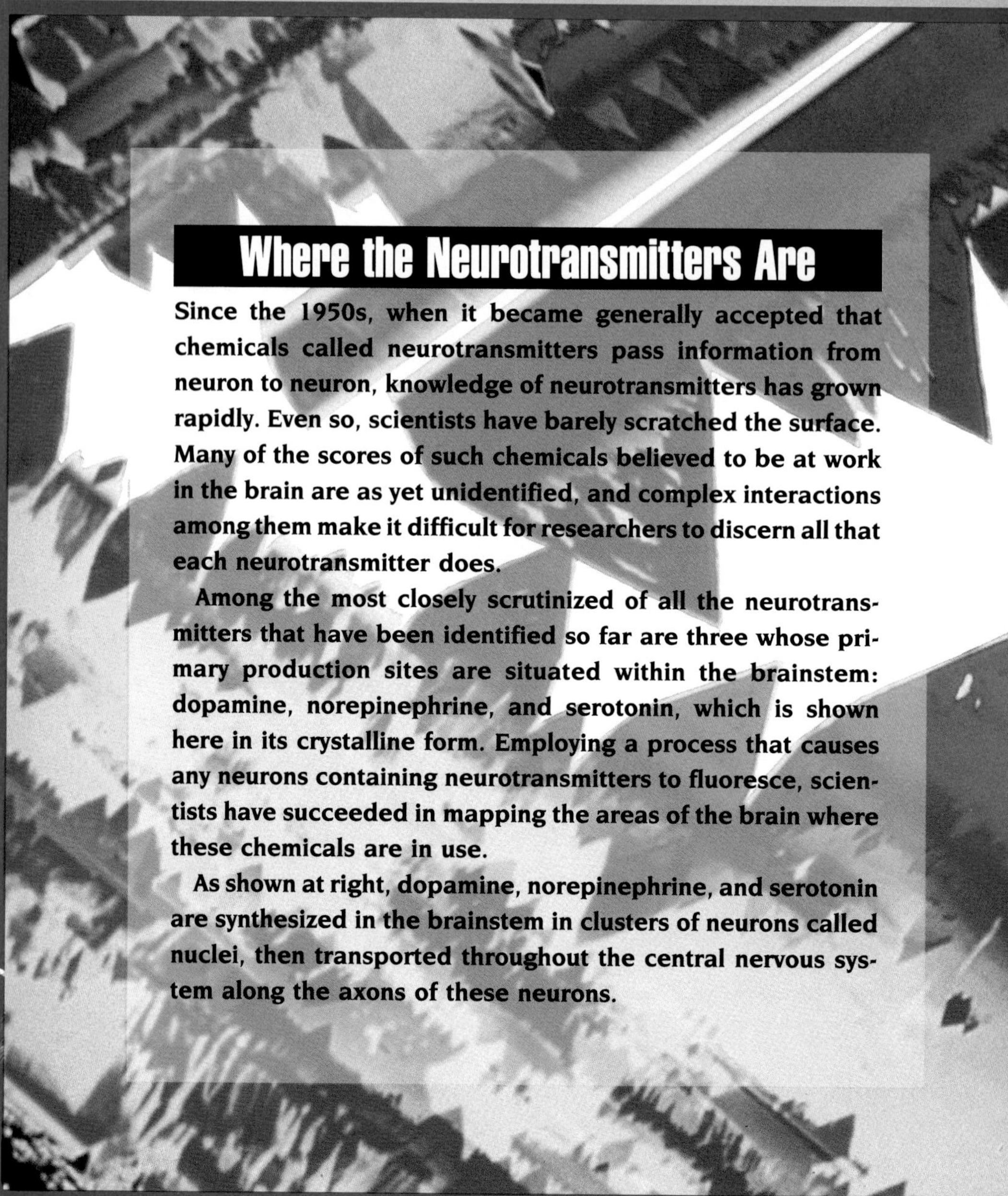

Where the Neurotransmitters Are

Since the 1950s, when it became generally accepted that chemicals called neurotransmitters pass information from neuron to neuron, knowledge of neurotransmitters has grown rapidly. Even so, scientists have barely scratched the surface. Many of the scores of such chemicals believed to be at work in the brain are as yet unidentified, and complex interactions among them make it difficult for researchers to discern all that each neurotransmitter does.

Among the most closely scrutinized of all the neurotransmitters that have been identified so far are three whose primary production sites are situated within the brainstem: dopamine, norepinephrine, and serotonin, which is shown here in its crystalline form. Employing a process that causes any neurons containing neurotransmitters to fluoresce, scientists have succeeded in mapping the areas of the brain where these chemicals are in use.

As shown at right, dopamine, norepinephrine, and serotonin are synthesized in the brainstem in clusters of neurons called nuclei, then transported throughout the central nervous system along the axons of these neurons.

ters. By the end of the decade, however, they recognized dopamine as a neurotransmitter in its own right. Shortly thereafter, three Swedish pharmacologists learned that 80 percent of the brain's dopamine supply is provided by the substantia nigra.

As with norepinephrine, one dopamine path leads to the limbic system, notably to centers for the sense of smell. Other dopamine-producing neurons fetch up specifically at the hypothalamus, which participates in the regulation of hormone production throughout the body. The full implication of these and other aspects of dopamine remains largely a matter of conjecture.

In 1960 an Austrian physician noticed during brain autopsies of a few deceased Parkinson's sufferers not only that the usually black substantia nigra was as pale as surrounding tissue but that dopamine levels were below normal. Neuroscientists already knew that dopamine-producing neurons of the substantia nigra ended in the basal ganglia. Putting two and two together, they concluded that when nerve cells in the substantia nigra die, for whatever reason, neurons in the basal ganglia become deprived of the dopamine they need to activate muscles properly. That, in turn, produces the jerky movements, tremors, and muscle weakness that plague patients with Parkinson's disease.

This affliction thus became the first illness attributed to a neurotransmitter deficiency, just as suspected 45 years earlier. Armed with this knowledge, physicians hoped to treat the disorder by giving their patients dopamine to make up for the deficit. However, they discovered that dopamine, when administered as medicine, will not cross the so-called blood-brain barrier, the tightly packed layer of cells that prevents many substances from entering the brain from the bloodstream.

It was 1967 before pharmacologists came up with a solution in L-dopa, which not only could cross the blood-brain barrier but on the other side was converted into dopamine by an enzyme found even in damaged sub-

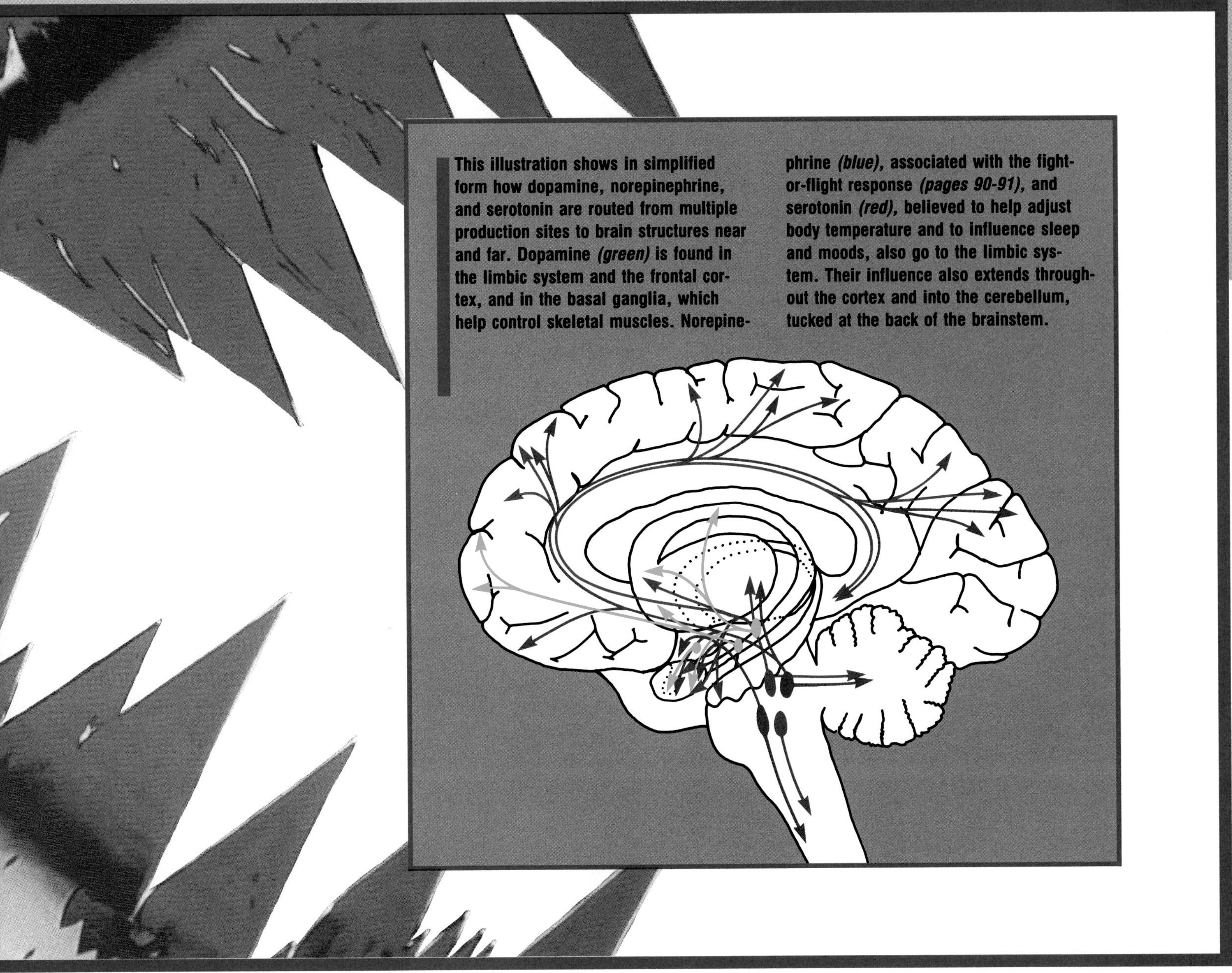

This illustration shows in simplified form how dopamine, norepinephrine, and serotonin are routed from multiple production sites to brain structures near and far. Dopamine *(green)* is found in the limbic system and the frontal cortex, and in the basal ganglia, which help control skeletal muscles. Norepinephrine *(blue)*, associated with the fight-or-flight response *(pages 90-91)*, and serotonin *(red)*, believed to help adjust body temperature and to influence sleep and moods, also go to the limbic system. Their influence also extends throughout the cortex and into the cerebellum, tucked at the back of the brainstem.

stantia nigra tissue. Yet the difficulties of the victims were far from over. L-dopa's side effects could be discouraging. Even after careful adjustment of the dose, the drug frequently caused nausea, anxiety, irritability, hyperactivity, dangerous clumsiness, and in extreme cases wild, uncontrollable movements and frightening hallucinations. But in general patients improved so remarkably that L-dopa took on the aura of a miracle cure.

Among the most dramatic and heartwarming transformations wrought by the new treatment were those described by neurologist Oliver Sacks in his 1973 book *Awakenings*, later made into a popular movie. Sacks's patients included a number of victims of a sleeping sickness pandemic that swept the world between 1916 and 1927. The disease killed millions and left millions of others in severe parkinsonian states similar to those of the "frozen" drug addicts in California. Some of Sacks's charges had spent half a century in a zombielike state, staring glumly and speaking little or not at all for day upon endless day. When the patients were treated with the newly available L-dopa, the results were truly miraculous. They began to speak, to walk without assistance, to evince joy.

Before the advent of L-dopa, Sacks had observed that one patient, a Mr. V., sometimes changed the position of one arm so slowly that it could never be seen to move. The man would start the day with his hand on his knee. By noon the hand would be fixed in midair halfway between knee and face, and several hours later it would arrive at his nose. After L-dopa had greatly alleviated Mr. V.'s condition, Sacks asked him about the "frozen poses." "What do you mean, 'frozen poses'?" the patient responded. When Sacks explained, Mr. V. was indignant. "I was merely wiping my nose!" he declared.

In disbelief, Sacks assembled 30 still photos that had been made of the patient in one day and had them converted to movie film. Running the film through a projector at 16 frames per second, he saw the patient was right. Mr. V. was simply wiping his nose, unaware that the action was taking 10,000 times as long as normal.

In time the massive doses of L-dopa required to overcome Parkinson's symptoms produced extremely unpleasant side effects for some of Sacks's patients, as they would later for the California addicts. For Californian George Carillo, it was a choice between being pursued by flames and terrifying snakes every night or giving up the L-dopa and once again becoming an unmoving statue; he decided to suffer the horrible hallucinations so he could continue to move his body. Though imperfect, L-dopa had proved it possible to correct a brain disorder by replenishing the supply of a missing neurotransmitter.

Meanwhile, a team led by Anders Bjorklund, a neuroscientist at Sweden's University of Lund, found a promising way to restore dopamine levels in the brain without unpleasant side effects. Working with rats, the Swedish group and other researchers harvested healthy substantia nigra tissue and implanted it in the brains of other rats whose substantia nigra cells had been destroyed to induce symptoms of advanced Parkinson's disease. The transplanted tissue soon began to produce dopamine, partially relieving the rats' symptoms, with no side effects noted.

For humans, healthy substantia nigra tissue is unavailable except from aborted fetuses. After much debate, the Swedish government instituted stringent safeguards to ensure that no abortions would be inspired by the demand for fetal brain tissue, and in the late 1980s, the University of Lund team began implanting fetal substantia nigra tissue in human Parkinson's sufferers. George Carillo and one other "frozen" Californian were among the earliest volunteers selected. Brain scans made several years later indicated that only a small portion of the new tissue had survived. Nonetheless, movement had improved significantly in these patients, although speech remained slurred. Moreover, the tissue transplants lowered the dose of L-dopa to a level that greatly reduced the drug's side effects.

Having established the existence of neurotransmitters and discerning that they are produced by neurons that also transport them along pathways of the central nervous system, scientists still were in the dark as to how the chemicals conveyed their messages to the receiving neurons. Finding the answer would follow a different avenue of research.

Scientists could see, as more of these agents were identified, that they were chemically different from one another. Moreover, that neurotransmitters participated in different functions implied that each affected some neurons but not others.

From this evidence, researchers theorized that each receiving nerve

Invaders at the Synapse

Virtually every type of illicit drug that affects the mind does so by interfering with the chemical transmission of impulses within the nervous system. For example, crack cocaine, shown here in vials against crystals of dopamine, meddles not only with that neurotransmitter but also with the neurotransmitter norepinephrine.

Under normal circumstances, these neurotransmitters are reabsorbed after use into the neurons that released them. Cocaine, however, appears to block this reabsorption process, leaving an excess of dopamine and norepinephrine in the tiny gap between neurons. The resultant surplus of these chemicals gives cocaine users heightened mental alertness, feelings of euphoria, and the illusion of great strength. But an overdose of cocaine can cause death by overwhelming the centers that control breathing and heartbeat.

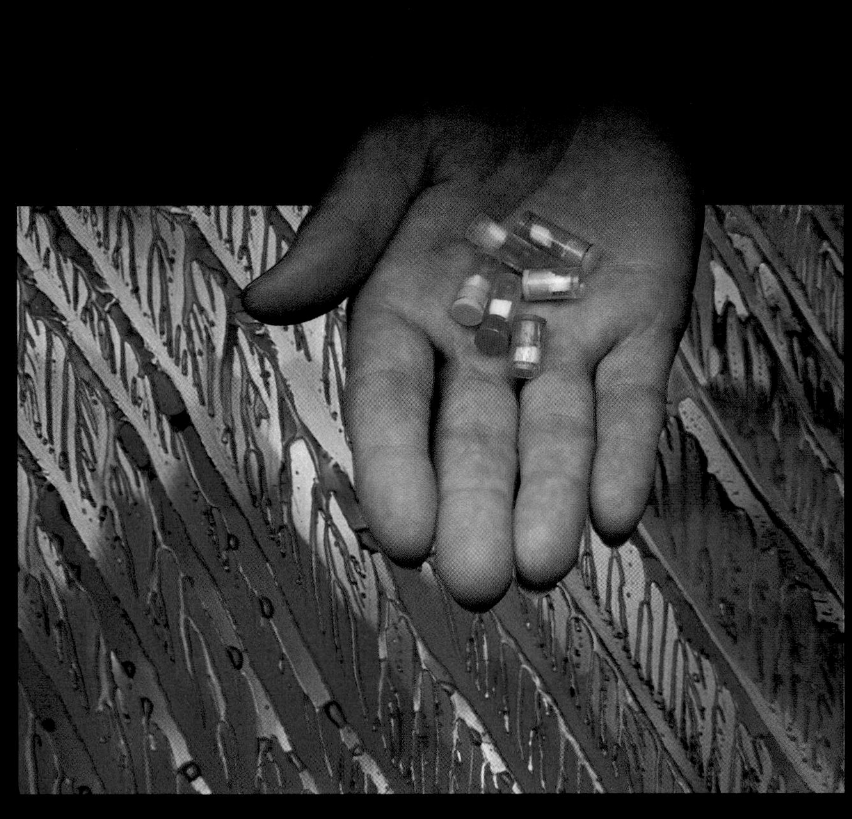

cell must have one or more cavities, each uniquely designed by nature to fit only one of the several neurotransmitters that might influence the cell. Either a neurotransmitter and one of these receptors fit together like two pieces of a jigsaw puzzle, or the chemical messenger is rejected. Thus only the right neurotransmitters, went the theory, would induce a response from a particular neuron—in some cases increasing the recipient cell's firing rate, in other cases slowing it or stopping it altogether.

There is no microscope powerful enough to reveal actual receptors, but by assuming that they exist, scientists have made great strides, including a life-saving treatment for heroin overdose and the discovery of a class of neurotransmitters called endorphins.

Unfortunately for heroin addicts, the blood-brain barrier presents no obstacle to that drug or to other opiates such as morphine. In too large quantities, these chemicals quickly shut down neurons in the medulla essential for breathing. Loss of consciousness comes quickly—and death follows inevitably—unless the victim gets an injection of a drug called naloxone, which reverses the effects of the opiate and restores normal breathing in a matter of seconds.

Naloxone was invented in 1960 by the application of the already-established principle that one substance may have a biologically antagonistic action on another if they are almost—but not quite—identical in their chemical structures. Naloxone was synthesized to be a replica of heroin's parent, morphine, except for having one extra carbon and one extra oxygen atom. It worked. If administered in time, naloxone rapidly returned breathing to normal.

At the time, no one knew just how naloxone accomplished this feat. One prominent theory was that, in a heroin overdose, molecules of the opiate attach themselves to neurotransmitter receptors in the brain. After a brief stay, heroin molecules, like those of neurotransmitters, become dislodged for a variety of reasons. When they drop off the receptors, the theory went, they are replaced by other heroin molecules—except when even small quantities of naloxone are present. Molecules of this drug were thought to have a much stronger attraction than heroin to these receptors and to remain coupled to them longer (though by no means permanently). Thus naloxone would quickly replace heroin, molecule for molecule, on neurons in the brain. Rather than causing them to shut down, the antidote enables the neurons to resume functioning.

In 1973 Candace Pert, then a graduate student at Johns Hopkins University, set out to prove this receptor theory of opiates and their effects on the body. In doing so, she and her colleagues began a chain of research that would not only confirm this hypothesis but would also lead to the discovery of other important neurotransmitters.

Pert chemically attached a radioactive tracer to some naloxone molecules, so that each one was radioactively "tagged." After adding a tiny amount of the tagged naloxone into a suspension of nerve-cell membranes, she thoroughly rinsed and filtered the mix to wash away as much naloxone as possible. Later readings of radioactivity showed that a fair number of the radioactive naloxone molecules remained in the slurry of membranes. The most plausible explanation of the strong attachment: Naloxone molecules were binding to receptors.

To prove that these receptors were the same ones that opiates use to achieve their drug effects, Pert repeated the experiment, each time pitting a different nonradioactive opiate against radioactive naloxone and using radioactivity readings to measure the proportion of receptors seized by the opiates. When a reading remained high, the opiate had claimed relatively few receptors from the radioactively tagged naloxone; a low radioactivity count meant that the opiate had locked into more receptors as they had been vacated by the radioactive naloxone. The relative abilities of the different opiates to compete for receptor sites matched their relative potencies as drugs. Further investigations would show that opiate receptors in the human brain are densely concentrated in the medulla's respiration center, which explains why breathing is so vulnerable to overdoses.

Proving the existence of specific receptors for opiates in the brain shed no light on why they should exist at all. The puzzle only deepened when scientists discovered that all vertebrates, even fish, have opiate receptors in their brains. This news implied that opiate receptors had appeared early during animal evolution. But why, researchers wondered, should there be a special receptor for a chemical produced by poppies, the only naturally occurring source of these substances and a plant that did not evolve until millions of years after the receptor first appeared on nerve cells in animal brains?

The answer came in 1975 when two researchers in Scotland, John Hughes and Hans Kosterlitz, discovered in the brains of pigs, rabbits, and other animals a molecule that would bind to an opiate receptor. Hughes and

Between Life and Death

At any given time, thousands of people are lost in the limbo of persistent vegetative state, or PVS. Characterized by chronic unconsciousness, PVS results from serious damage to the cerebral hemispheres, which are responsible for thinking and for instructing muscles to move. Victims sleep and wake up; heartbeat and breathing are maintained by the brainstem, and the eyes may move reflexively toward sound or motion. Yet PVS individuals are unaware of their surroundings. They cannot speak, feel, or initiate movement. Recovery is exceedingly rare; odds have been estimated at less than one in 1,000. Thus, many experts in medical ethics agree that, on a case-by-case basis, it is permissible to let such patients die.

Unfortunately, PVS can resemble another affliction, the locked-in syndrome, in which the victims, though unable to move, are conscious and alert. For example, although locked-in patients can neither move nor speak, many can demonstrate awareness by answering yes or no questions with eye blinks.

PET scans, better than any other means, can reliably distinguish between these two tragedies. As shown at right, a locked-in brain (*bottom*) is as dynamic as a healthy brain (*top*) and is markedly more so than the brain of a PVS patient (*middle*), as indicated by the higher proportion of yellow and red zones. PET-scan evidence can provide solace to relatives of PVS patients, helping to reassure those who wish to allow a loved one in such circumstances to slip away.

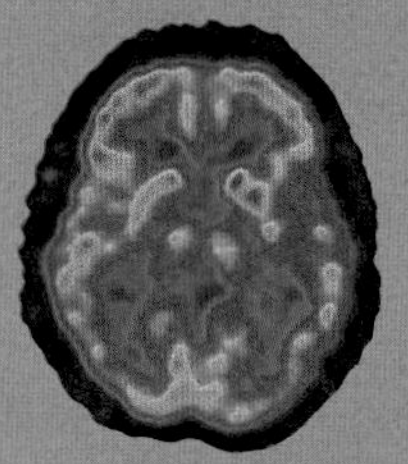

Healthy Brain

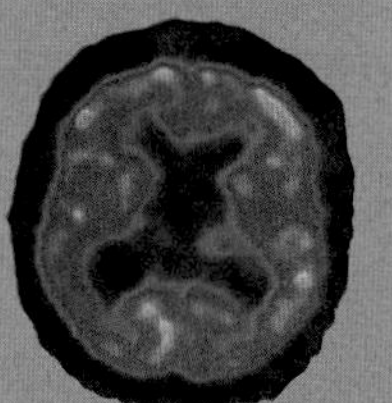

PVS Brain

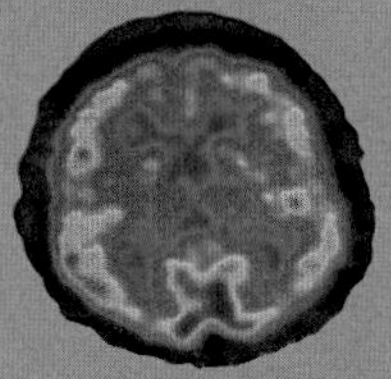

Locked-in Brain

Kosterlitz added naloxone to brainstem tissue taken from laboratory animals, allowing the opiate antagonist to bind to the opiate receptors. They then added extracts from the same brain tissue to see if they could find any naturally produced substance that could displace the naloxone from the receptors.

Indeed there was, and after a long series of purification steps, Hughes and Kosterlitz eventually isolated the brain's own opiates and named them enkephalins, meaning "in the head." Neurobiologists called these neurotransmitters endogenous morphine-like substances—commonly shortened to endorphins.

These neurotransmitters and others similar to them in their effects are produced naturally in the brainstem, the medulla, and other regions of the brain that are vulnerable to opiates. The body uses endorphins and endorphin-like neurotransmitters to help regulate breathing, to release pleasurable emotions, and also to relieve the pain of unusual stress, which explains the "runner's high" experienced by athletes and the ability of soldiers to fight on when they are wounded.

Considerable experimental evidence has led to the conclusion that molecules of heroin and the other opiates are similar in shape to endorphins and thus fit endorphin receptors. Beyond that, opiates have effects on the body much like those of endorphins. If the drugs are used often, most endorphin-making neurons soon cease production and depend instead on the opiate to do the natural substance's job.

The result is addiction. If a drug addict cannot get a fix, the neurons are deprived suddenly of the neurotransmitter they require. Until they begin making endorphins once again—or get another dose of opiate—those neurons will not function properly. Their malfunctioning is what produces the terrible symptoms of withdrawal: cold sweats, nausea, severe abdominal cramps, and uncontrollable kicking as leg muscles contract involuntarily.

By displacing heroin molecules from endorphin receptors in the respiratory center of the medulla and allowing neurons there to reassert control over breathing, naloxone saves many an overdose victim's life. But with no neurotransmitter effects of its own, naloxone cannot lessen the agony of withdrawal.

That treatment at the neurotransmitter level in the brain succeeds with ailments as diverse as heroin overdoses and Parkinson's disease explains in part why researchers pursue these chemicals so resolutely. A complete map of neurotransmitters, showing their sources and their pathways through the brain, could point the way to tempering all kinds of debilitating and even fatal illnesses. No longer would Alzheimer's disease, for example, suck the joy from old age.

Such rewards could still be a long way off, however. Although neurotransmitters have been identified at a fairly rapid rate since the 1950s, figuring out exactly what they do proceeds at a far slower pace. Thus decades may pass before a comprehensive neurotransmitter map is drawn. In the meantime, serendipitous discoveries will no doubt lead to remedies for afflictions that today, for all practical purposes, lie beyond the reach of medicine.

THE BODY'S AUTOPILOT

Settled into his seat on an airplane, a business traveler ponders the journey ahead of him, perhaps wondering what he will be served for lunch, whether his flight will depart late because of an approaching thunderstorm, or if the seat next to him will remain unoccupied.

The ruminations, speculations, and meditations that might occupy his mind are countless, but there are entire classes of thoughts that will never enter his mind. He will not, for example, focus any mental energy on keeping his heartbeat or his breathing steady or on the head and eye movements that are involved in, say, glancing idly around the cabin.

All such basic physical activities are primarily the responsibility of the brainstem and the cerebellum, or little brain. As explained on the following pages, these brain components function as a we-never-sleep control center, handling vital body functions automatically—and freeing the conscious mind from the minutiae of muscle contractions and relaxations involved in even the simplest of actions.

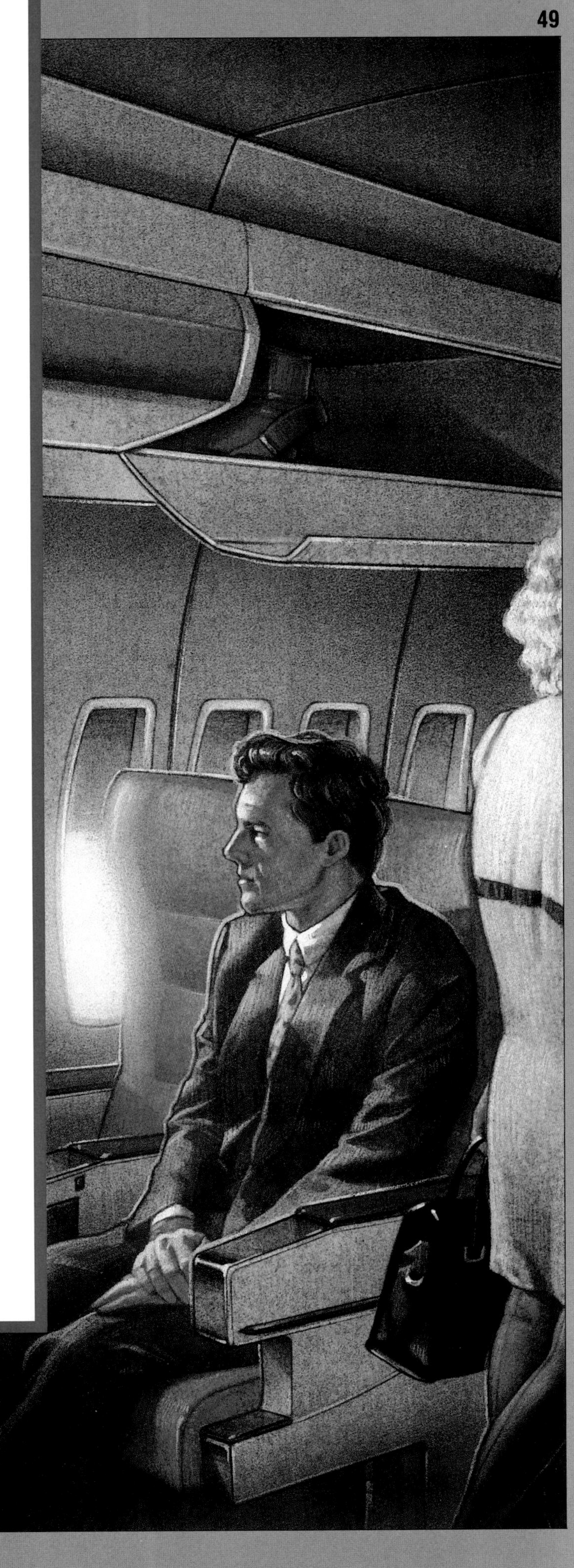

MAIN PLAYERS IN THE BRAINSTEM

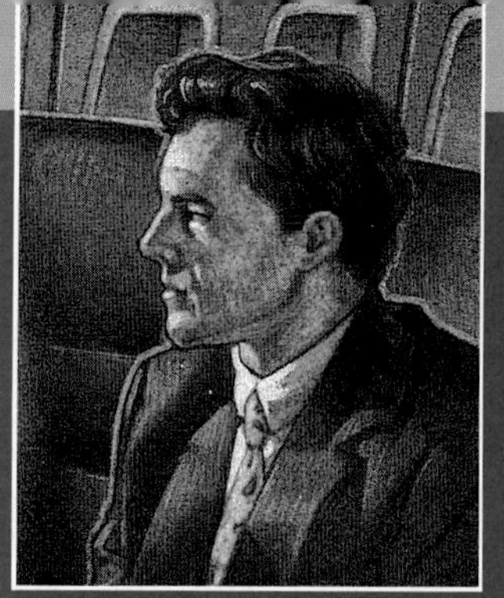

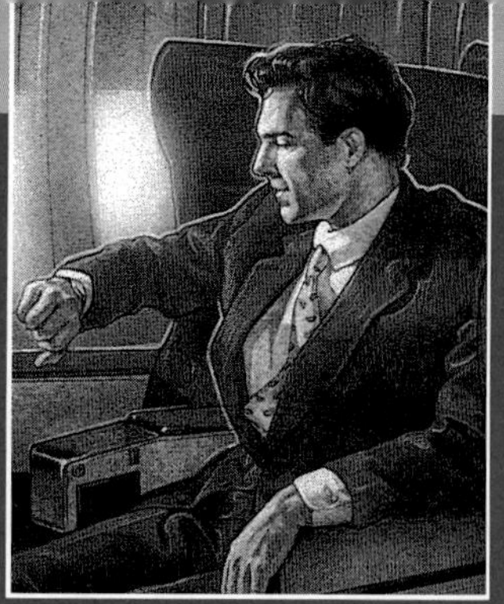

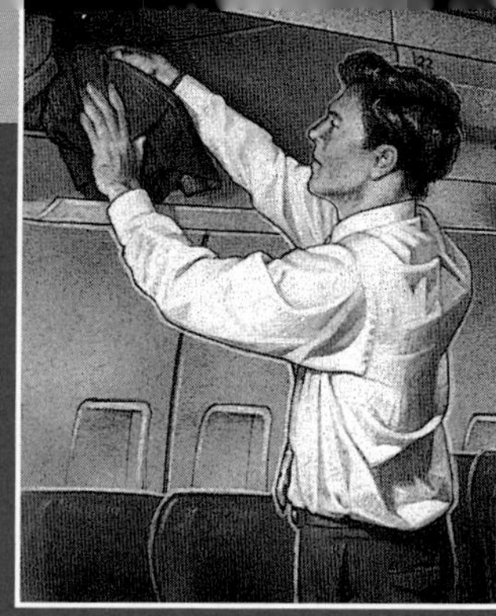

At the base of the traveler's brain, the spinal cord widens into a structure called the brainstem, shown with the cerebellum at right. The lowest part of the brainstem—the medulla—is crucial to life: Among other things, it controls the muscles that fill the lungs with air. The pons serves largely to relay signals between the cerebrum and other parts of the central nervous system and to trigger some eye movements. Atop the pons sits the midbrain, which functions in hearing and in other eye movements, as well as in additional aspects of vision.

At the core of the brainstem lies the reticular formation (*purple dots*). With neurons that extend upward into the cerebrum and downward to the spinal cord, this network processes signals from every part of the central nervous system. Clusters of neurons within the reticular formation play roles in the perception of pain, in muscle control, in breathing and heartbeat, and in reflexive actions such as swallowing and vomiting.

From the brainstem emerge 10 of the body's 12 pairs of cranial nerves, numbered III to XII. (I, the olfactory nerve, and II, the optic nerve, deliver information from the nose and eyes for processing in the cerebral cortex.) As detailed on the opposite page, these nerves spread to the head, neck, and torso, activating glands and muscles—both voluntary and involuntary—and returning a wealth of sensory information to the brain.

THE TRIGEMINAL NERVE (V), a large, three-part conduit, both controls muscles and passes sensory information from the head to the brain. The trigeminal nerve governs jaw muscles used for chewing and carries sensations from skin, eyes, nose, mouth, and teeth.

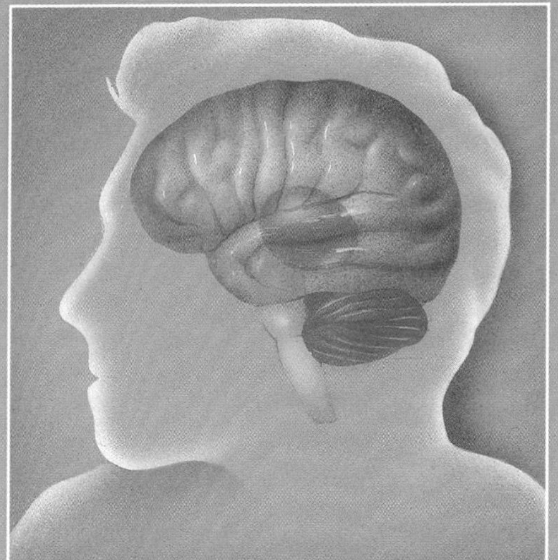

THE GLOSSOPHARYNGEAL NERVE (IX) complements the facial nerve by carrying taste sensations from the back of the tongue. This nerve also helps work some of the muscles in the throat that are needed for swallowing and relays information about blood pressure and respiration to the brain.

THE VAGUS NERVE (X), named with the Latin word for wandering, branches into the chest and abdomen where it detects such visceral sensations as breathing and "butterflies" in the stomach. The vagus nerve also helps govern respiration, heartbeat, and digestion. Furthermore, it transmits commands to muscles of the throat and larynx—where the vocal cords are—essential to speech.

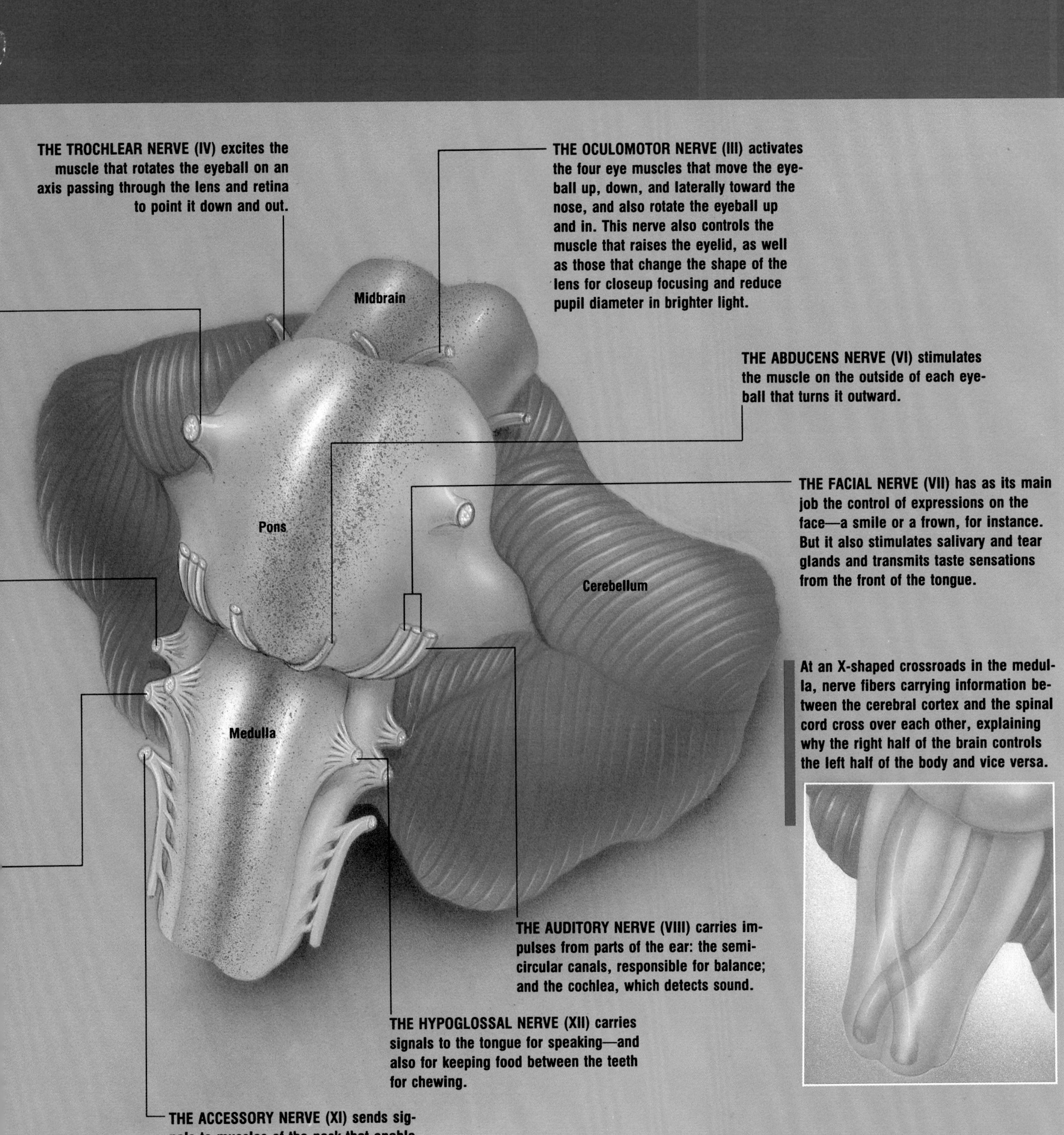

At an X-shaped crossroads in the medulla, nerve fibers carrying information between the cerebral cortex and the spinal cord cross over each other, explaining why the right half of the brain controls the left half of the body and vice versa.

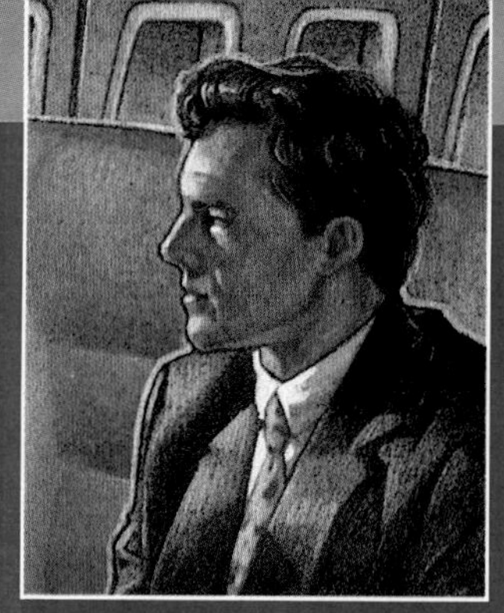

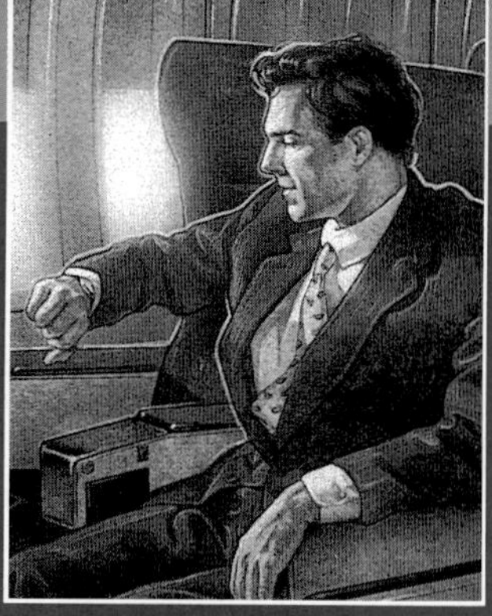

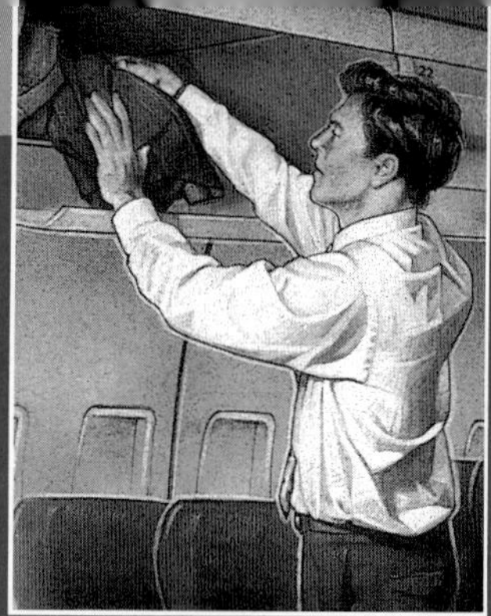

AN ESSENTIAL CUSTODIAN

Content to sit quietly after boarding, the traveler is likely unaware of subtle changes in his respiration and heart rates. They are controlled unconsciously in the brainstem, chiefly by the medulla in clusters of neurons that are called the cardiovascular center (for heartbeat) and the respiratory center (for breathing). Both functions slow down as his body adapts from the exertion of taking his seat, small as the effort may be.

Measures of this adaptation include blood pressure and—in some situations—levels of oxygen and carbon dioxide in the body. As explained at right, neural sensors tell the cardiovascular center and the respiratory center when blood pressure, oxygen, or carbon dioxide deviates from normal levels called setpoints. Restorative action is then taken.

Although the brainstem polices heartbeat and breathing automatically, these functions can be influenced by signals coming from the cerebral cortex. Strong emotions can boost heart rate, while depression or meditation can slow it somewhat. Human beings can stop breathing at will, of course, but only for a short period of time. When levels of oxygen and carbon dioxide in the blood become too unbalanced, the medulla reestablishes normal breathing.

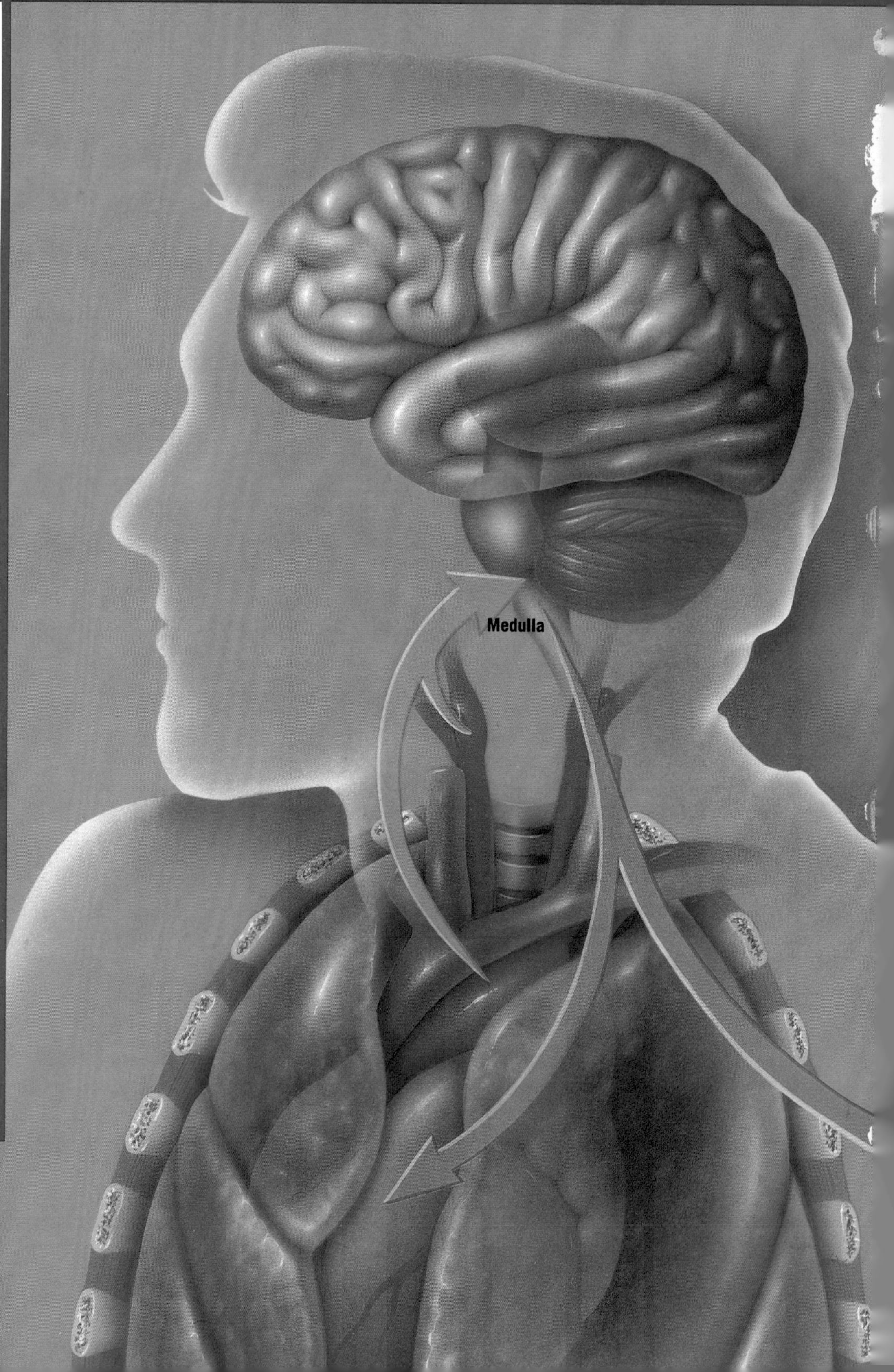

REGULATING BLOOD FLOW. To keep blood pressure stable, the medulla receives blood-pressure information from two major arteries, one near the heart and one in the neck *(blue arrow)*, then uses the data to send signals *(orange arrows)* to the heart and blood vessels that raise or lower blood pressure as required. The pressure information comes from special nerve cells in the wall of each artery. Called baroreceptors, the cells fire off impulses that travel to the cardiovascular center in the medulla. The rate of firing depends on tension in the artery walls. If blood pressure rises, increasing tension, the baroreceptors fire more rapidly, triggering signals from the cardiovascular center that slow the heart and weaken its beat. Other signals tell muscles in blood-vessel walls to relax, further helping to lower blood pressure. Low pressure causes baroreceptors to send fewer impulses to the medulla. This triggers signals that speed up the heart and make it beat more strongly; other signals constrict blood vessels slightly, increasing blood pressure.

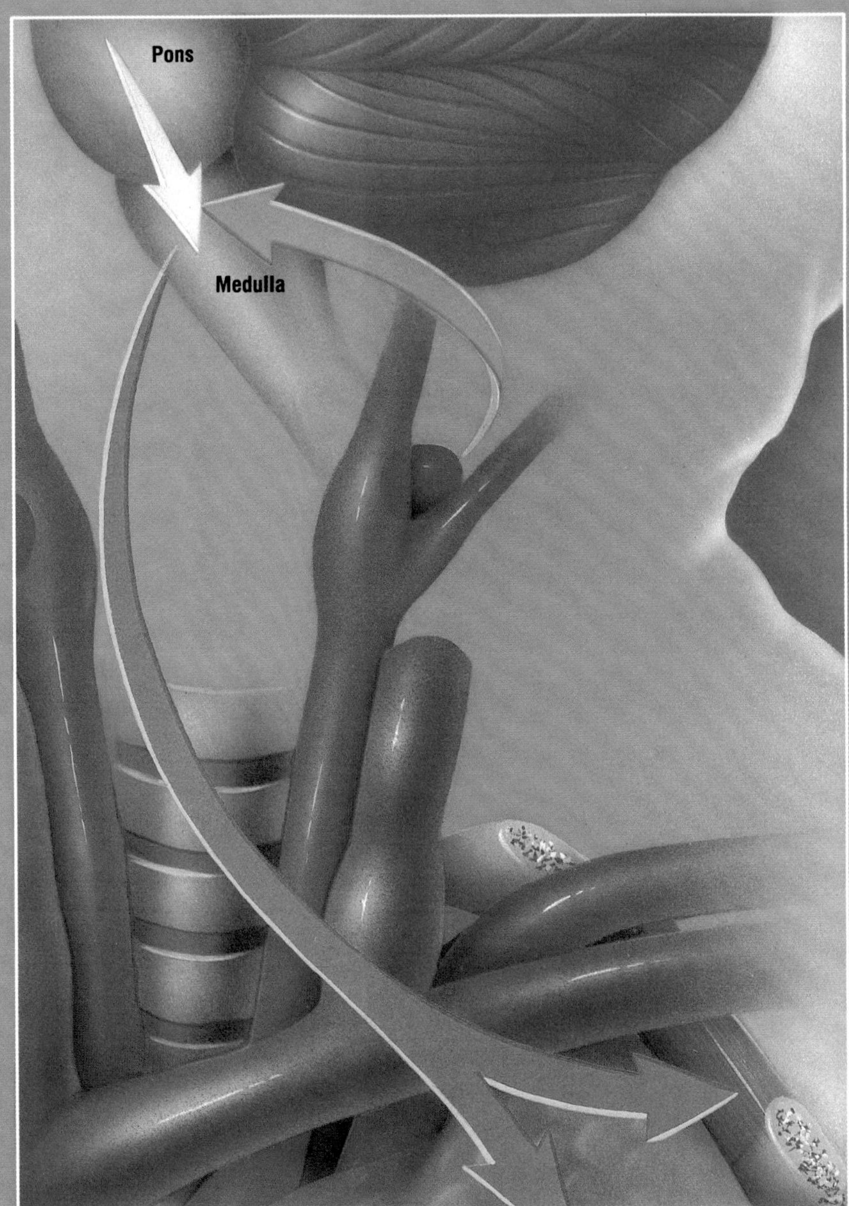

BREATH CONTROL. Aided by the pons *(yellow arrow)*, the medulla's respiratory center makes breathing muscles contract *(orange arrows)*, drawing air into the lungs—then lets these muscles relax to exhale. Nerve cells of the carotid body *(red)*, which is positioned at the fork in the carotid artery, send oxygen data to the respiratory center *(blue arrow)*. When there is a low level of oxygen, the neurons send more pulses to the respiratory center, which then calls for faster, deeper breathing. Neurons situated near the surface of the medulla are sensitive to carbon dioxide, a normal waste product of animal metabolism that is expelled from the body by breathing. Even a slight rise in the level of this chemical has the same effect as a low oxygen level.

THE INTRICACY OF A GLANCE

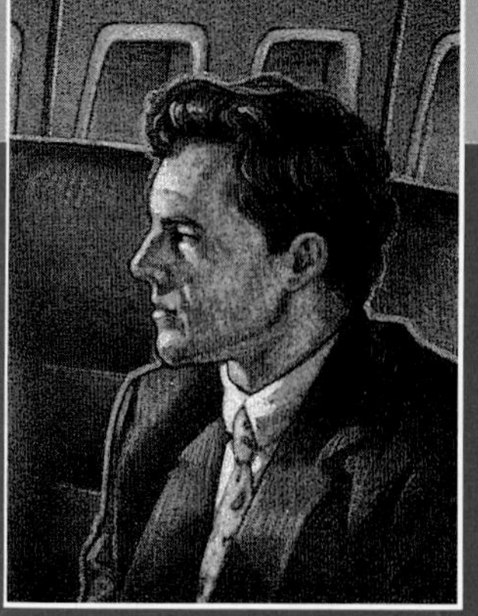

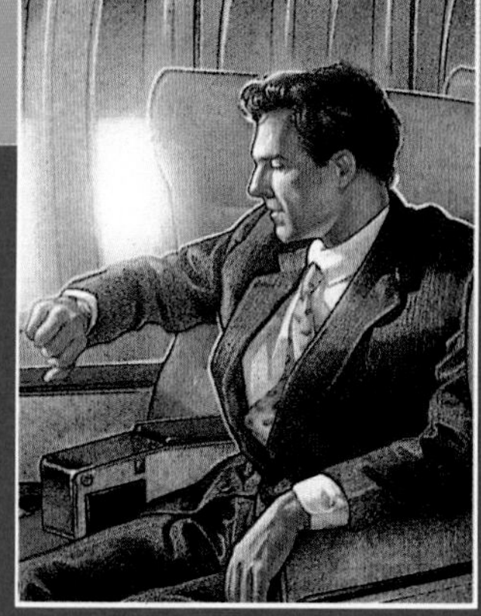

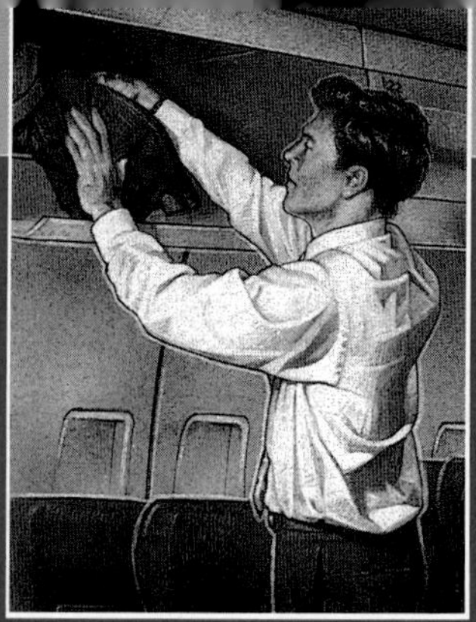

The airline passenger, curious about how much longer he might have to wait for takeoff, glances down at his watch. The idea arises in the cerebral cortex, but responsibility for activating the muscles involved in any eye movement, voluntary or not, falls to the pons and the midbrain, which handle the intricate task automatically.

This seemingly simple act has a number of components: lightning-quick adjustments of several muscles that move the eyes and refocus both lenses on his watch. The six muscles moving each eye within its socket—some of the fastest and most precisely controlled in the body—oppose each other in pairs to keep the eye stable and on target. As one muscle of a pair contracts, its opposite relaxes. Both eyes must move in concert to stabilize the image of the watch on the retina at the back of each eye. Without this coordination, double vision would result. Thus, even the simplest eye movement requires simultaneous control of all 12 muscles.

The illustrations at right explain just one part of this complexity: how the brain makes the left eye look down and to the right at the watch. Similar actions move the right eye in sync with the left.

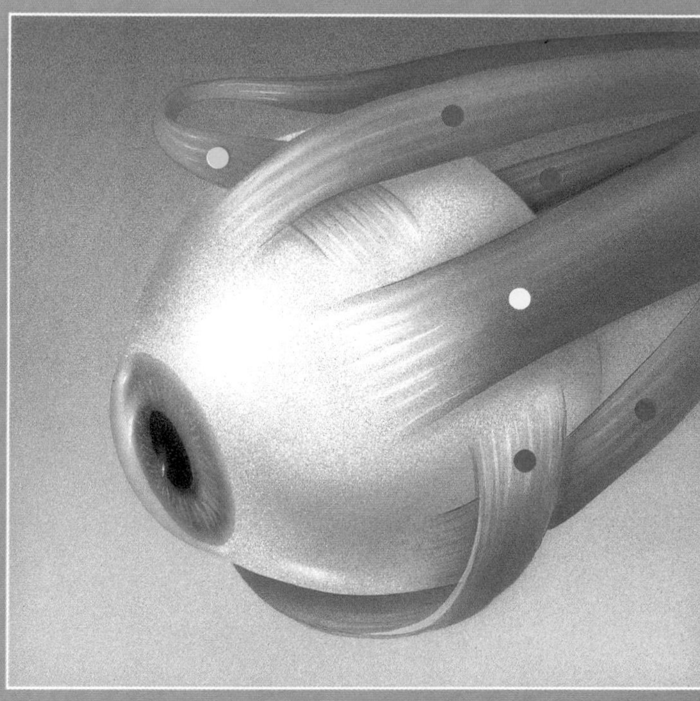

AIMING THE EYES. The airline passenger's decision to consult his watch sets off a flurry of brainstem activity *(right)* that stimulates the eye muscles, coded with color dots in this illustration to match the cranial nerves that activate them. Arising in the cortex, the thought to look at the watch travels to the brainstem *(purple arrow)*. The oculomotor nerve *(pink arrow)* carries messages that, in this instance, change the shape of the lens to focus on the watch face, constrict the pupil if necessary, lower the gaze, and move it toward the watch. The abducens nerve *(yellow arrow)* contributes by reducing impulses to the muscle that, if stimulated, would move the eye laterally, away from the watch. The trochlear nerve *(green arrow)* plays an equally minor role, abetting the action mostly by allowing the muscle it serves to relax.

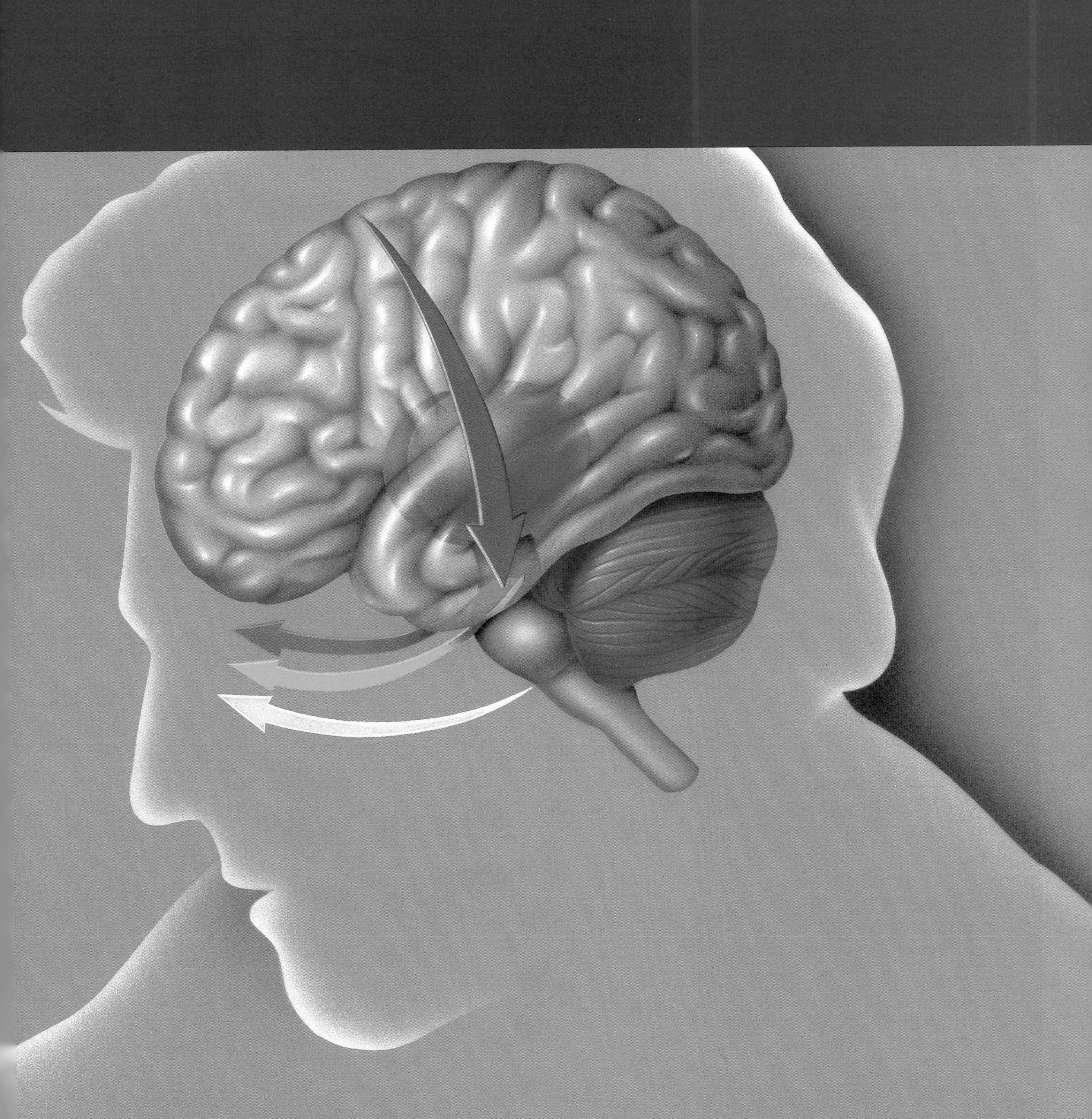

UNCONSCIOUS MASTERY OF MOVEMENT

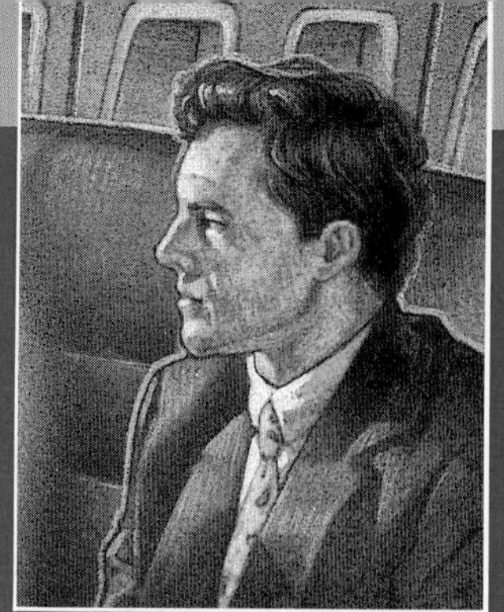

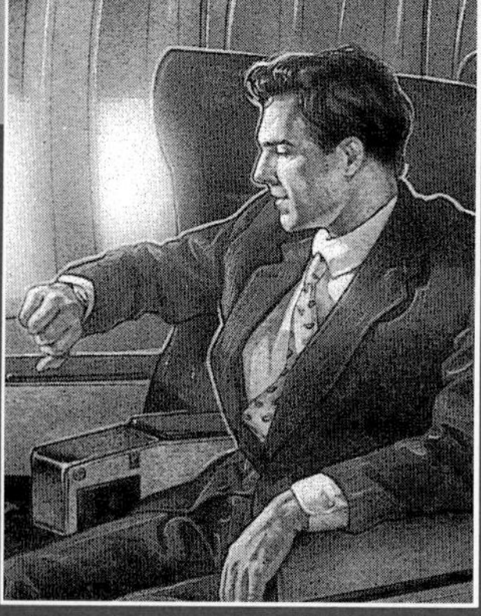

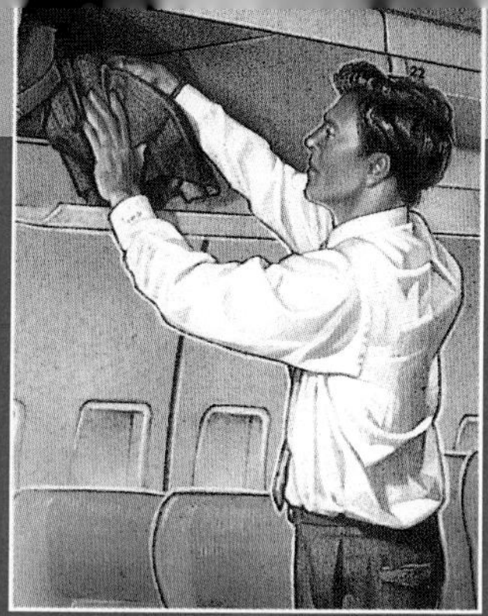

Noting that departure is several minutes away, the traveler decides to stow his coat in the compartment overhead, a mundane feat that requires complex coordination between brain and muscles. This synchronization falls largely to the cerebellum, which makes up more than 10 percent of the brain's weight and contains nearly half of all its neurons.

The cerebellum receives input from many parts of the nervous system, but its output reaches only those parts that are important for the control of movement. Functionally, the cerebellum can be divided into three zones: the vestibulocerebellum, which chiefly helps to maintain equilibrium and synchronize head and eye movements; the spinocerebellum, which orchestrates the muscle activity responsible for limb movements of the kind needed to stuff a coat into an overhead rack; and the cerebrocerebellum, which plays a role in the planning of movement.

As explained in much simplified form at right, the cerebellum receives a wealth of input to perform these tasks. Processing this information automatically and unconsciously, it compares motion instructions from the cerebral cortex with movements in progress, optimizing them as needed. The cerebellum is also thought to store details of how to walk, swim, or shoot a basketball. It is where practice enhances performance in such activities and why, once we learn to ride a bicycle, we never forget.

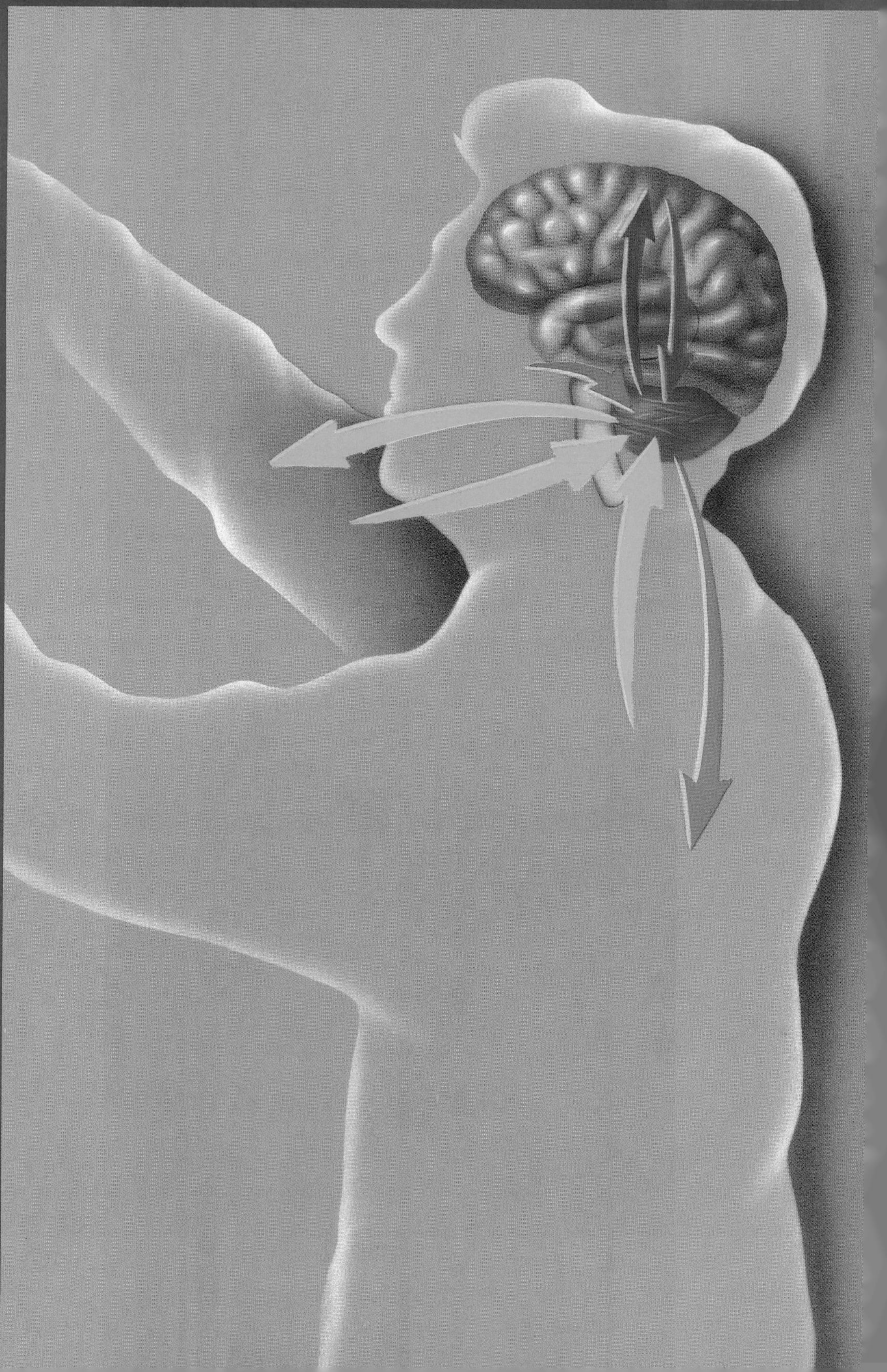

AN ARBITER OF MOTION. Three functional zones in the cerebellum *(blue, green, orange, at right)* communicate with various parts of the body and the cerebral cortex to coordinate motion. The cortex signals impending movement *(blue arrows, left)* to the cerebrocerebellum, which advises the cortex when a motion—reaching beyond arm's length, for example—cannot be performed without some other preparatory movement. Dialogue between the spinocerebellum and peripheral muscles *(green arrows)* includes feedback on joint position and muscle stretch. Orange arrows show balance and head-position information from the inner ear going to the vestibulocerebellum to coordinate head-eye movements. Working through back and shoulder muscles among others, this zone also enables us to stand erect.

A DENSE NETWORK OF NEURONS. Overlying the white matter of the cerebellum, as shown below, is a cortex with three layers of nerve cells. One layer consists entirely of the cell bodies of Purkinje cells, the output neurons of the cerebellar cortex that influence movement. Two types of impulse pathways called fibers—actually long axons of distant nerve cells—bring a variety of muscle and sensory information to the cerebellar cortex, causing Purkinje cells to fire. Climbing fibers are each connected directly to a single Purkinje cell; mossy fibers are linked to Purkinje cells by way of one or more granule cells, whose axons rise into the molecular layer of the cerebellar cortex to become parallel fibers that individually influence thousands of Purkinje cells.

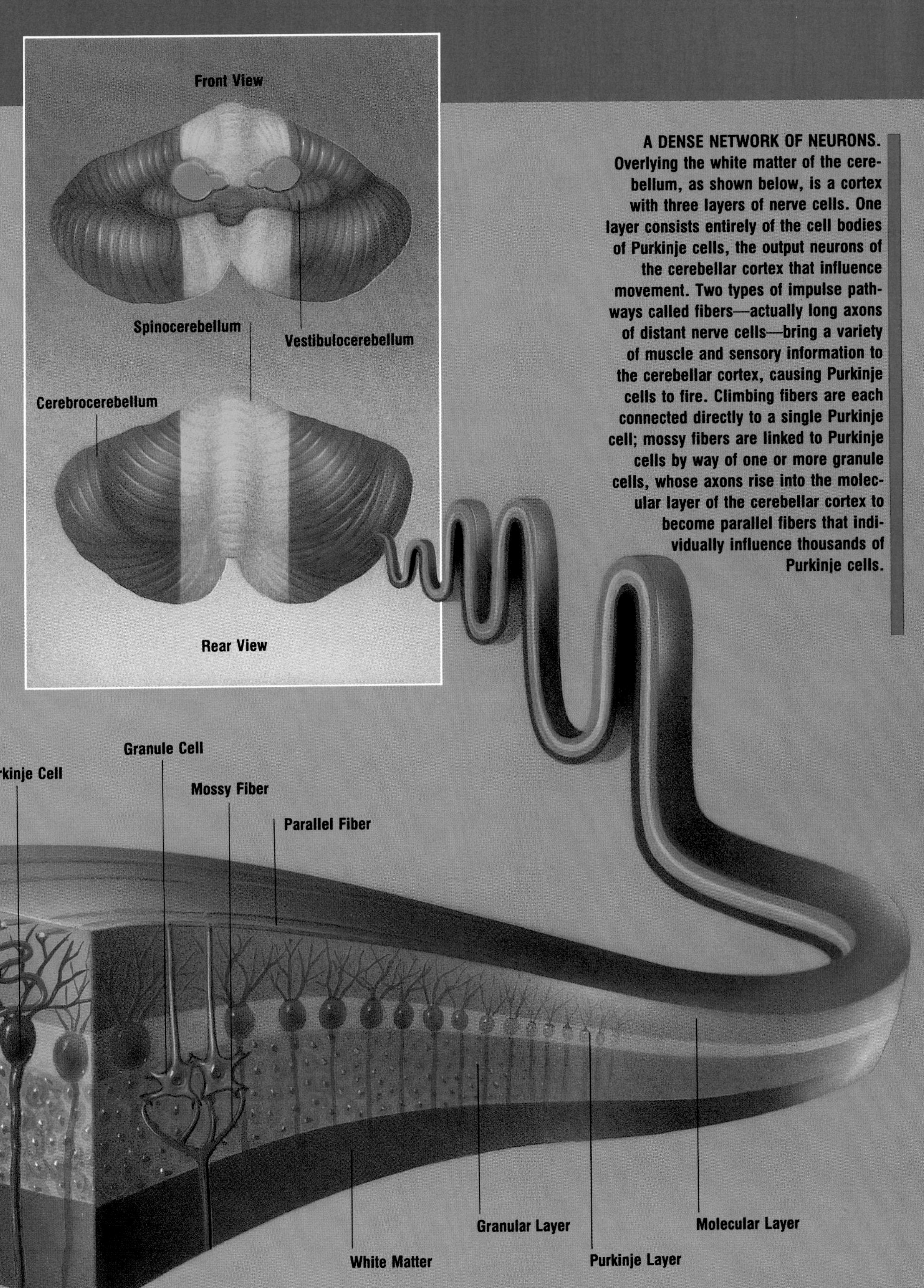

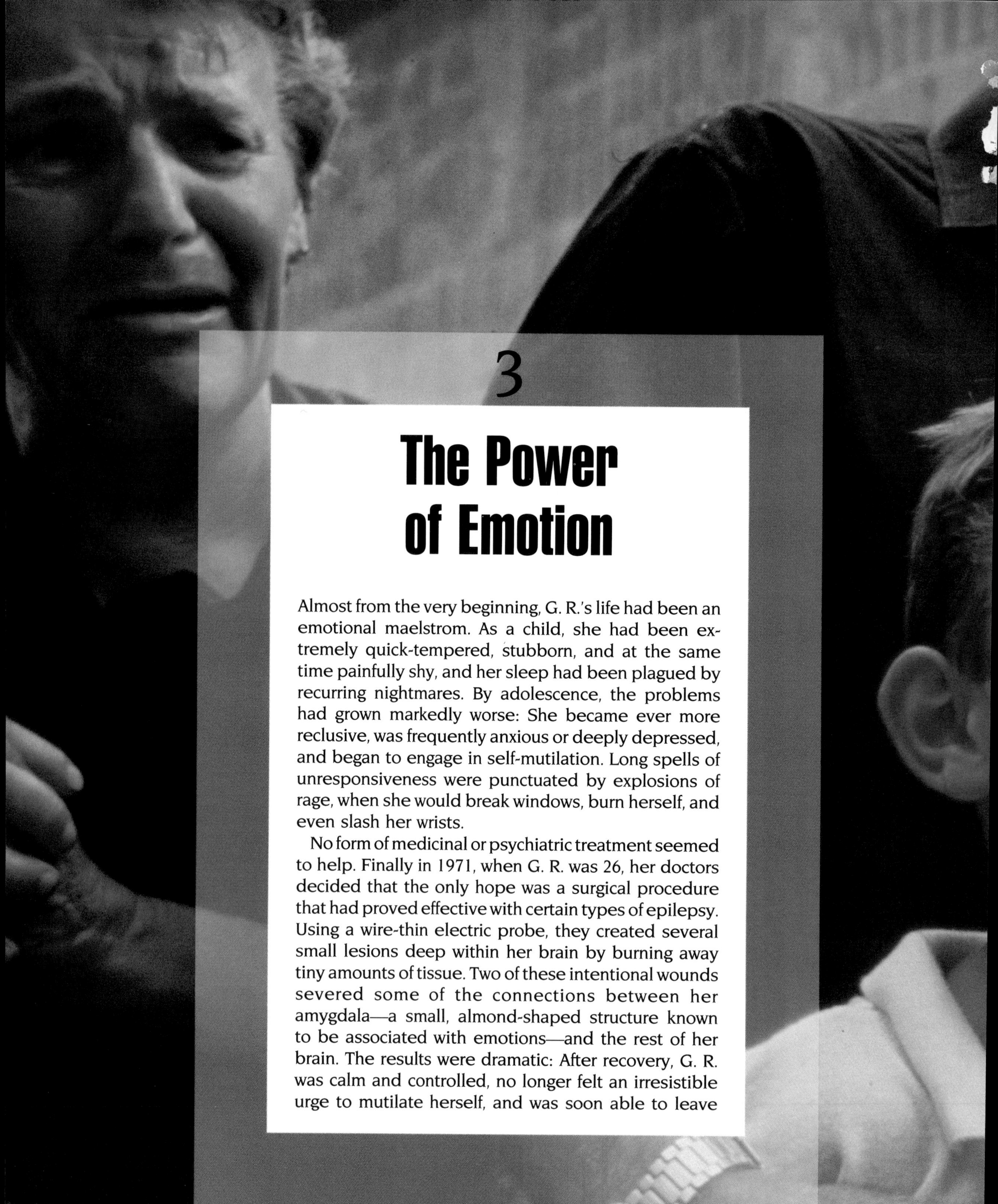

3

The Power of Emotion

Almost from the very beginning, G. R.'s life had been an emotional maelstrom. As a child, she had been extremely quick-tempered, stubborn, and at the same time painfully shy, and her sleep had been plagued by recurring nightmares. By adolescence, the problems had grown markedly worse: She became ever more reclusive, was frequently anxious or deeply depressed, and began to engage in self-mutilation. Long spells of unresponsiveness were punctuated by explosions of rage, when she would break windows, burn herself, and even slash her wrists.

No form of medicinal or psychiatric treatment seemed to help. Finally in 1971, when G. R. was 26, her doctors decided that the only hope was a surgical procedure that had proved effective with certain types of epilepsy. Using a wire-thin electric probe, they created several small lesions deep within her brain by burning away tiny amounts of tissue. Two of these intentional wounds severed some of the connections between her amygdala—a small, almond-shaped structure known to be associated with emotions—and the rest of her brain. The results were dramatic: After recovery, G. R. was calm and controlled, no longer felt an irresistible urge to mutilate herself, and was soon able to leave

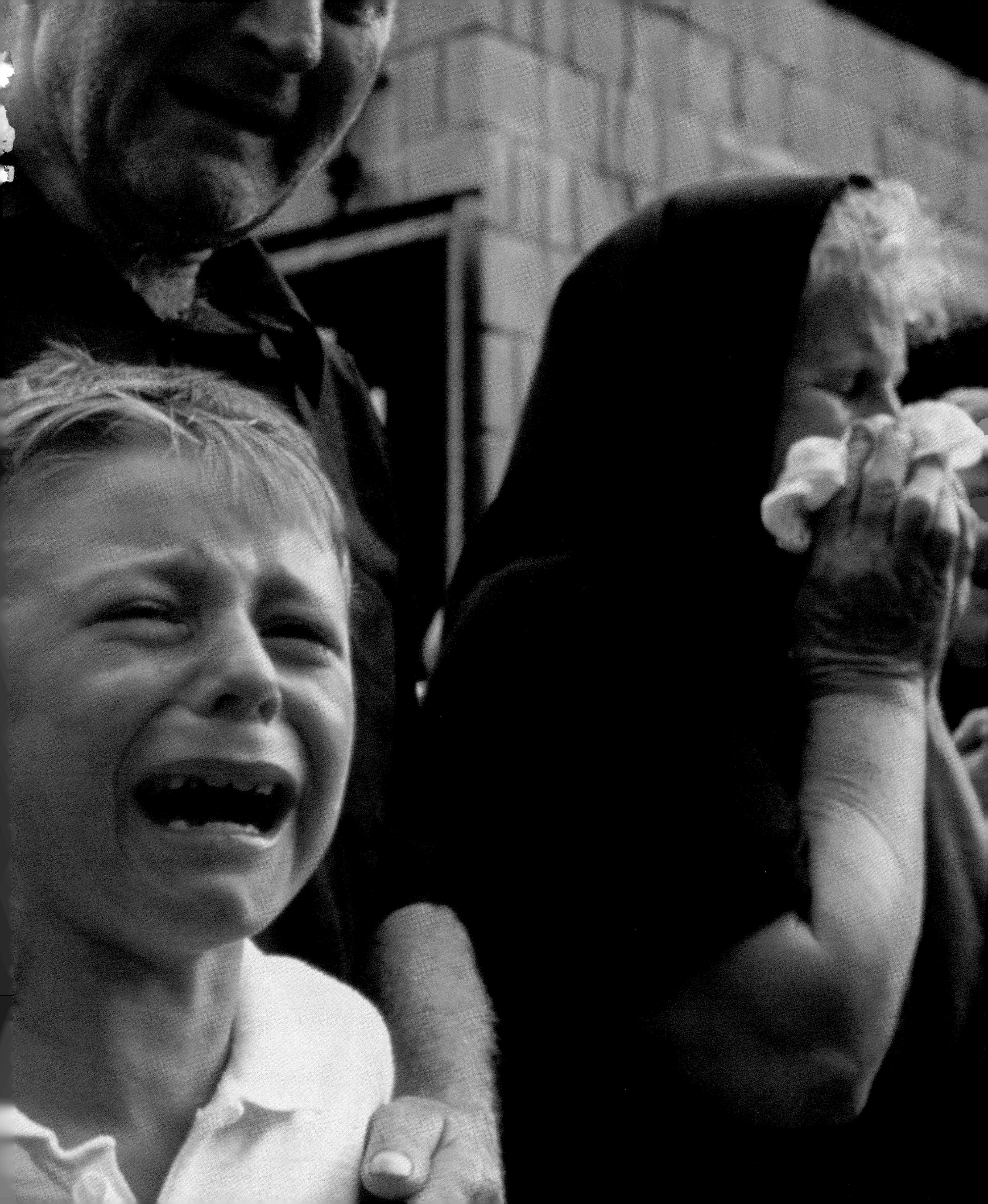

the hospital, eventually getting a job as an occupational therapist.

But while her behavior appeared relatively normal—if somewhat passive—the surgery had created some unusual side effects that manifested themselves over the course of the next 10 years. For one thing, she found it extremely difficult to remember faces or to recognize their emotional expression. Furthermore, she would often report feeling very anxious and afraid even though her pulse remained normal and she showed no outward signs of fear.

Strangest of all, some of G. R.'s emotions seemed completely unfamiliar to her. She talked of feeling these emotions very strongly but could describe them in only the vaguest of terms, noting that they could not be, as she put it, "pigeonholed into any familiar category." For all the apparent good the surgery had done, in many ways G. R.'s emotional experience of the world remained as much in turmoil as it had ever been.

G. R.'s case points to the difficulties of trying to understand how the brain goes about generating emotions and how those emotions, whatever they are, translate into subjective experience. Much of the research in this area has focused on the complex of structures lying at the very core of the brain—encompassing elements generally referred to as the limbic system (from the Latin word for "border," because the components here border the corpus callosum, which links the brain's two hemispheres). Evidence suggests that several of these structures, including the amygdala, are intimately involved in the generation of emotional states.

The temptation of such findings is to think of the limbic system as the seat of emotions. But as G. R.'s sad story reveals, the interpretation of any given feeling is obviously essential to the overall experience of an emotion, and that interpretation involves conscious activity at the level of the cortex. In fact, as today's neuroscientists have come to realize, the brain's circuitry is so complex, its various elements so interconnected, that identifying any one part of the brain as the source of a particular behavior is fundamentally misleading.

Nevertheless, much has been gleaned from examining the critical role that certain structures do indeed play in emotions. For example, investigators have found that key physiological aspects of emotional experience—from the chill of fear to the warm glow of desire—are clearly traceable to components in the limbic area. In addition, the discovery that some memory processing also takes place here has helped explain the close relationship between emotions and memory—why our most vivid recollections of the past seem always to be tinged with deep feelings. Little wonder, then, that as research into the neurological processes behind emotions has developed throughout the 20th century, studies have turned again and again to these various elements that conveniently—if not entirely accurately—have come to be called the emotional brain.

The notion that there might be a specific part of the brain responsible for emotions traces back to a bizarre accident in the middle of the 19th century that has become famous in the annals of brain science. Near the end of the day on September 13, 1848, Phineas Gage, a personable young man who worked as a foreman of a railway blasting crew, was manning the tamping rod used to pack gunpowder into holes drilled into the bedrock. One hole had been filled with powder, and Gage had just told an assistant to add a layer of sand, which would prevent any sparks from igniting the powder prematurely.

But at that moment, a fateful noise distracted the two of them. When Gage turned back to his task, assuming the sand had been poured, he rammed the three-and-a-half-foot,

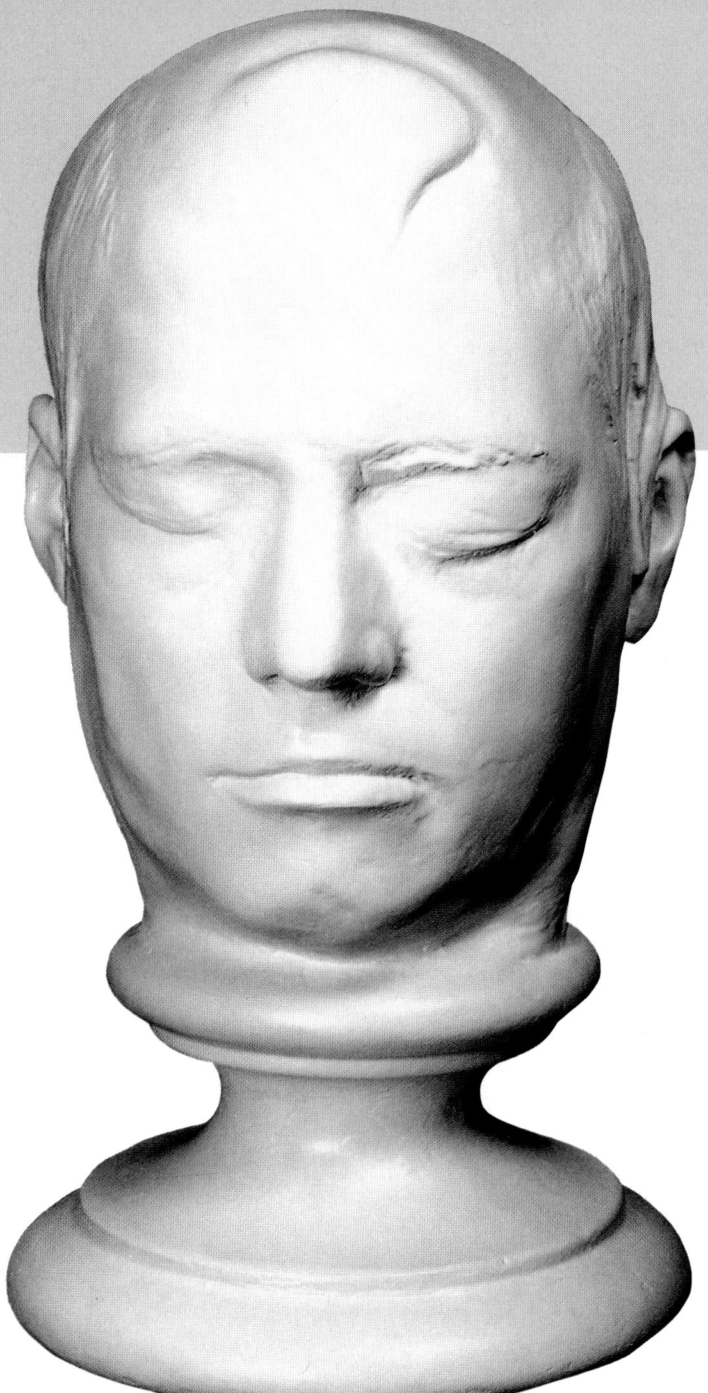

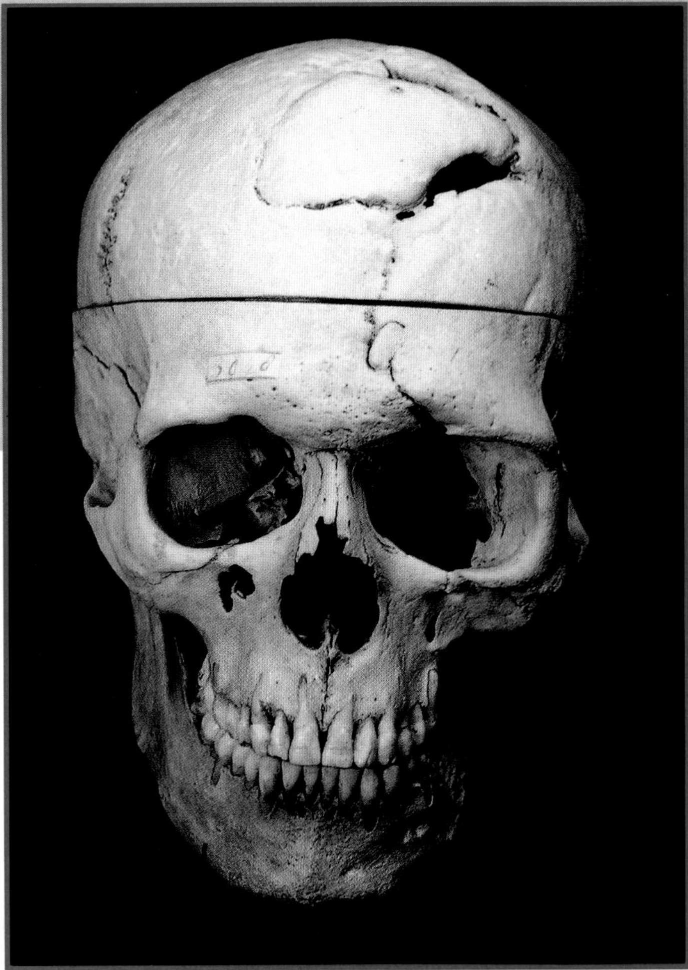

A LIFE TRANSFORMED. Although Phineas Gage's death mask *(left)* shows relatively minor scarring, his skull reveals the gaping holes in cheek and forehead caused by the tamping rod that pierced his head. He lost the sight in his left eye as a result but had few other physical problems. However, the damage to his brain altered his personality, leaving him unable to control childish behavior and outbursts of cursing. He tried to get his old railway job back, but his employers and friends shunned him, declaring that he was "no longer Gage." Drifting for some years, he worked as a stable hand in New Hampshire and a coach driver in South America, and also appeared as a sideshow freak with P. T. Barnum's circus—tamping rod in hand. He died at the age of 37 in San Francisco in 1861, nearly 13 years after the accident.

inch-thick length of iron into the hole. As the rod scraped against the flinty rock, a shower of sparks fell onto the unprotected powder. The explosion blew the 13-pound rod out of the hole like a modern whale hunter's spear. Its pointed end ripped through Gage's left cheek, behind his eye, up through the left frontal lobe of his brain, and out at the hairline, then flew 50 feet farther through the air.

Gage flew as well, flattened by the impact. He writhed on the ground for a few minutes, apparently mortally wounded. But suddenly, miraculously, he sat up, clamping his hand to his bleeding head. The stunned crew carted Gage to a local hotel, where two doctors were soon attending him. When the first physician arrived, Gage—who had begun to speak almost as soon as the initial

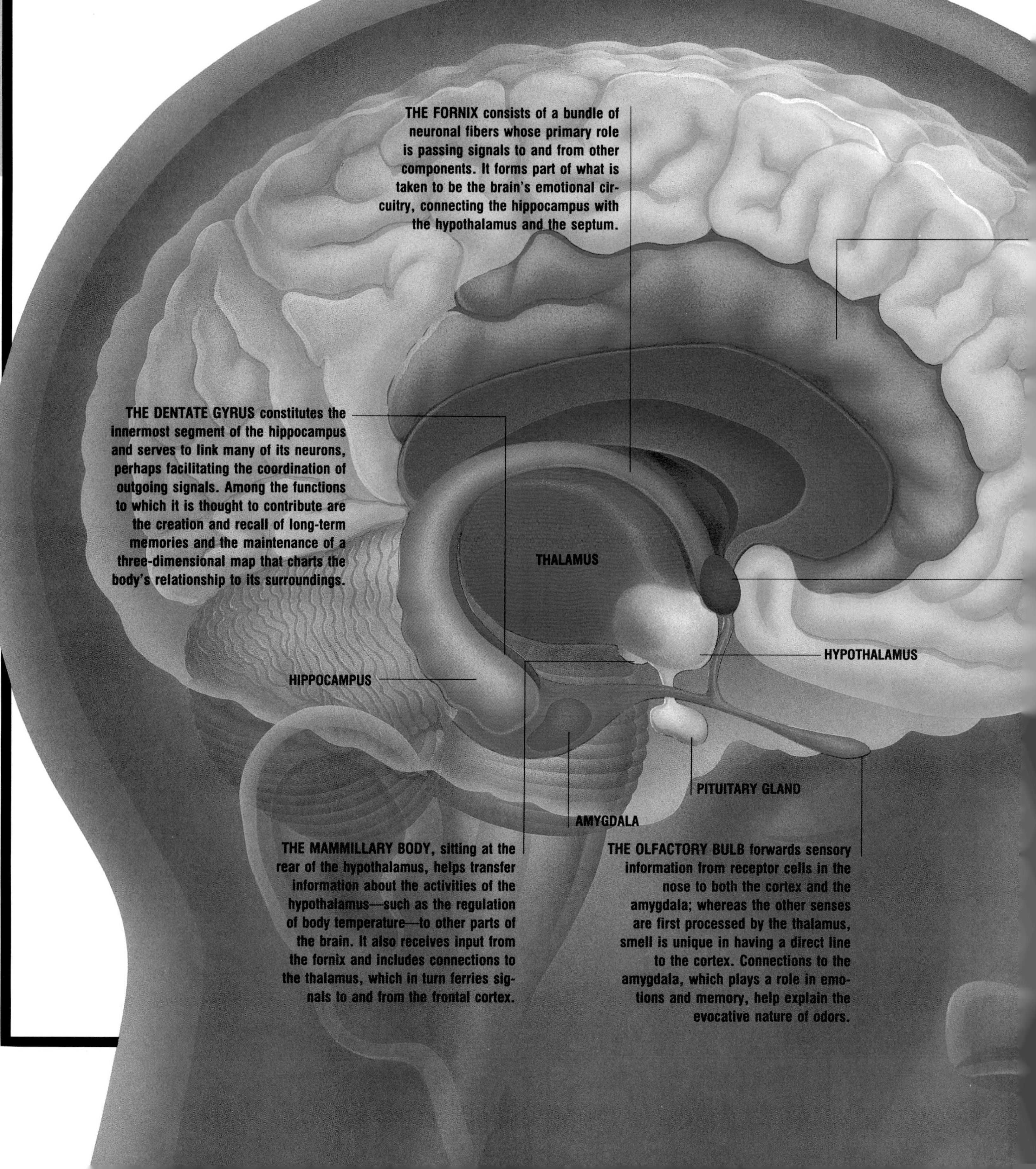

THE FORNIX consists of a bundle of neuronal fibers whose primary role is passing signals to and from other components. It forms part of what is taken to be the brain's emotional circuitry, connecting the hippocampus with the hypothalamus and the septum.

THE DENTATE GYRUS constitutes the innermost segment of the hippocampus and serves to link many of its neurons, perhaps facilitating the coordination of outgoing signals. Among the functions to which it is thought to contribute are the creation and recall of long-term memories and the maintenance of a three-dimensional map that charts the body's relationship to its surroundings.

THALAMUS

HYPOTHALAMUS

HIPPOCAMPUS

PITUITARY GLAND

AMYGDALA

THE MAMMILLARY BODY, sitting at the rear of the hypothalamus, helps transfer information about the activities of the hypothalamus—such as the regulation of body temperature—to other parts of the brain. It also receives input from the fornix and includes connections to the thalamus, which in turn ferries signals to and from the frontal cortex.

THE OLFACTORY BULB forwards sensory information from receptor cells in the nose to both the cortex and the amygdala; whereas the other senses are first processed by the thalamus, smell is unique in having a direct line to the cortex. Connections to the amygdala, which plays a role in emotions and memory, help explain the evocative nature of odors.

THE CINGULATE GYRUS acts as a relay station between many cortical regions and such structures as the hippocampus and hypothalamus. Its cells are arranged in three layers—a relatively simple organization that distinguishes it from other portions of the cortex.

THE SEPTUM has been associated particularly with feelings of pleasure and euphoria but is now considered to be only one element in a network of structures that give rise to these and other emotions. It incorporates some of the fibers of the fornix and assists in routing neuronal impulses between the hippocampus and the hypothalamus.

Complexity at the Core

Nestled deep within the brain—atop the brainstem and between the two hemispheres of the cerebrum—lie a host of components that play vital roles in many different types of brain activity, from the processing of sensory input and the storing and retrieving of memories to the generating of emotional reactions. Earlier this century, neuroscientists grouped some of these elements together as a unified assemblage called the limbic system, from the Latin word *limbus*, or "border." But researchers have become increasingly reluctant to describe these features as forming a system, a term that in scientific circles implies a structural arrangement with clearly delineated boundaries, both anatomically and functionally.

In reality, the neuronal connections throughout the brain are so widespread and so intricate that functions once thought to be the sole purview of the limbic system—such as emotional responses—are now considered to arise from much more complex interactions involving many different areas. However, each element in this middle region does have a definable part to play, and investigators have been able to identify many of those contributions—not only for such components as the thalamus, hypothalamus, pituitary gland, amygdala, and hippocampus (*pages* 14-15), but also for the assortment of other structures detailed below and at left. As it turns out, relaying information may be the most significant task of all.

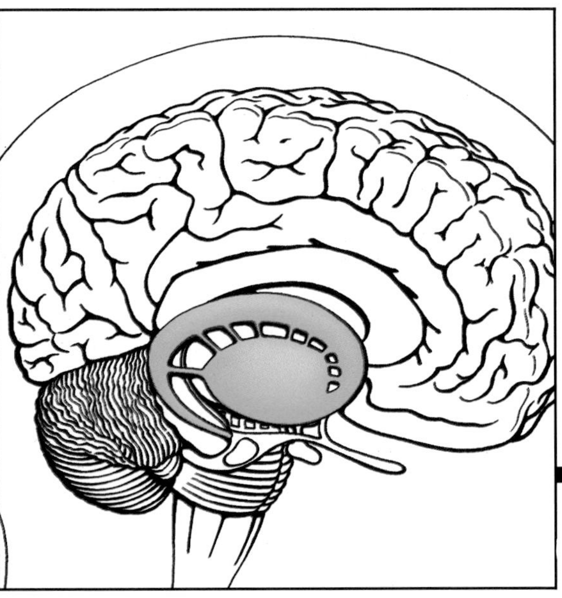

AN ADDITIONAL LAYER OF CIRCUITRY. Lying just outside the components at far left is a complex of structures called the basal ganglia, portions of which are shown in green at left with the thalamus; other segments are hidden within the brainstem. Scientists have discovered myriad connections between the basal ganglia and other parts of the brain, including all four cortical lobes. As a result, they now believe that the basal ganglia perform many duties—starting and stopping movement, as was originally assumed, but also processing emotions and memories, and even taking part in planning motor activities.

convulsions stopped—calmly said to him, "Doctor, here is business enough for you." He was even able to describe how the rod had passed through his head.

Gage survived the injury and subsequent infections despite, rather than because of, the medical treatments of the time: liberal doses of calomel, castor oil, and rhubarb. But the wounding totally transformed the polite and proper foreman. Like Dr. Jekyll turned permanently into Mr. Hyde, Gage became childish, obstinate, and crude. John Harlow, one of the two doctors who had been first on the scene and who continued to treat Gage, kept track of his behavior, noting instances of gross profanity, capriciousness, and an abundance of what Harlow called "animal passions." Dr. Harlow's conclusion was that "the equilibrium, or balance, between his intellectual faculties and animal propensities seems to have been destroyed."

Although there was little hard science behind Harlow's deduction, the damage to Gage's left frontal lobe did seem to have ripped away a veneer of civilized behavior, allowing raw, underlying emotions to erupt to the surface. And if the frontal lobe could thus be said to play a role in constraining emotional impulses, the question now was whether some other part or parts of the brain—working beneath the level of conscious control—could be identified as the source of those emotions.

The first inklings of such a possibility emerged around the turn of the 20th century from a study of brain tissue by a German neurologist named Korbinian Brodmann. He had dissected samples from an area in the center of the brain that had earlier been dubbed the limbic lobe. Examining the samples under a microscope, Brodmann noticed that the cellular organization of this deep-seated tissue was much simpler than that of the cerebral cortex, already known to be the locus of such complex functions as thought. This limbic region, then, was taken to be an older part of the brain, in charge of more basic activities and behaviors—although precisely what those might be remained unclear.

A few decades later, neuroanatomist James Papez of the Cornell Medical School in New York began to sketch in at least some of the details. During a 1930s study of patients with rabies, Papez realized that there was probably a connection between one of the chief manifestations of the disease—feelings of extreme terror and displays of rage—and the fact that the rabies virus damages tissue in the hippocampus, one of the structures in the limbic area. Naturally enough, he reasoned that the site of the viral attack must be strongly associated with the darker emotions. In a 1937 paper on his findings, he went on to propose that the mechanism behind such emotions was an intricate circuit of neurons connecting several limbic structures and a part of the cortex. He called the flow of signals through this circuitry the "stream of feeling." Papez even suggested that some forms of mental illness, especially those such as manic-depressive disorders that represent a drastic tipping of emotional balance, must arise from malfunctions in this network.

At about the same time, two neurophysiologists at the University of Chicago set about exploring the role of this part of the brain through experiments on monkeys. Heinrich Klüver and Paul Bucy operated on wild animals, removing their amygdalas, hippocampi, and portions of the temporal cortex overlying these structures. In a startling turnaround, the monkeys—which were normally terrified in the presence of humans—became docile and tame after the procedure, tolerating handling and even deliberate provocation. They showed no fear of large snakes—one of their natural enemies—or of other monkeys that had attacked them in the past.

The results were clear-cut, but the surgical targets certainly had not been. Later, more refined experiments seemed to indicate that removal of the amygdala alone had been the chief reason for the changes in behavior that Klüver and Bucy had produced. But in the meantime, researchers continued to try to figure out which brain components controlled which emotional responses. As the data piled up, the picture became more and more complicated.

One particularly fruitful avenue of investigation involved not the removal but the stimulation of selected structures. Among the most important researchers in this area was Swiss physiologist Walter Hess, who had perfected a method of exciting small parts of the brains of cats with electricity. Originally, Hess's goal had been to study how the hypothalamus regulates such physiological functions as heart rate and blood pressure, but as his experiments continued through the decade of the 1930s, he became increasingly intrigued by the effects on the behavior of his animals.

Time and again, when Hess turned on a weak current in an electrode that was implanted in the hypothalamus of domesticated cats—which were awake and unrestrained—the mild-mannered creatures would suddenly arch their backs, hiss, and spit, their drooling mouths stretched wide, the very archetype of an enraged feline. Because they were not caged or held down in any way, the stimulated cats were also able to put their apparent rage into action and would lunge at practically anything that moved, whether it was a laboratory rat or one of Hess's assistants.

Although some of his fellow scientists contended that the so-called rage was purely mechanical, Hess was convinced that the electrical stimulation was eliciting a natural emotional state. His belief rested partly on his observation that the behavior seemed to persist even after the current had been turned off.

"It often happens," Hess later wrote, "that after prolonged stimulation the cat proceeds to attack and strike out in a well-directed fashion or jump upon a nearby observer. A certain attitude of defense remains after cessation of stimulation. There is no reason to consider it different from natural rage." He concluded that a center for angry, defensive behavior existed in the hypothalamus.

Hess won the Nobel Prize in physiology and medicine in 1949 for his work, but by that time additional observations had called into question just how natural electrically elicited rage was. For example, when researchers removed a cat's entire cortex and then stimulated the hypothalamus, the cat would exhibit all the signs of rage, but it was never directed at a specific target. Furthermore, some cats would purr, preen, lap milk, or lick a researcher's face between fearsome hisses and snarls. The cats, it seemed, did not experience anger—at least as humans understand the term—even though they went through all the physiological motions of rage.

From these observations grew the notion of what became known as sham rage—in effect, an acknowledgment that a real emotional reaction must involve the coordinated activity of more than one part of the brain. The hypothalamus might indeed be responsible for the mechanics of an emotion like rage, but it could not really lay claim to being a center for the emotion.

To make matters more confusing, surgical experiments around the same time were producing data that directly contradicted what Hess, as well as Klüver and Bucy, had found. In one case, injury to the hypothalamus caused tame cats to become wild and fierce, and in another, destruction of the amygdala resulted in rage rather than passivity. One suggested possibility was that the loss of these structures had somehow interfered with the natural responses to certain stimuli, so that once-tame animals now reacted inappropriately to the world around them. But to this day, no definitive explanations have emerged.

The intriguing and sometimes conflicting results of laboratory experiments did not always involve such unpleasant emotions as fear and anger. In the early 1950s, researchers quite accidentally stumbled upon data that hinted at a neurological basis for an opposite emotion—pleasure. But here, too, the evidence has turned out to be far from conclusive.

At the beginning of the decade, Canadian neuroscientists Peter Milner and Seth Sharpless of the psychology department at McGill University, in Montreal, had started an investigation into the mechanisms of arousal—in simple terms, the state of being alert—and were trying to use an electrode implanted in a rat's brainstem as a training aid. They theorized that by stimulating what was then thought to be an arousal system located there, they could mimic the motivational urge that occurred when a rat was aware that a food reward could be found at the end of a maze. Unfortunately, all of the rats they tested avoided parts of the maze that became associated with brainstem stimulation. Discouraged, Sharpless and Milner turned to other research.

But in the fall of 1953, an American social psychologist named James Olds joined the department and began to learn about physiology and brain anatomy from Milner. Casting about for a technical training project for Olds, Milner taught him how to implant electrodes in the rat brainstem.

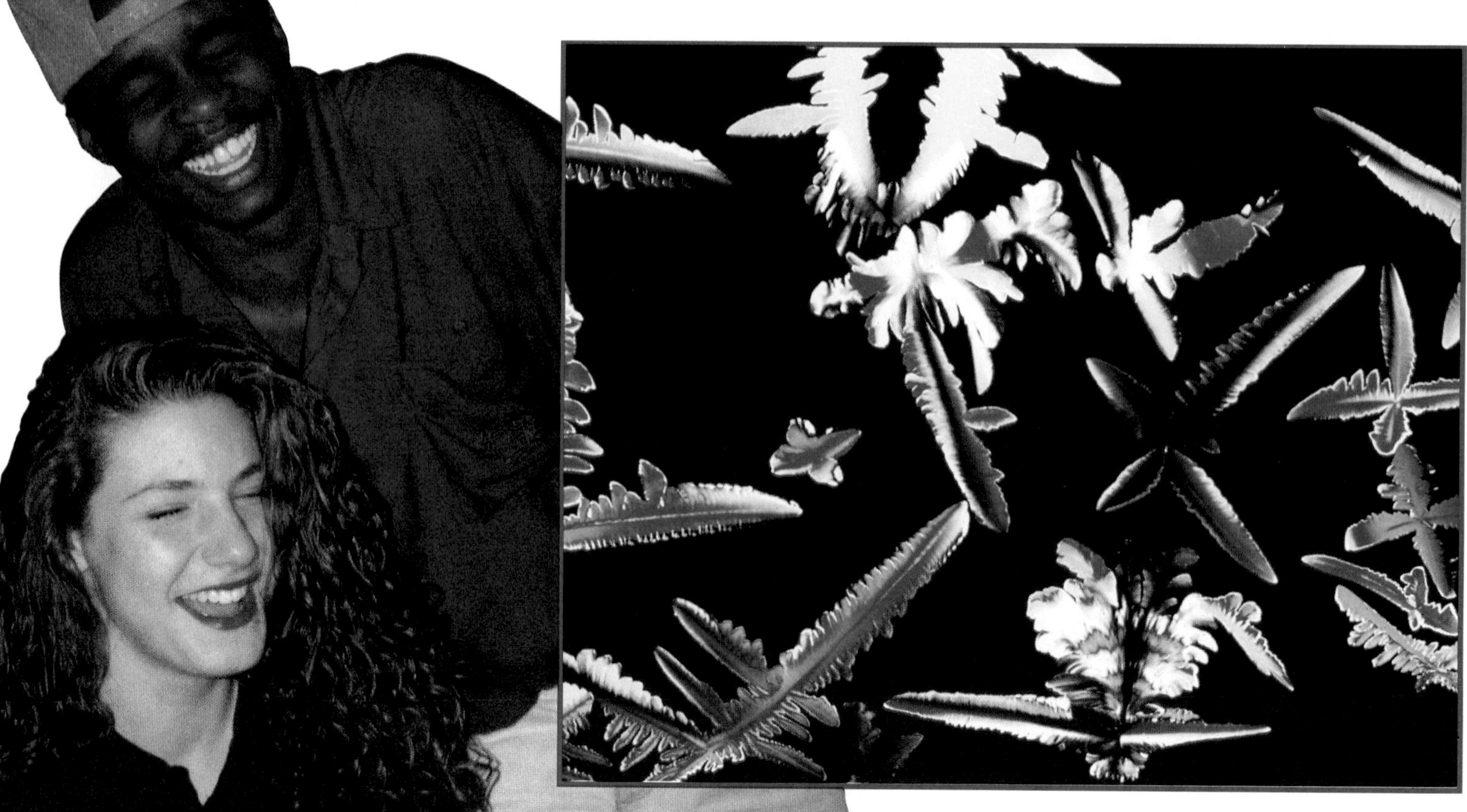

One day, Olds inserted an electrode and set up the stimulator to run a test similar to the ones Milner and Sharpless had performed earlier.

The rat was placed in an enclosure measuring slightly more than three feet by three feet and was free to move around to a degree that would allow Olds to gauge whether it was attracted to or repelled by any given area. He then sent a brief current through the electrode every time the rat moved to one particular corner, expecting that it would learn to avoid that spot. To Olds's surprise, however, as he later wrote, "the animal did not stay away from that corner, but came back quickly after a brief sortie that followed the first stimulation, and even more quickly after a briefer sortie that followed the second stimulation. By the time the third stimulation had been applied, the animal seemed indubitably to be 'coming back for more.' "

THE BEST MEDICINE. Hearty laughter has distinct physiological effects involving portions of the brain's emotional circuitry. By a mechanism not yet fully understood, laughter apparently causes the hypothalamus to initiate a process that reduces blood levels of such hormones as cortisol *(crystallized, at left)*, which can be overproduced under conditions of chronic stress.

In subsequent trials with the same rat, Olds found he could guide it around a tabletop cage with a burst of current every time it turned in a particular direction. According to Milner, teaching the rat any sort of behavior in this manner was "incredibly easy." Perhaps most astounding of all, the rat ignored food and headed to a spot associated with the stimulation —even after having been deprived of food for 24 hours.

Almost unable to believe that this rat was actively seeking out the same kind of stimulation that other rats in earlier experiments had so consistently avoided, the researchers connected the stimulator to a switch located in the rat's cage. Reaching the high lever required the rat to stretch, but it nonetheless immediately began to pull the lever again and again, each time giving itself a tiny jolt in the brain.

Milner repeated the experiment with several rats, each with an electrode carefully implanted in the part of the brainstem he had targeted in his first trials. None acted pleased with the stimulation. Milner began to suspect that Olds had misplaced the electrode in his rat.

Not wanting to kill this valuable animal, they carried it to the experimental surgery department in the Montreal Neurological Institute for a head x-ray. On the film, they saw a bent electrode, its tip lodged not in the brainstem but close to the front portion of the hypothalamus and another nearby structure known as the septum (*pages* 62-63); however, before they could determine the exact location, the rat managed to dislodge the electrode. Subsequently, though, Milner and Olds succeeded in repeating the experiment in a number of other rats, with electrode placements in or near the same region. Only then did they publish their results.

Given how inherently rewarding the stimulation seemed to be, Olds chose to refer to the hypothalamus and the septum as "pleasure centers." The concept caught on, and soon other labs set out to duplicate Olds and Milner's experiment, with electrodes targeting either the septum or the hypothalamus. After a little fine-tuning, the rats almost always became completely fixated on the stimulation. The animals gave up eating, drinking, sleep, and even sex as they focused only on pressing the lever—sometimes up to 10,000 times an hour and often to the point of total exhaustion.

Hundreds of experiments using the same kind of stimulation followed, in species ranging from dogs to dolphins and guinea pigs to goldfish. All of these animals would perform unnatural and exhausting feats for the sake of a few seconds of brain stimulation.

Psychologist Elliot Valenstein of the University of Michigan at Ann Arbor spoke for many when he said of Olds's fortuitous misplacement of that original electrode: "No single discovery in the field of brain-behavior interactions can rival the finding that animals could be highly motivated to stimulate certain areas of their own brain." Not only did Olds and Milner's work generate a flood of experimentation along new lines, but it also stirred theorists to reevaluate their understanding of a fundamental aspect of behavior.

For some time, the prevailing opinion had been that pleasure is a by-product of the satisfaction of some need or drive, such as hunger, thirst, or sex—that when an urge is fulfilled, the resulting absence of that urge is the feeling of pleasure. But Olds, Milner, and others had apparently demonstrated that pleasure is a thing in itself, unrelated to the satisfaction of any urge. The rats, for example, presumably never reached a point of satiety, and when the lever was disconnected from the current, they quickly learned that there was no reason to keep pressing it: They seemingly felt no need for the stimulation when it was no longer available.

If pleasure, then, was an emotional state of the same nature as fear or rage, all the more reason to attempt to link it to actual physical components of the brain. Indeed, much of the testing spurred by Olds and Milner's discovery aimed to pinpoint the so-called pleasure centers that they had tentatively identified in the original experiments.

As had happened with studies of rage, however, continued research did more to cloud than to clarify the picture. Soon, investigators were finding that stimulation of many different areas of the brain—from parts of the thalamus to regions of the frontal cortex—could give rise to apparently pleasurable sensations. Once again, the appealing simplicity of a localized center for emotion had to give way to the undeniable complexities of the brain's circuitry. Olds himself eventually dropped the term "pleasure center" in the face of the evidence, and it has since all but disappeared from the literature of brain science.

Of course, linking a concept such as pleasure to the behavior of laboratory animals was in itself problematic. As Walter Hess's experiments with cats and the issue of sham rage had indicated, a complete understanding of the mechanisms of emotion had to take into account subjective experience—what it feels like to react angrily or fearfully or joyfully. So, despite the obvious limitations, scientists seeking to fathom the neural basis of emotion have whenever possible studied the only subjects who can tell them what is going on inside their own heads—human beings.

Although researchers cannot tamper with healthy human brains, they have been able to learn a great deal from people whose brains—for one reason or another—are not functioning properly. For example, attempts to treat patients with severe mental illness have often incidentally provided vital information on the anatomical underpinnings of emotion. One of the first scientists to gain new insights into this aspect of the brain's workings was Robert Heath, who began his investigations in the 1950s as chairman of the psychiatry department at Tulane University in New Orleans.

Heath experimented with human brain stimulation primarily in an effort to help dangerously psychotic patients. He employed two basic tactics: By electrically bringing on the rage that his patients exhibited in the throes of psychotic fits, he hoped to pinpoint the faulty part of their brains; and by stimulating areas that Olds and Milner's animal experiments seemed to indicate were associated with pleasure, he thought he might be able to short-circuit the explosions of anger. His procedure involved implanting electrodes during surgery and leaving them in place. At first, he left them for only a few days, but as the technique proved itself, some patients retained electrodes for years.

Heath was partially successful in both searching for rage and seeking to turn it off. In one particularly frightening episode, stimulation caused a young man who was peaceful a moment before to bristle with hatred. As Heath described the incident, "All of a sudden he wanted to kill. He would have, too, if he hadn't been tied down." At one point, the patient made a particularly significant connection between the electrode-induced emotion and an event from his past. "He started remembering a time when he lost his temper," Heath noted, "when his shirts weren't ironed right and he wanted to kill his sister. That showed us we'd activated the same circuit that was fired by his spontaneous rage attacks."

Numerous similar tests led Heath to delineate what he called an aversive, or "punishment," system that included, among other components, parts of the amygdala, hippocampus,

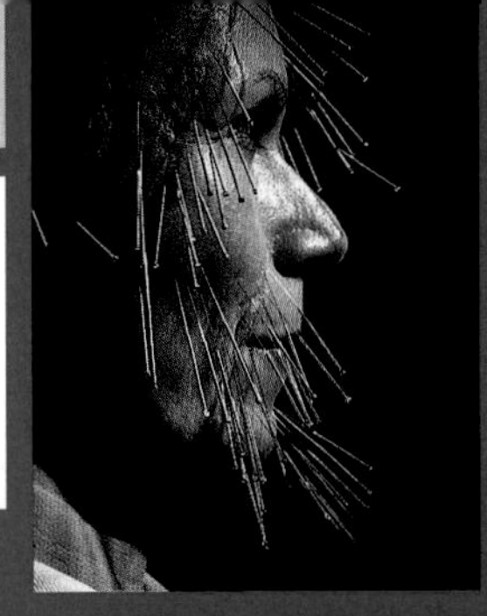

The Workings of Pain

Pain speaks in a thousand voices—sometimes subtle, sometimes savage, sometimes alternating between extremes. Like any sensation, it is partly shaped by the mind, varying according to fears, hopes, and other expectations. The felt pain of childbirth, for instance, tends to be far greater in some societies than in others, depending on whether the experience is viewed as an ordeal or not. War, too, reveals how pain is bound up with its perceived meaning: A wounded soldier, relieved that he will escape the battlefield alive, may experience far less pain than a civilian with an identical injury.

The mind can also be enlisted for therapy. Hypnosis affords relief in some cases, and placebos—treatments that depend entirely on the patient's belief in their efficacy—promote the production of neurotransmitters called endorphins, the body's natural painkillers. Some evidence shows that the Asian practice of acupuncture (*above*) also causes the release of endorphins. But how sugar pills and needle pricks might boost endorphin secretion remains a mystery.

Pain is sensed through an intricate, versatile system of specialized neurons, messaging routes, and molecules that convey or block signals. Pain begins when neuronal detectors are stimulated in some way—by pressure, for example, or heat, or the release of chemicals associated with tissue damage (*overleaf*). The special nerve cells are found in skin, in the sheathing of muscles, in organs, and in the membranes around bones—and they often respond to more than one kind of stimulus.

Signals are transmitted first to junctions in the spinal cord. One hypothesis for what happens there is known as the gate theory of pain—an interplay of chemical traffic controls that is explained on page 71. From the spinal cord, pain travels to the brain by one of two pathways. The first is very fast; messages on that route reach the brain in about a tenth of a second, and they identify the location and degree of the trouble, but they do not elicit much of an emotional reaction. The other path is slow; the signal takes at least a second to reach the brain. This is the persistent, throbbing, emotionally unpleasant pain that encourages rest and recuperation.

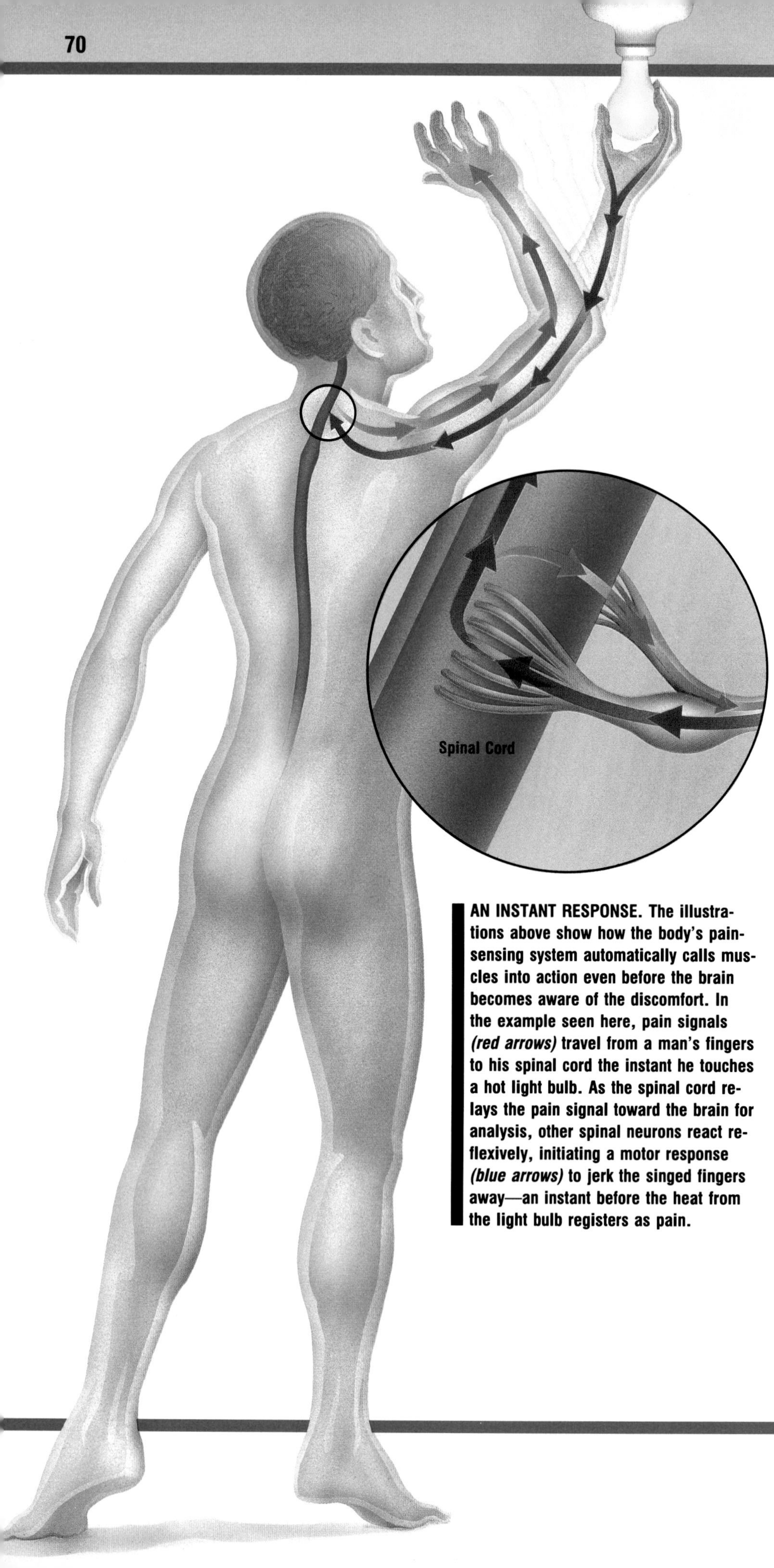

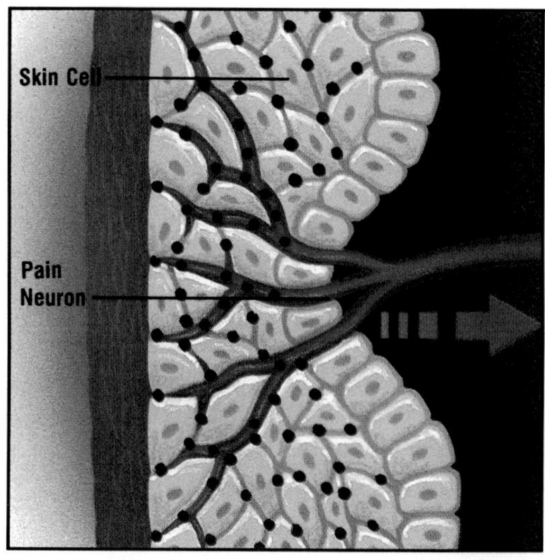

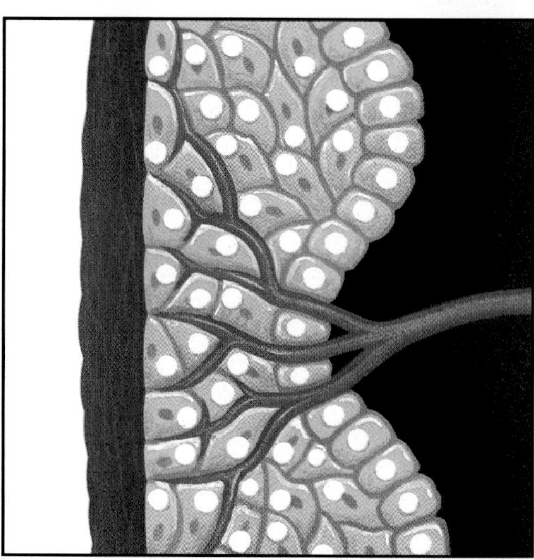

AN INSTANT RESPONSE. The illustrations above show how the body's pain-sensing system automatically calls muscles into action even before the brain becomes aware of the discomfort. In the example seen here, pain signals *(red arrows)* travel from a man's fingers to his spinal cord the instant he touches a hot light bulb. As the spinal cord relays the pain signal toward the brain for analysis, other spinal neurons react reflexively, initiating a motor response *(blue arrows)* to jerk the singed fingers away—an instant before the heat from the light bulb registers as pain.

WHAT ASPIRIN DOES. In registering pain, neurons in the skin respond first to heat or pressure, then to chemicals released by damaged cells. For example, when skin is burned, injured cells produce various chemicals, including compounds called prostaglandins *(top picture, black dots).* Along with other chemicals, prostaglandins cause pain neurons to fire more often, intensifying the sensation. Aspirin works against pain by halting the production of prostaglandins. Aspirin molecules *(white dots, above)* are absorbed by skin cells, where they interfere with the enzyme needed to make prostaglandins. As a result, the neurons fire at a reduced rate and transmit less pain.

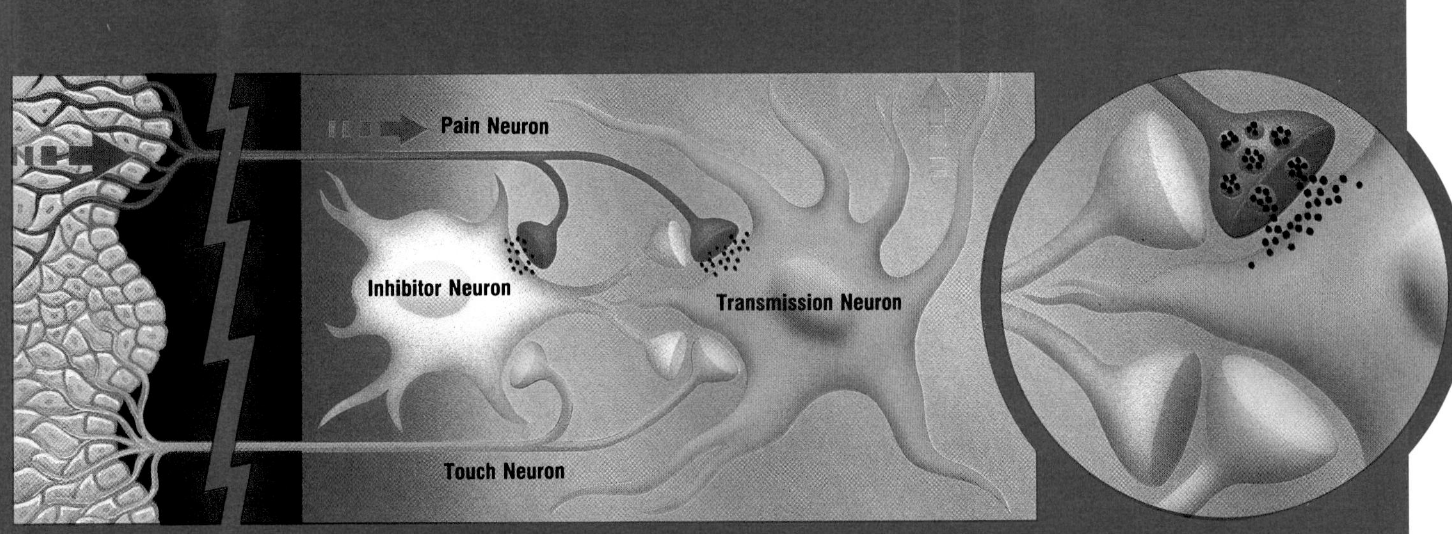

OPENING THE GATE FOR PAIN. In the spinal cord, a pain signal *(red arrows)* may be either blocked or passed on to the brain. As shown in the illustrations on this page, the outcome depends on several kinds of nerve cells: sensory neurons (chiefly for pain and touch); inhibitor neurons; and pain-transmission neurons that send the message to the brain. In the absence of pain, inhibitor neurons in the spinal cord release an endorphin-like chemical that prevents the nearby transmission neurons from firing. To get its message to the brain *(green arrow)*, a pain neuron *(red)* turns off the inhibitor neuron with a neurotransmitter cascade of its own *(above)*. Then, as seen in the closeup, synaptic vesicles in the pain neuron shower the transmission neuron with neurotransmitters that make it fire.

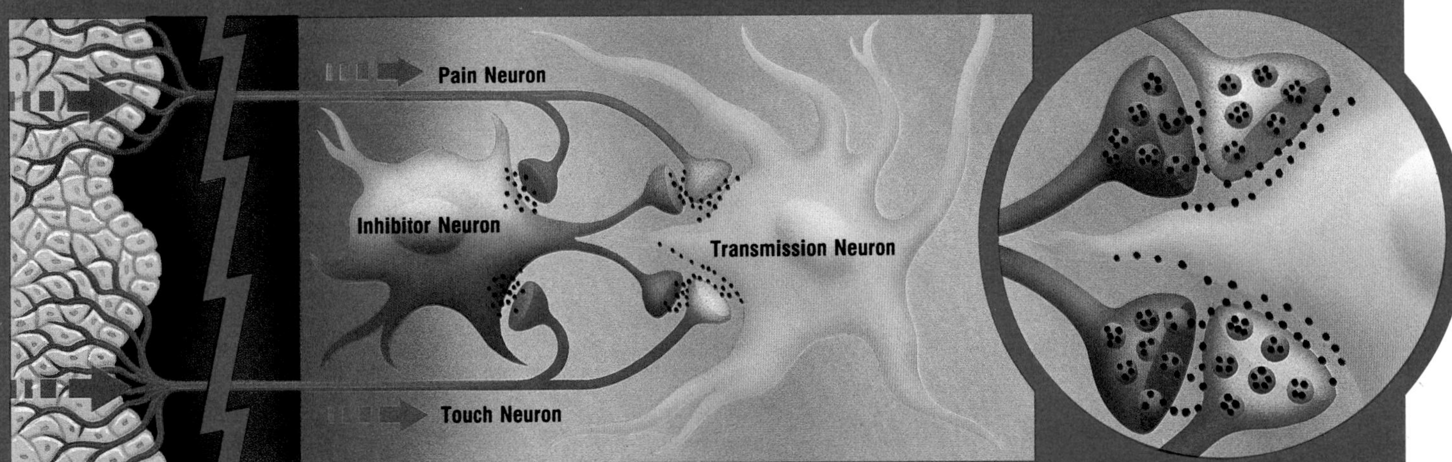

SHUTTING THE GATE. Rubbing an injury often eases pain because inhibitor neurons react to messages from sensory cells other than pain neurons. In the sequence above, an inhibitor neuron is showered with neurotransmitters triggered by both the pain signal and a touch signal from rubbing *(red and purple arrows)*. Neurotransmitters from the touch neuron counteract those from the pain neuron. The inhibitor cell switches on, releasing an endorphin-like substance into the synapses between the pain and transmission neurons *(closeup at right)*. This inhibitory chemical quenches the flow of neurotransmitters to the transmission neuron, checking the pain message. The rubbing sensation that accompanies pain relief comes from touch neurons that activate touch-transmission nerve cells.

and thalamus. This network was, it turned out, surprisingly close to other limbic-system circuits forming what Heath dubbed pleasure systems—the interconnected structures that animal experimenters were also discovering at about the same time.

Heath's attempts to short-circuit this punishment system focused on schizophrenics. He reasoned that schizophrenics suffer from some kind of imbalance between pleasurable and painful emotions. With a dysfunctional pleasure system, he argued, they remain charged with fear and rage. In many cases, Heath's brain stimulation of pleasure circuits seemed to work, if only temporarily.

"If we stimulated their pleasure systems, violent psychotics stopped having rage attacks," Heath reported. Over the years, he learned that a single stimulation of pleasure systems was a cure of the moment only. Patients might need occasional stimulation for years to stay well. To improve the technique, Heath developed a battery-powered, self-contained automatic stimulator. Instead of inserting long electrodes through the cortex into the underlying limbic system itself, he arranged a more stable array of tiny electrodes in a narrow strip less than an inch long that could be positioned on the surface of a certain section of the cerebellum, at the back of the head. Every few minutes, the stimulator would launch a volley of signals into the cerebellar cells, which Heath had discovered would relay the impulses to the appropriate limbic-system circuits, switching pleasure on and rage off.

The first recipient of the new device was, according to Heath, "the most violent patient in the state." But the stimulation worked like a charm, eliminating the man's horrific outbursts. The experiment worked so

The Neurochemistry of Depression

In its extreme form, depression is among the most crippling of emotional disorders. It was once treated solely through such techniques as psychotherapy, but in the 1950s, investigators discovered that certain drugs alleviated its symptoms. There is now a growing consensus that clinical depression may stem from imbalances in brain chemistry and may, in particular, be related to low levels of the neurotransmitters norepinephrine and serotonin, both normally highly concentrated in neurons of the brain's emotional circuits. Treatment nowadays includes antidepressant drugs that boost the levels of these chemicals in two ways. Some inhibit the breakdown of neurotransmitters within neurons, while others prevent their reabsorption by neurons, increasing concentrations in synapses and improving the transmission of neuronal impulses.

well, in fact, that a short time after getting his stimulator, he was released from the mental hospital and allowed to go home. Later, however, he suddenly launched a murderous rampage, attempting to kill his parents and severely wounding a neighbor. Back at the hospital, x-rays revealed the problem: broken battery wires. Once his stimulator was repaired, the man was able to enter and succeed in a vocational rehabilitation program.

Other researchers were also gathering information from humans about emotional changes wrought by brain stimulation. Working at Yale University in the early 1960s, the Spanish-born physiologist José Delgado duplicated some of Heath's results and identified other emotional nuances related to the limbic system as well.

One of Delgado's patients was a normally calm and cheerful woman who was prone to sudden violent outbursts, having one time stabbed a nurse in the chest with a pair of scissors. Suspecting that abnormal activity in her amygdala might be involved in the unpredictable rage, Delgado implanted an electrode there and then supplied a small dose of current. After seven seconds of stimulation, the woman, who had been quietly playing her guitar, suddenly slammed down the instrument and launched a furious attack against the wall.

Stimulating various other parts of the limbic system in other patients, both Delgado and Heath elicited all sorts of reactions. One person described the sensation as "like the feeling of just having been missed by a car"; another reported a wave of overwhelming dread. When it came to those networks associated with pleasure, the reactions ranged from a glow of well-being to outright ecstasy. One patient said the electrode-induced experience was "better than sex."

To the researchers who were able to turn these reactions on and off with the flick of a switch, the cause-and-effect relationship between brain stimulation and behavior was obvious. But Heath's and Delgado's patients often made no such connection: According to their reports, stimulus-provoked movements or emotions sprang from within; they sought wherever possible to find a rationale for their actions, some real-world connection. For example, a patient who mechanically rocked his head back and forth in response to stimulation said he was "looking for his slippers," or he "heard a noise." A severely depressed, blank-faced woman who would suddenly break into a fit of the giggles after stimulation tried desperately to rationalize her glee: "I don't usually sit around and laugh at nothing," she insisted. "I must be laughing at something."

Researchers and philosophers alike have been deeply impressed by the attempts of test subjects to explain artificially evoked physiological states. These efforts imply that what we consider to be genuine sentiments, aspects of our own unique personalities arising from our individual minds, may in some degree be grounded in purely physical processes. Even our value systems can be traced to this neurological activity. As Edward Wilson, a noted biologist at Harvard, has written, structures of the limbic system "flood our consciousness with all the emotions—hate, love, guilt, fear, and others—that are consulted by ethical philosophers who wish to intuit the standards of good and evil." Robert Heath himself is perhaps even more forthright on the matter: "All moral learning is ultimately based on the pain and pleasure circuitry in your brain—on your internal reward and punishment system."

Some of the most significant insights garnered by Heath, Delgado, and others came not from experiments with

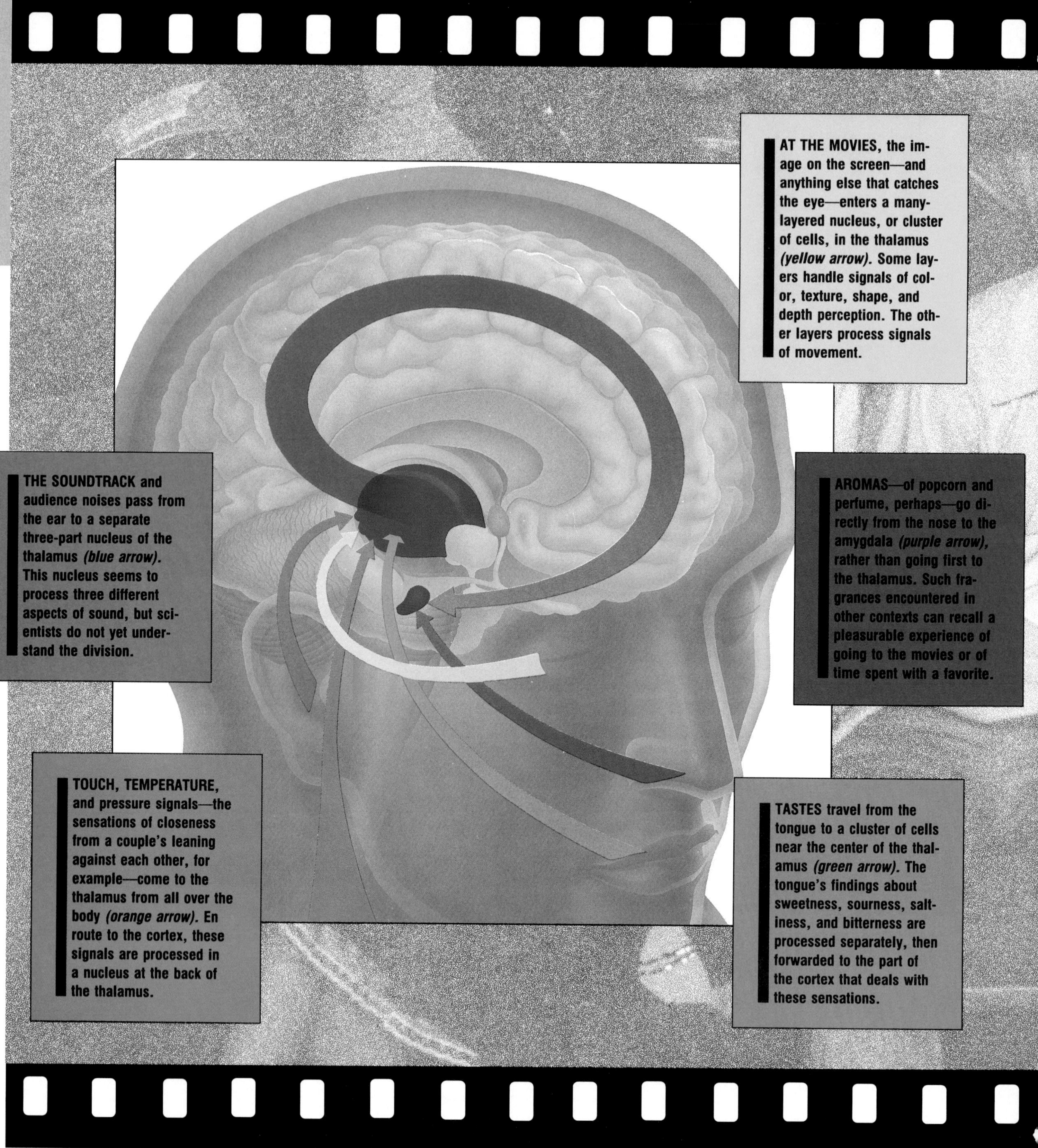

AT THE MOVIES, the image on the screen—and anything else that catches the eye—enters a many-layered nucleus, or cluster of cells, in the thalamus *(yellow arrow)*. Some layers handle signals of color, texture, shape, and depth perception. The other layers process signals of movement.

THE SOUNDTRACK and audience noises pass from the ear to a separate three-part nucleus of the thalamus *(blue arrow)*. This nucleus seems to process three different aspects of sound, but scientists do not yet understand the division.

AROMAS—of popcorn and perfume, perhaps—go directly from the nose to the amygdala *(purple arrow)*, rather than going first to the thalamus. Such fragrances encountered in other contexts can recall a pleasurable experience of going to the movies or of time spent with a favorite.

TOUCH, TEMPERATURE, and pressure signals—the sensations of closeness from a couple's leaning against each other, for example—come to the thalamus from all over the body *(orange arrow)*. En route to the cortex, these signals are processed in a nucleus at the back of the thalamus.

TASTES travel from the tongue to a cluster of cells near the center of the thalamus *(green arrow)*. The tongue's findings about sweetness, sourness, saltiness, and bitterness are processed separately, then forwarded to the part of the cortex that deals with these sensations.

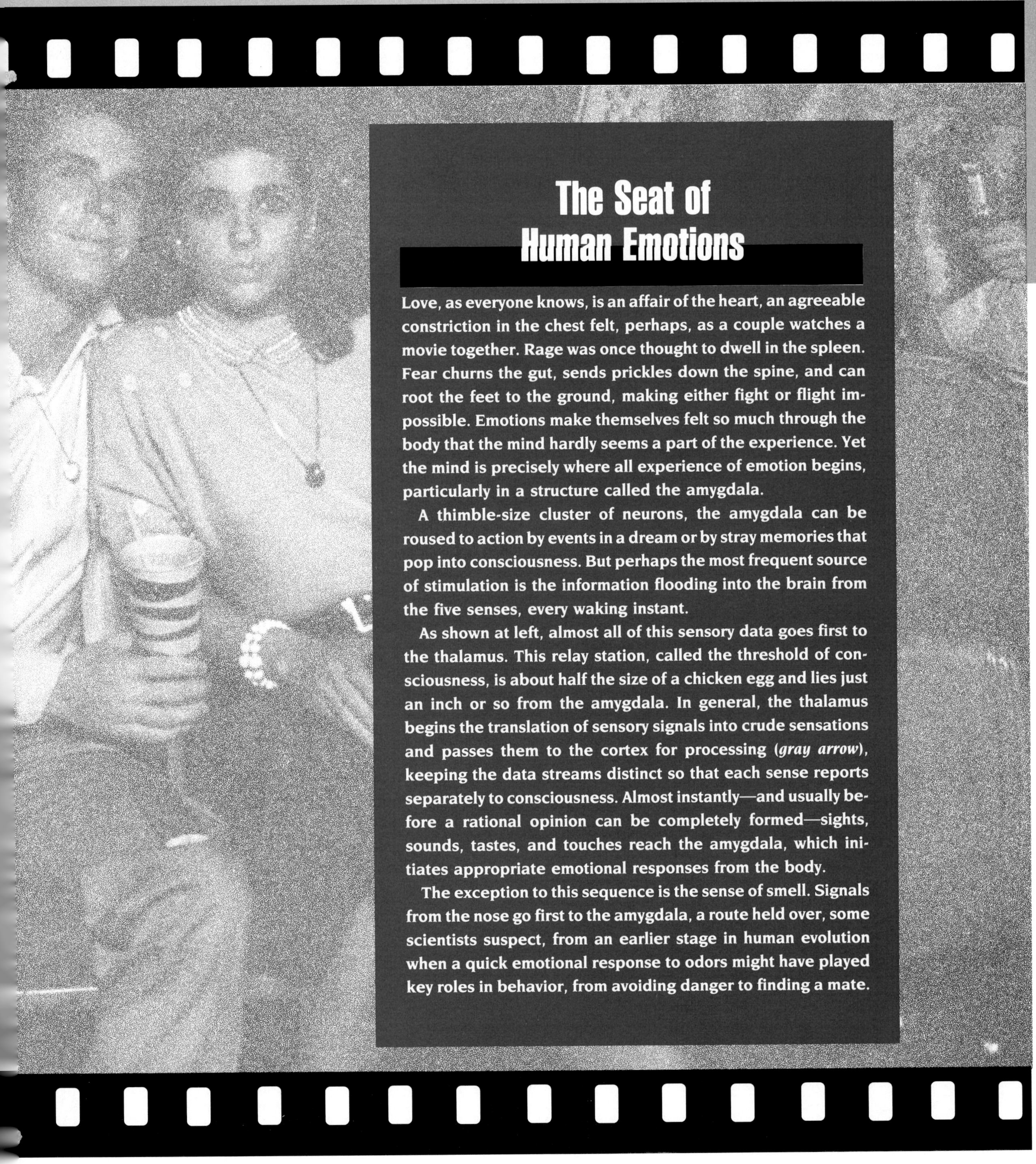

The Seat of Human Emotions

Love, as everyone knows, is an affair of the heart, an agreeable constriction in the chest felt, perhaps, as a couple watches a movie together. Rage was once thought to dwell in the spleen. Fear churns the gut, sends prickles down the spine, and can root the feet to the ground, making either fight or flight impossible. Emotions make themselves felt so much through the body that the mind hardly seems a part of the experience. Yet the mind is precisely where all experience of emotion begins, particularly in a structure called the amygdala.

A thimble-size cluster of neurons, the amygdala can be roused to action by events in a dream or by stray memories that pop into consciousness. But perhaps the most frequent source of stimulation is the information flooding into the brain from the five senses, every waking instant.

As shown at left, almost all of this sensory data goes first to the thalamus. This relay station, called the threshold of consciousness, is about half the size of a chicken egg and lies just an inch or so from the amygdala. In general, the thalamus begins the translation of sensory signals into crude sensations and passes them to the cortex for processing (*gray arrow*), keeping the data streams distinct so that each sense reports separately to consciousness. Almost instantly—and usually before a rational opinion can be completely formed—sights, sounds, tastes, and touches reach the amygdala, which initiates appropriate emotional responses from the body.

The exception to this sequence is the sense of smell. Signals from the nose go first to the amygdala, a route held over, some scientists suspect, from an earlier stage in human evolution when a quick emotional response to odors might have played key roles in behavior, from avoiding danger to finding a mate.

"You all, healthy people, cannot imagine the happiness which we epileptics feel during the second before our fit."

—Fyodor Dostoyevsky

psychotic patients but from research into another brain-related malady—epilepsy. This affliction turned out to be particularly revealing not only of the link between limbic areas and emotion but also of a three-way conjunction that also encompasses certain kinds of memory.

Epilepsy, with its characteristic convulsive seizures, had been observed since ancient times—Julius Caesar is thought to have been one of its victims—and had been recognized early on as a disease of the brain. But it was not until the advent of EEG monitoring in the 1930s that scientists began to understand what goes on inside the brain during an attack. Normally, the overall electrical activity of the brain's neurons is relatively random, analogous perhaps to low-level electrical "white noise." But at the onset of an epileptic seizure, a few cells—often near the site of a lesion or other injury—begin to fire simultaneously. This trigger group excites nearby cells, and the pattern spreads, sometimes sweeping across the entire brain, as if every member of an orchestra was blaring out a single note on the beat.

Those interested in understanding epilepsy had long been fascinated by sufferers' descriptions of how they felt just before an attack. Fyodor Dostoyevsky, the great Russian novelist of the 19th century, had vivid emotional reactions preceding seizures—not an uncommon phenomenon. But perhaps surprisingly, these feelings led Dostoyevsky to consider the malady almost more of a blessing than a curse: "You all, healthy people," he once commented to friends, "cannot imagine the happiness which we epileptics feel during the second before our fit." Describing the sensation, he noted, "I feel a complete harmony within myself and in the world, and this feeling is so strong and so sweet that for a few seconds of this enjoyment one would readily exchange 10 years of one's life—perhaps even one's whole life."

Other victims of epilepsy have detected strange smells or tastes, and even had visions or auditory hallucinations just before a seizure struck. Another reported phenomenon is a powerful sense of déjà vu—the feeling that a present experience has actually occurred before, detail by detail. By all indications, this had to have something to do with a misfiring of memory circuits.

Given that many epileptic seizures arise in the temporal lobes and the underlying limbic system, the strong bursts of emotion prior to an attack were not surprising to researchers focusing on this part of the brain. The strange sensory experiences also conformed with the discovery that the thalamus is crucial to the processing of sensory information (*pages* 74-75). But among the most fascinating stories is the way brain scientists began to learn how involved certain limbic components are in the formation of memories. The déjà vu experiences were only a hint of what investigators would unearth.

One of the first breakthroughs in this regard owes to the work of the Canadian neurosurgeon Wilder Penfield, founder of the Montreal Neurological Institute. From the 1930s through the 1950s, Penfield operated on numerous epileptic patients in efforts to remove damaged tissue and so alleviate their symptoms. He introduced the technique of keeping patients conscious during surgery and stimulating parts of their brains in order to identify and then avoid healthy tissue. As he probed, his electrode would elicit a toe twitch here, a phantom buzzing sound there. In the temporal lobe, however, patients reported entirely different reactions. Here, Penfield elicited memories, some in startling detail. (Although Penfield stimulated only the cortex, he later felt sure his results came from current spreading to the underlying limbic system—a conclusion confirmed by more recent

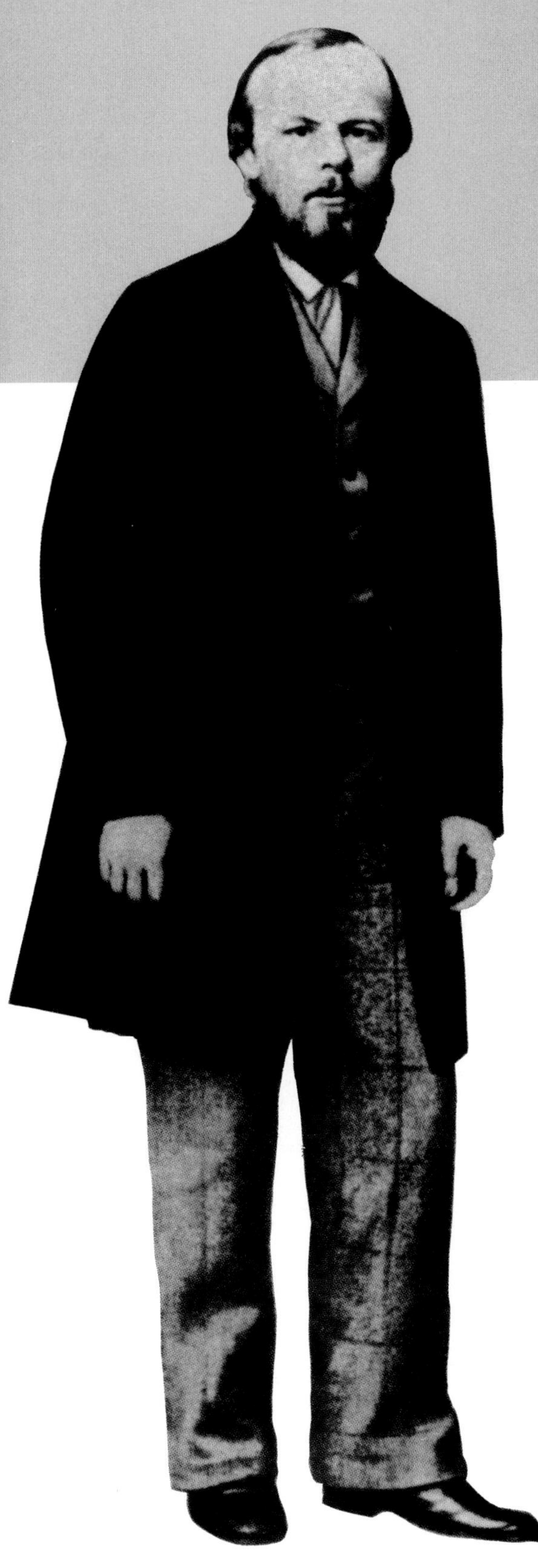

The Mood Swings of Epilepsy

During the more than 30 years that he suffered from epilepsy, the Russian writer Fyodor Dostoyevsky (*left*) often reflected on the emotional turmoil that the affliction had brought to his life. He was thrilled by the almost religious ecstasy that engulfed him moments before the onset of a seizure but was tormented by the periods of deep depression that set in afterward. These contradictory strains seemed to fuel his creativity, becoming a central theme in many of his works. Immediately after an attack, Dostoyevsky could neither write nor speak well, an indication that he may have had temporal lobe epilepsy in the left hemisphere, which houses language functions. The overhead-view PET scans below reveal the effects of this type of epilepsy on brain activity. During a seizure (*left*), the left lobe is more active, as shown by the graph (*bottom*) of the boxed area; between seizures (*right*), the left temporal lobe is actually quieter than other areas.

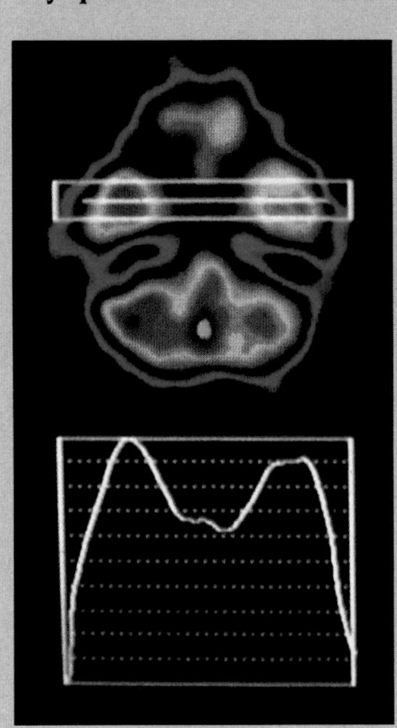

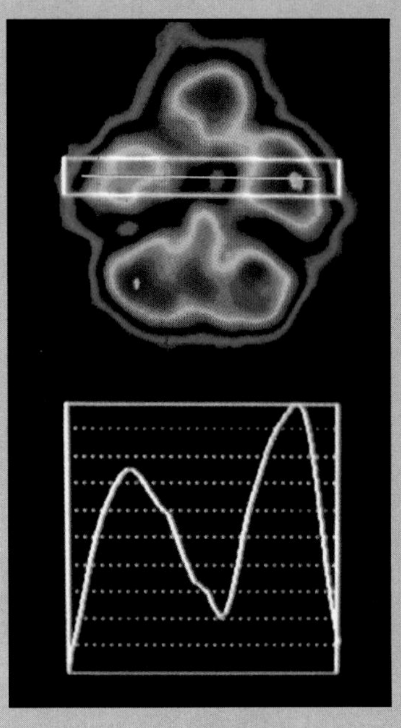

experiments with electrodes reaching into this area.)

One of Penfield's subjects spoke of hearing the voices of a man and a woman by a river and even seeing the river; stimulation at another point brought back a distinct memory of an office, and "a man leaning on the desk with a pencil in his hand." With several patients, music memories seemed to predominate, some so clearly expressed as to make them identifiable by operating-room attendants. One woman heard instruments playing a melody. Penfield actually stimulated the same point 30

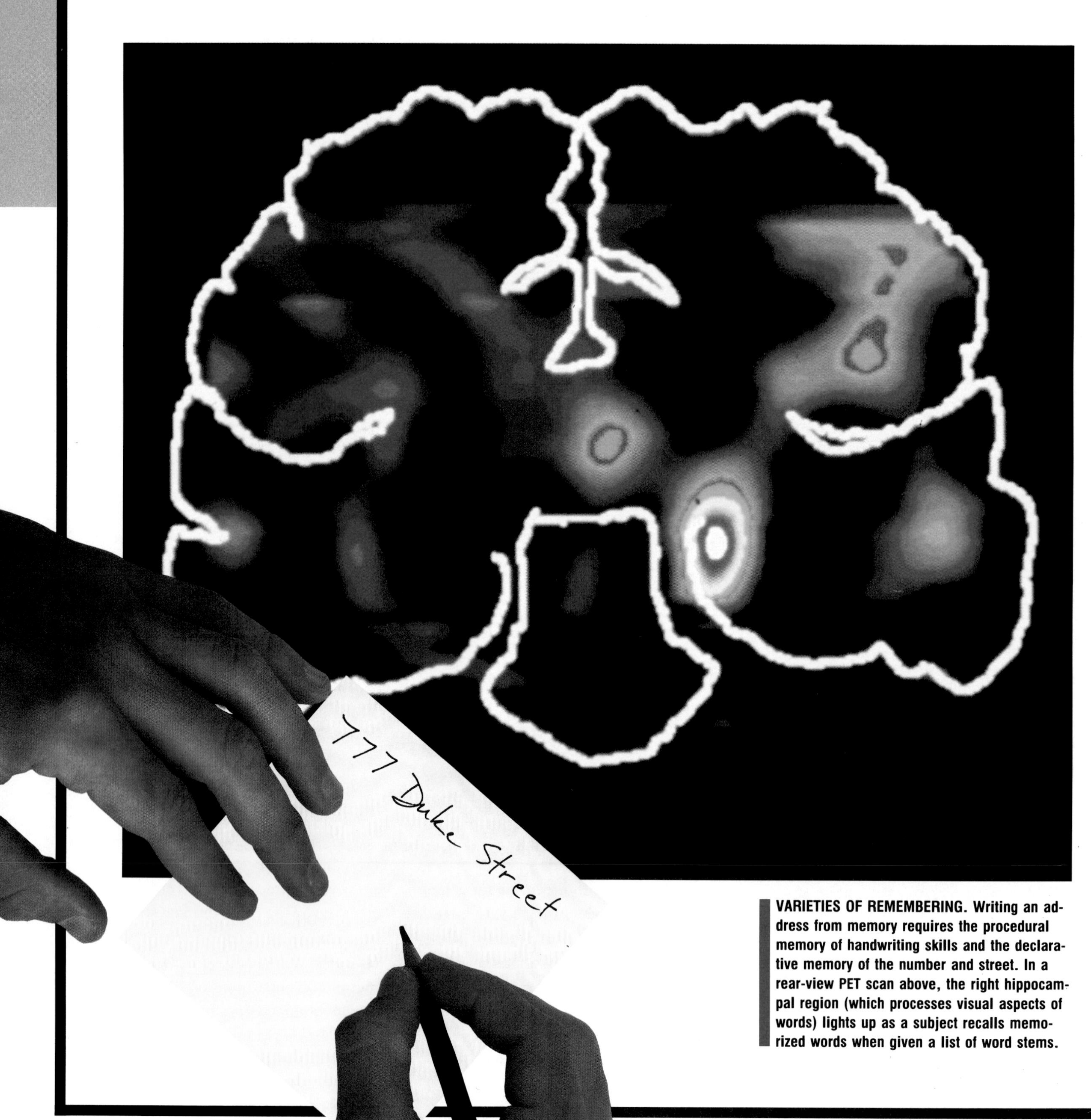

VARIETIES OF REMEMBERING. Writing an address from memory requires the procedural memory of handwriting skills and the declarative memory of the number and street. In a rear-view PET scan above, the right hippocampal region (which processes visual aspects of words) lights up as a subject recalls memorized words when given a list of word stems.

Remembering How, Remembering What

Studies of the brain suggest that it performs at least two kinds of remembering, mixed seamlessly in most behavior. Procedural memory is the repository of such skills as handwriting or driving and involves the cerebellum and basal ganglia. Declarative memory consists of information—an address, roads to a destination, words, faces, and other knowledge thought to be stored in the cerebral cortex.

Information entering the brain is processed in the cortex as it is experienced. Temporary links among neurons persist for a few minutes as a place for a short-term memory. This allows us to recall a phone number long enough to dial it or to address a person by name several minutes after an introduction.

For such memories to become more durable, a process called long-term potentiation (LTP) is thought to be important. LTP is the tendency of nerve cells exposed to a rapidly repeated stimulus to respond more strongly long after the intense exposure than beforehand. One theory suggests that dendrites of neurons excited in this way may sprout new growth that greatly improves existing connections, perhaps explaining the long life of the improved performance.

According to the LTP hypothesis, the making of a long-term declarative memory begins as the cortex sends information to the hippocampus and nearby structures (*pages* 62-63). Evidence suggests that the hippocampus then strengthens the memory by rapidly and repeatedly exciting the neural circuit in the cortex. Initially, the hippocampus also seems to take part in the deliberate retrieval of facts from the cortex (*left*) but plays a lesser role in jogging the memory as time passes.

One implication of this theory of memory is that LTP can be invoked voluntarily—as when striving to memorize a telephone number—or unintentionally; most people can also remember, without even trying, what they had for breakfast the day before. Emotion, too, plays a role. Recollections of a close call or a first love are often more vivid than others of similar vintage.

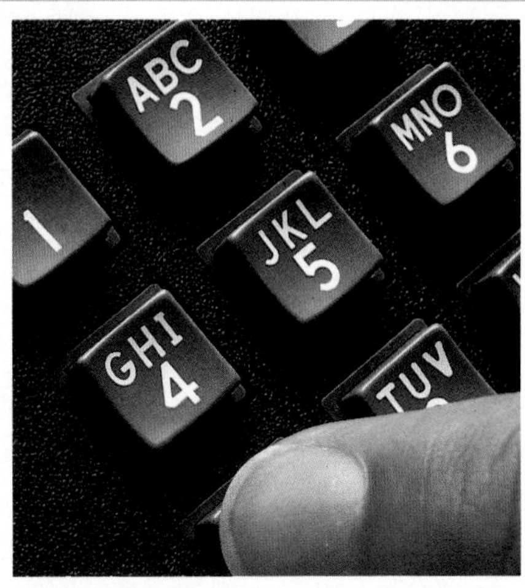

Secrets of a Sharper Memory

A time-honored tactic for anchoring facts permanently in memory is "chunking"—reducing unwieldy data into fewer pieces. The need can be acute with short-term memory, which generally holds from five to nine distinct items: Even a seven-digit phone number may be unmanageable for many people. To reduce the number of elements, Europeans, for example, typically write such numbers in groups of two or three, which are easier to recall than the three- and four-digit parts of phone numbers in the United States. An advertiser seeking telephone orders might urge customers to dial "1-800-BUY THIS," converting seven digits into easy-to-remember words. Mnemonic rhymes are yet another trick: "Thirty days has September, April, June, and November . . ." condenses the information into a ditty with proven sticking power.

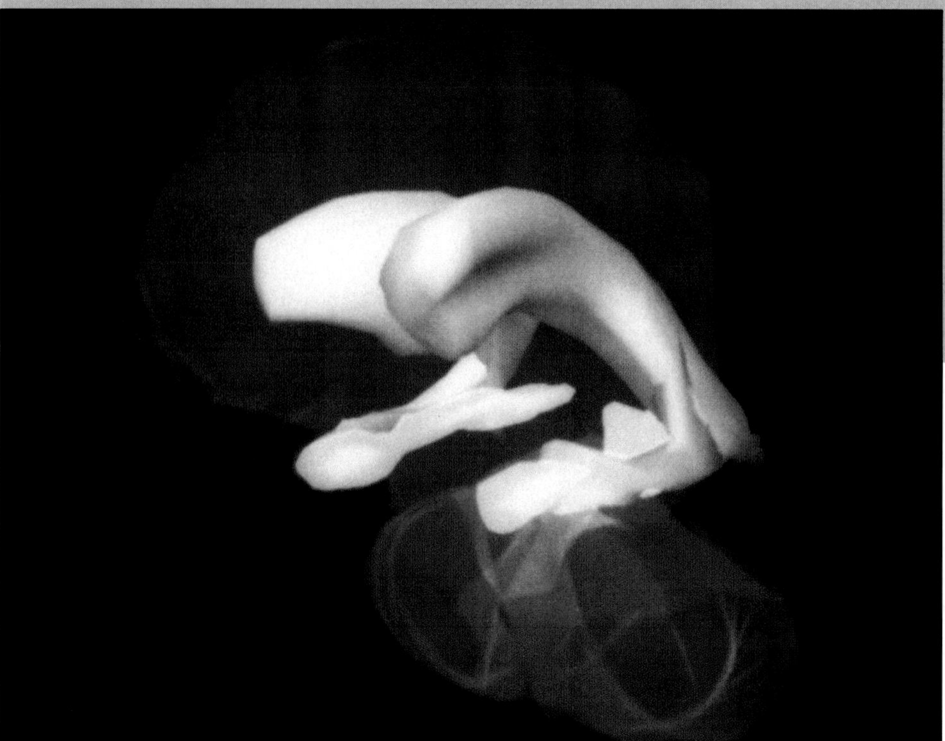

Constructed from a series of MRI scans, this computer-generated three-dimensional image highlights sections of the hippocampus in yellow. (The large bluish gray structures are fluid-filled cavities called ventricles.) Investigators have found that Alzheimer's disease may destroy more than half of the neurons in the hippocampus, severely impairing the brain's ability to form long-term memories. Alzheimer's also causes certain proteins to accumulate in the hippocampus and parts of the cortex associated with memory, further interfering with normal neuronal activity.

times to test the response, and "each time I restimulated, she heard the melody again. It began in the same place and went from chorus to verse."

Penfield was incredulous at first. Eventually he came to believe not only that the memories were real, but also that the mental record contained every single thing that had ever happened to the patient, in detail well beyond what is normally available to consciousness.

"It was evident," he concluded, "that these were not dreams. They were electrical activations of the sequential record of consciousness, a record that had been laid down during the patient's earlier experience." He further postulated that the electrode activated random samples of this filmstrip of the past, and "since the most unimportant and completely forgotten periods of time may appear in this sampling, it seems reasonable to suppose that the record is complete and that it does include all periods of each individual's waking conscious life."

This was, of course, a bold supposition, one that almost begged to be challenged. Penfield himself was troubled by one aspect of such a superaccurate memory system. He happened to espouse the notion, originally proposed by Sigmund Freud, that experiences become memories only when firmly linked with emotions. "It would be very difficult to imagine," Penfield noted, "that some of the trivial incidents recalled could have any possible emotional significance to the patient, even if one is acutely aware of this possibility." What, then, was going on in these people's minds? Had they really recorded every event in their lives, even when they had made no conscious effort to do so?

Psychologists Elizabeth and Geoffrey Loftus thought not. In the late 1970s, they reexamined records of more than 1,000 patients whom Penfield had tested with electrode stimulation: Only 40 had reported memory-like experiences. Most of these so-called reminiscences consisted only of vague voices, snatches of music, or disconnected thoughts. And the most complete "memories" were difficult to believe in retrospect. One patient had seen herself being born. Another described visiting a lumberyard but also confessed to never having been in a lumberyard. The Loftuses and other scientists were led to conclude that Penfield's "memories" were hallucinations or generic reconstructions of many similar events. Penfield's patients appeared to be fitting strange feelings produced by brain stimulation into a rational train of thought, just as Delgado's and Heath's patients had done with induced emotional reactions.

AGING VERSUS ALZHEIMER'S. During the normal course of aging, the brain loses neurons—as many as a fifth in the hippocampus. Those that remain send out longer dendrites, to some extent compensating for the loss of connections that support such functions as memory. As shown in the drawings of neurons below, this process is particularly evident between the ages of 50 and 70. However, the neurons of a 70-year-old Alzheimer's victim typically show no such growth and are equivalent to those of a 90-year-old—by which age even a healthy individual's neurons have begun to shrink.

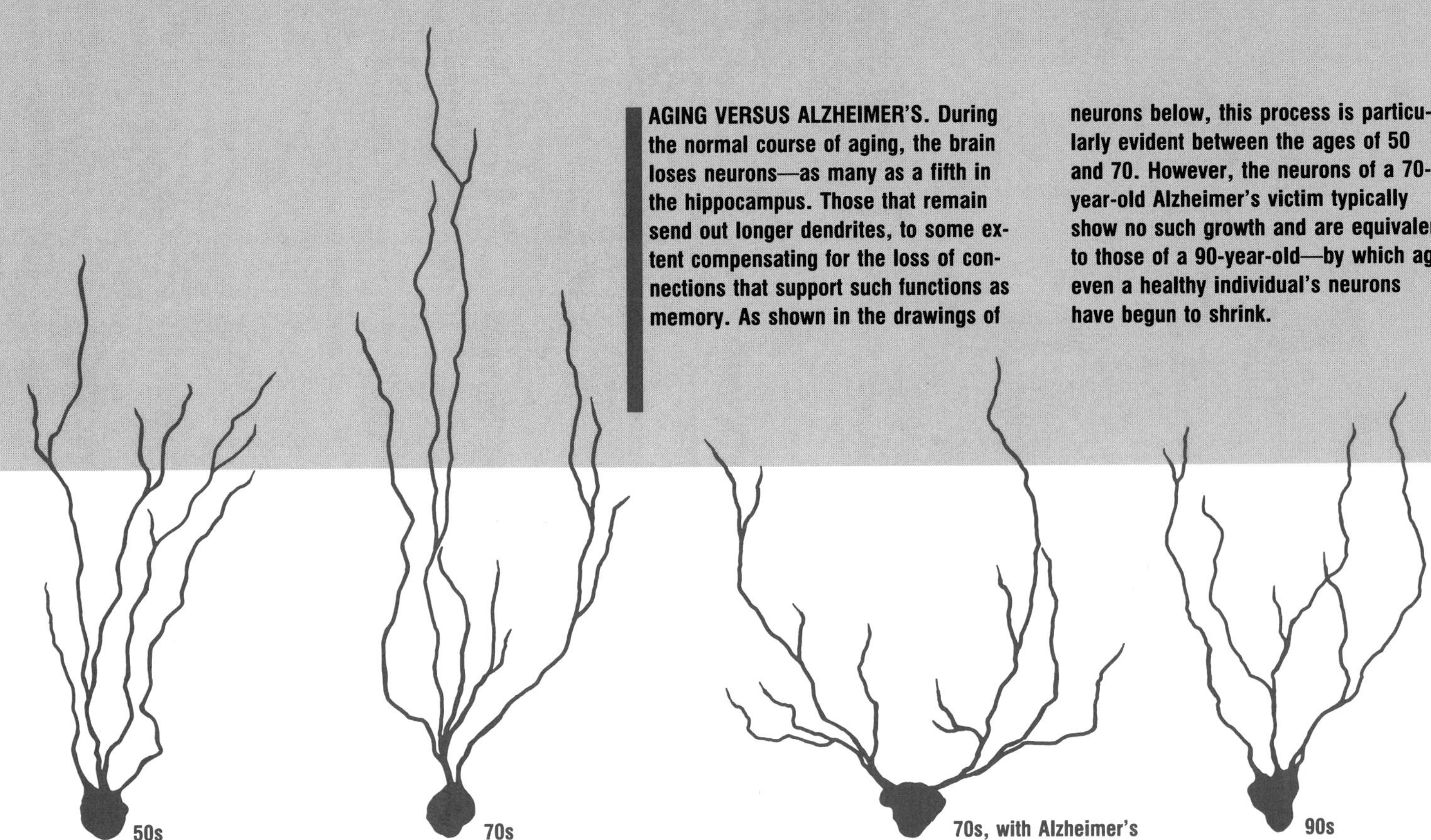

This was not to say that the limbic system was unassociated with the processing of memories. In fact, during the time Penfield was conducting his stimulation experiments, one of the most famous cases in the study of human memory was beginning to shed new light on the subject.

In 1953 neurosurgeon William B. Scoville, who had a practice in Hartford, Connecticut, decided to perform a particularly extreme form of surgery, as a last resort, on one of his epileptic patients, a former assembly-line worker known in the brain science literature only as H. M. For 10 years, the victim had suffered crippling seizures that began in his temporal lobe and then spread devastation throughout his brain, leaving him unable to work. During the surgery, Scoville removed the suspected source of the seizures, tissue under the temporal cortex on each side of H. M.'s brain, and he also excised much of the limbic system, including the hippocampus and the amygdala.

The results were decidedly mixed. Scoville's operation succeeded in controlling H. M.'s seizures, but it also robbed the patient of his ability to remember new events. Indeed, the supposed cure so adversely affected his life that few patients since have undergone the radical procedure.

In the years that followed, neuropsychologist Brenda Milner, at the Montreal Neurological Institute, conducted an extensive study of H. M.'s memory loss, which seemed to take a strangely specific form. In the short term—for periods ranging up to 10 minutes—he remembered perfectly well, and he was able to recall events before the operation clearly. He could even learn difficult dexterity tasks, such as drawing while seeing his hand only in a mirror. He chatted normally with Milner and retained a hearty and sharp sense of humor. But if Milner repeated a joke word for word after a 15-minute wait, H. M. laughed just as hard as he had the first time he heard it. And every time Milner, attendants, or nurses left the room, H. M. would have no idea who they were when they returned a few minutes later.

Today, the reasons behind such deficits are well known in the medical profession—to the extent that, in the case of a stroke victim like George (*Chapter* 1), doctors know precisely which brain structures have been affected and what sort of memory mechanisms are involved. But those working with H. M. had no such advantages. In fact, it was up to them to elaborate new theories of memory in order to explain H. M.'s situation.

A few details could be straightforwardly deduced. For one thing, the areas where H. M.'s long-lasting memories resided (now thought to be throughout the cerebral cortex) were clearly intact. And the first brief recording of information (also nowadays considered to be a cortical function) seemed equally unaffected. However, there was something definitely wrong with the transfer of information between short-term and long-term storage. The natural assumption was that the limbic components removed from H. M.'s brain carried out this memory transfer function.

But one aspect of H. M.'s behavior hinted that this relatively simple hypothesis of how the memory system works did not tell the whole story. Not only could H. M. learn new skills, but he also got better at those skills day by day.

Following up on Brenda Milner's original investigations, several neuropsychologists, including Neal Cohen at the University of Illinois and Larry Squire at the University of California in San Diego, pursued this intriguing feature of H. M.'s memory beginning in 1981. In one test, Cohen asked H. M. to learn a puzzle called the Tower of Hanoi, in which the object is to transfer a set of five rings, each of a different diameter, from one peg to another according to certain rules: moving only one ring at a time, never placing a larger ring on top of a smaller one, and finishing with the rings arranged in order by size, the largest on the bottom.

Both H. M. and another patient with a similar form of memory impairment learned to solve this puzzle as easily as did control subjects who had no brain damage. And with practice both H. M. and the other patient improved, eventually managing to complete the tower in the minimum 31 moves. Yet from their point of view, each time they tried the puzzle was the first. Somehow they had mastered the procedure involved in solving the puzzle, but they had no conscious memory of learning it.

This and similar tests that demonstrated the unconscious learning of skills led Squire and other researchers to the notion that there are two distinctly different kinds of memory, beyond the familiar division of short- and long-term. The first—which H. M. had apparently retained—was dubbed procedural memory, and it encompassed the so-called muscle memory that enables a person to ride a bicycle without consciously remembering how to. The memory ability that H. M. had lost became known as declarative memory—the conscious recollection of facts and experiences. H. M.'s case indicated that structures in the limbic system play an absolutely essential role in the formation of declarative memories.

The damage to H. M.'s brain had been so extensive, however, that researchers could not with confidence identify which specific component took care of this memory process. New information, including images produced by the most advanced brain-scanning techniques, has pinpointed the hippocampus as the crucial structure. What remains to be fully understood are the neuronal mechanisms through which the hippocampus takes a short-term memory and turns it into a recollection that can last for decades.

The discoveries stemming from H. M.'s condition reconfirm the intimate relationship between the limbic area of the brain and the overlying cortex. With certain forms of memory, as with emotions, the mind's experience depends on elaborate exchanges of information through neuronal circuits that continue to stymie researchers' efforts to understand them. This should, of course, be of little surprise: Among this dazzling system's skills are the ability to recognize all the fine nuances that form the palette of human emotions, and to store—ready for almost instantaneous recall—the reminiscences of a lifetime.

WHERE THE BODY MEETS THE MIND

Although it is scarcely the size of an olive, the hypothalamus is the grand master of virtually all of the body's involuntary, or autonomic, functions. It maintains the general state of bodily equilibrium known as homeostasis. As an internal thermostat, it works to keep the body temperature within an optimum range for organ function. It also regulates the flow of various hormones involved in human reproduction, among other things. Even in times of stress, when the body must abandon this equilibrium, the hypothalamus remains in command.

As part of the complex known as the limbic system, the hypothalamus is the broker between mind and body, giving physical form to thoughts and emotions. When other parts of the limbic system and the cerebral cortex signal love, anger, or fear, for instance, the hypothalamus produces the familiar—and remarkably similar—symptoms, such as a racing pulse and the increased blood pressure that brings on a pounding head, flushed face, and constricted feeling in the chest. These sensations then feed back to the rest of the brain largely through the hypothalamus, creating the sometimes confusing, often exhilarating, and uniquely human interplay among our physical, emotional, and rational selves.

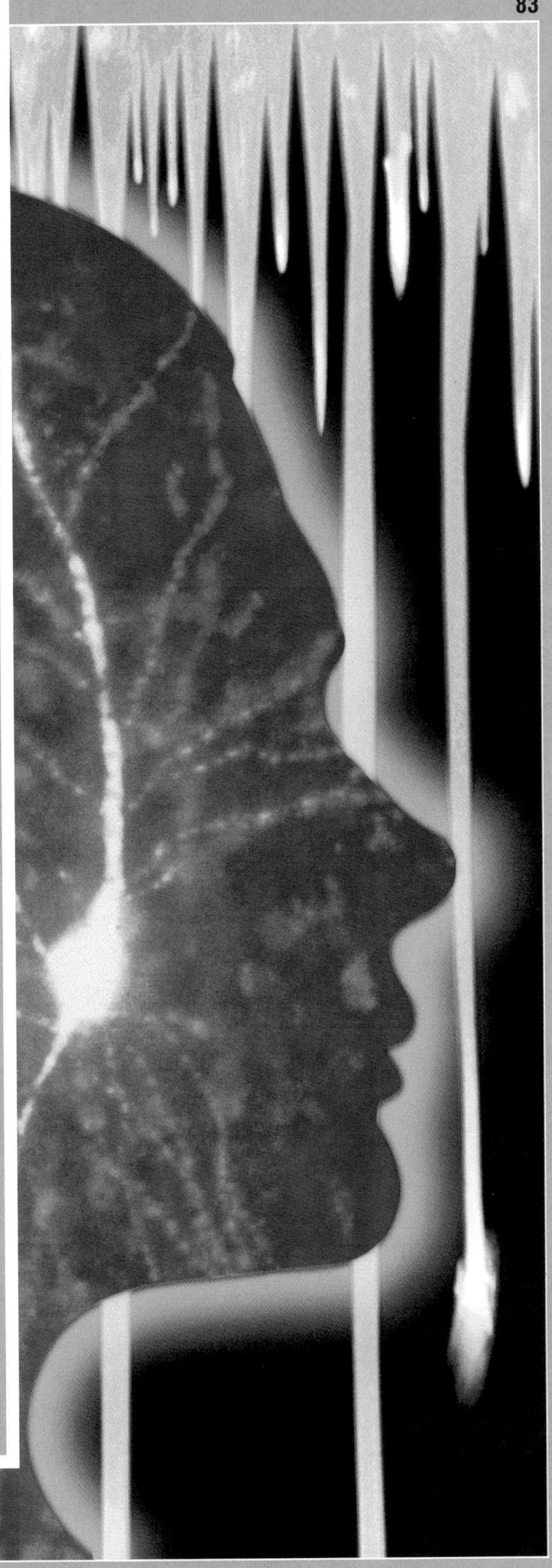

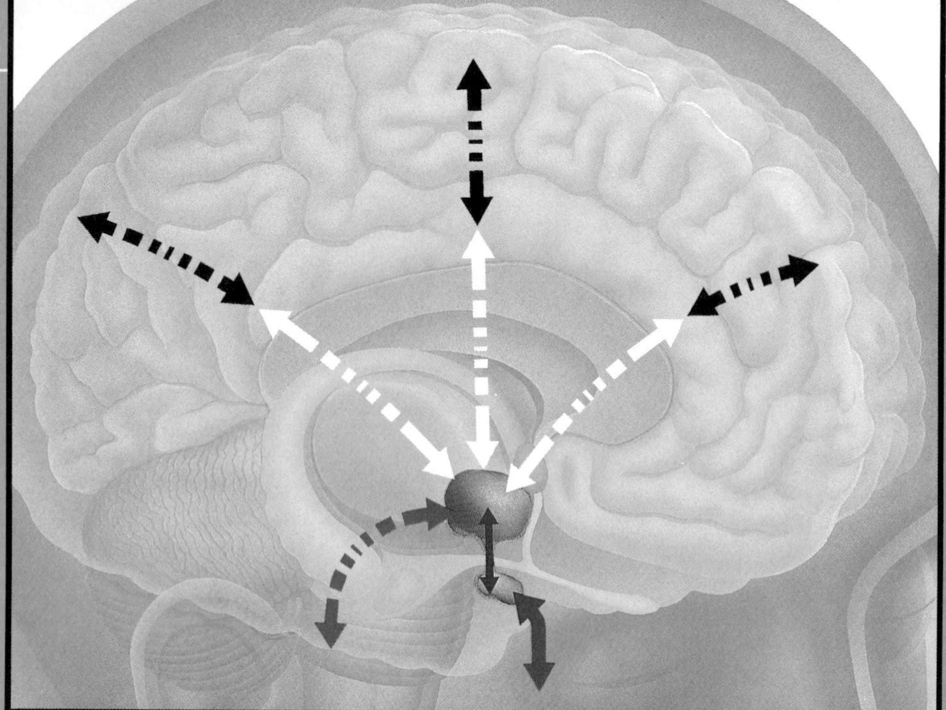

RULING A VAST DOMAIN

Strategically sited in the center of the brain, the hypothalamus carries on a constant dialogue with neighboring structures and regions. As depicted above, it communicates directly with other parts of the limbic system (*white*) and, via that complex, exchanges information with the cerebral cortex (*black arrows*). A neural pipeline to the brainstem (*blue arrows*) serves as the conduit through which the hypothalamus controls the autonomic nervous system.

The hypothalamus also governs the endocrine system, a network of glands distributed throughout the body. By secreting hormones, these organs regulate growth, sexual development, and a host of other functions. Hormones, which are carried by the blood through the body, sometimes have the same chemical makeup as neurotransmitters, substances that transport impulses across the synaptic gaps between neurons. The endocrine system includes other hormone-secreting organs, not technically considered glands, that perform a variety of duties. The stomach, for example, produces a chemical that regulates digestion. Hormones from the liver help promote cell growth in the body.

Although the hypothalamus releases a few hormones on its own, for the most part it rules the endocrine system through the pituitary gland, a structure measuring about one-third its size. Prompted by the hypothalamus (*orange arrows*), this "master gland" produces as many as nine different hormones. Some influence the body directly; most act as triggers that activate other glands (*green arrows*).

To achieve homeostasis, the hypothalamus stages a nonstop balancing act between the autonomic nervous system and the endocrine system. The two sometimes perform solo, but as shown on the following pages, most bodily functions require both systems to work as a team.

A WIDESPREAD INFLUENCE. In the figure at right, areas controlled by the autonomic nervous system are tinted pink; glands and other hormone-secreting organs of the endocrine system are shown in purple. Sex hormones are the same in males and females, although quantities and target glands differ. Males also have no mammary glands and develop testes *(inset)* instead of ovaries. The adrenal glands help establish the body's metabolic rate—the rate at which the cells burn energy. Oddly, their hormone-producing components answer to different masters. The adrenal cortices, part of the endocrine system, take orders from the pituitary gland, but the adrenal medullas, within the adrenal cortices, respond mainly to the autonomic nervous system.

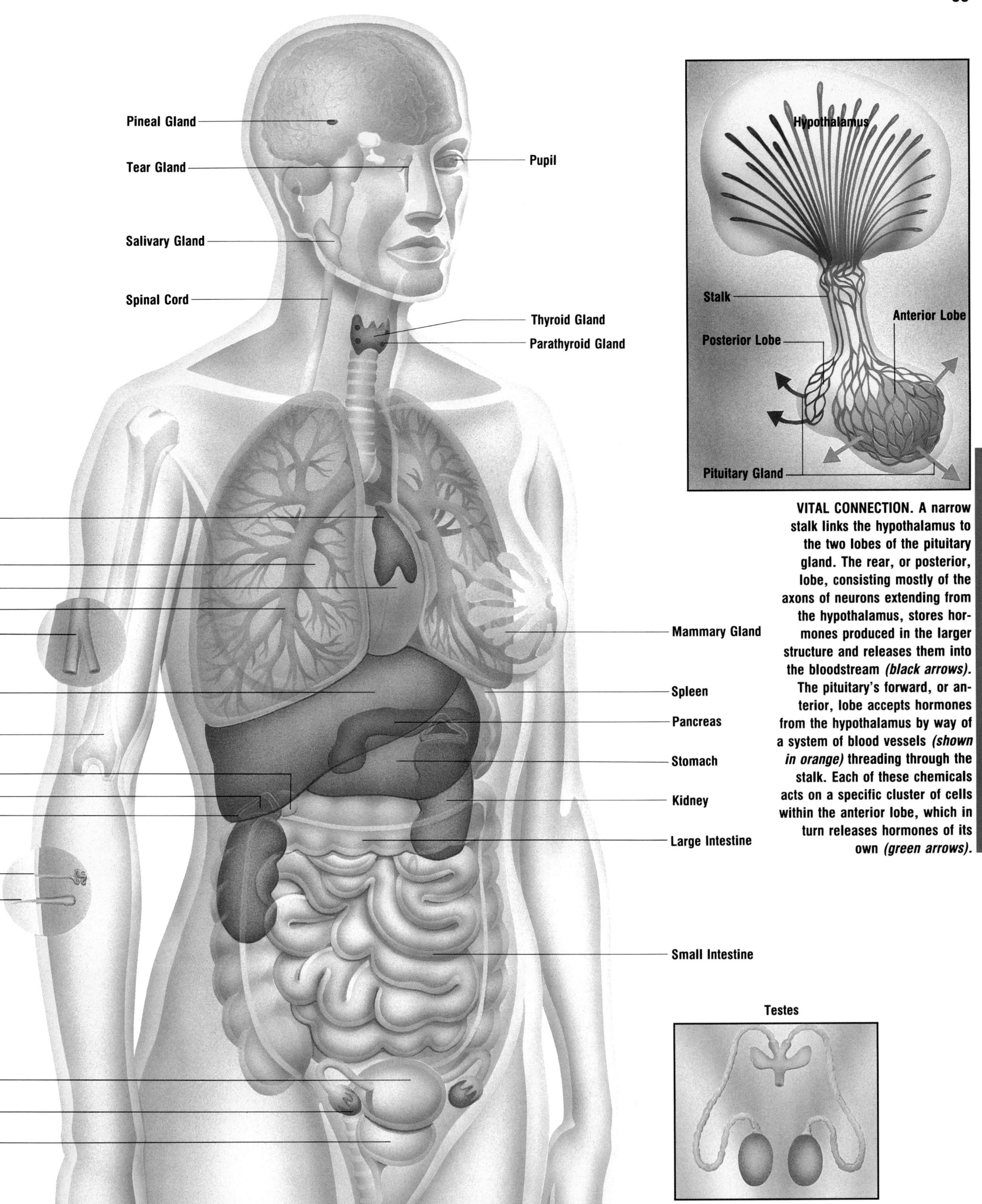

VITAL CONNECTION. A narrow stalk links the hypothalamus to the two lobes of the pituitary gland. The rear, or posterior, lobe, consisting mostly of the axons of neurons extending from the hypothalamus, stores hormones produced in the larger structure and releases them into the bloodstream *(black arrows)*. The pituitary's forward, or anterior, lobe accepts hormones from the hypothalamus by way of a system of blood vessels *(shown in orange)* threading through the stalk. Each of these chemicals acts on a specific cluster of cells within the anterior lobe, which in turn releases hormones of its own *(green arrows)*.

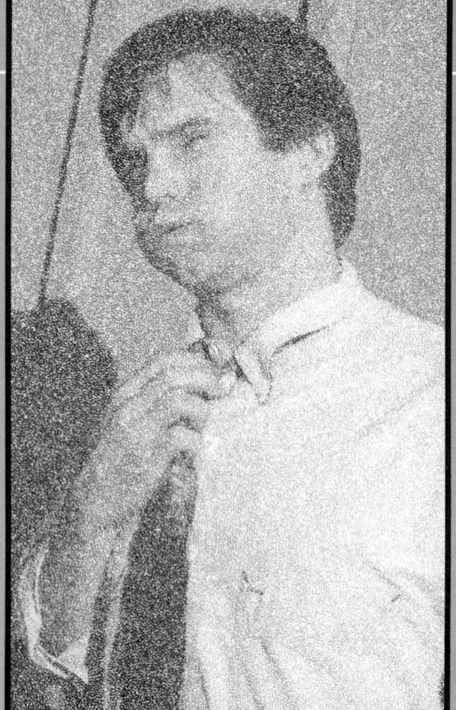

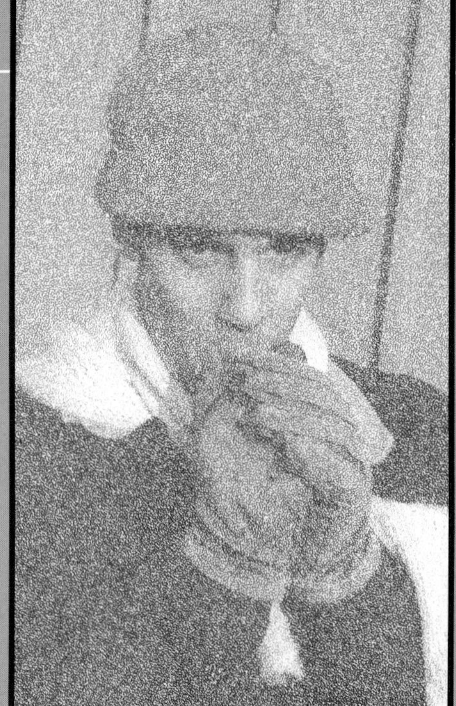

COOLING OFF. When the hypothalamus detects rising blood temperatures *(red arrows in figure at right),* it sends signals *(light blue arrows)* all over the body. Some impulses *(purple arrows)* activate cooling processes, such as the production of sweat *(A, below),* which cools as it evaporates, and the dilation of tiny vessels called bronchioles *(B)* in the lungs, allowing heat to escape with every exhalation. Other commands *(dark blue arrows)* inhibit activities that conserve or generate heat—stifling signals to constrict peripheral vessels *(C),* for example, bringing more blood to the skin so heat can radiate away, and instructing adrenal medullas to turn down the metabolic furnace *(D).*

THE BODY'S THERMOSTAT

Regulating adult body temperature is the job of the autonomic nervous system. Within the hypothalamus, specialized neurons called thermoreceptors constantly monitor the temperature of blood, comparing each reading to an internal standard, or setpoint—an element crucial to the maintenance of homeostasis. Setpoints vary from one person to the next around a general average.

During the course of the day, the hypothalamus repositions the setpoint many times, allowing blood temperatures to fluctuate from a morning low of approximately 96° Fahrenheit to about 99.9° in the evening. If the measurement deviates from an individual's prevailing setpoint, the hypothalamus adjusts the body's heating or cooling system accordingly, as shown opposite.

When body temperature dips too low, for example, hypothalamic nerves signal blood vessels near the skin to constrict. Less blood flow close to the surface means less heat loss through radiation. Meanwhile, other sets of nerves signal skeletal muscles to shiver, producing heat-generating kinetic energy. Skeletal muscles are usually under voluntary control, which is overridden when body temperature drops severely.

When the body needs to cool down, the hypothalamus sends out countervailing signals. Peripheral vessels dilate, for example, to promote heat loss. And because cells generate heat as they consume nutrients, the body also may slow down its metabolic rate.

Besides temperature setpoints, the hypothalamus establishes standards to regulate hormone production as well as the mix of salt, sugar, and water in the blood, both of which help preserve homeostasis. In each case, the hypothalamus takes whatever steps necessary to bring a given variable—temperature, rate, or concentration in the blood, for instance—into line with its predetermined standard.

A

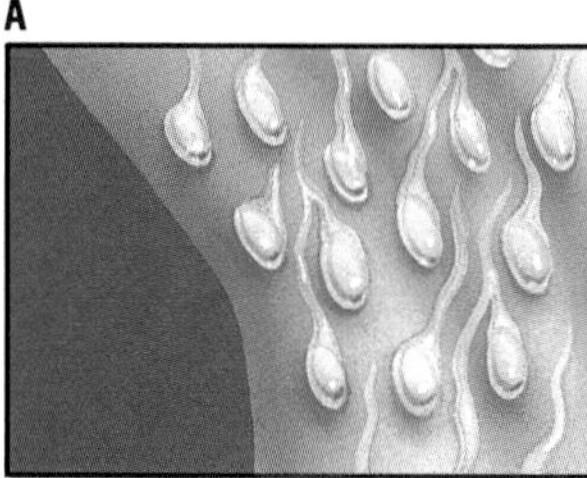

B

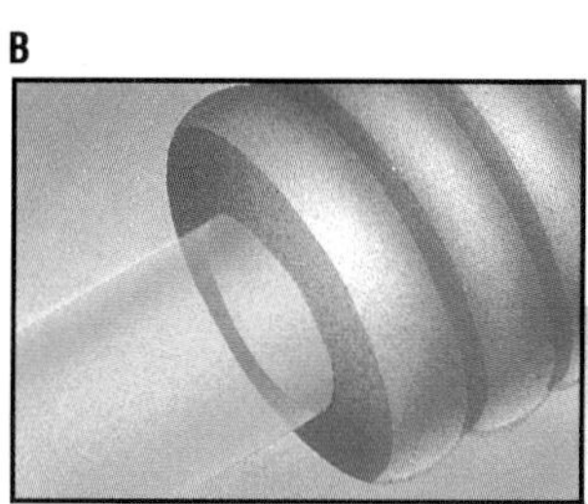

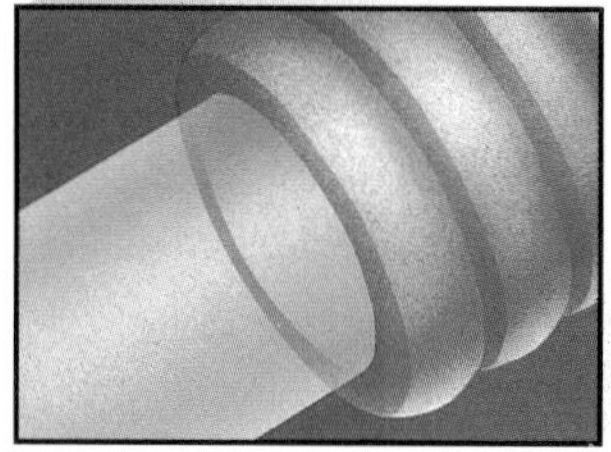

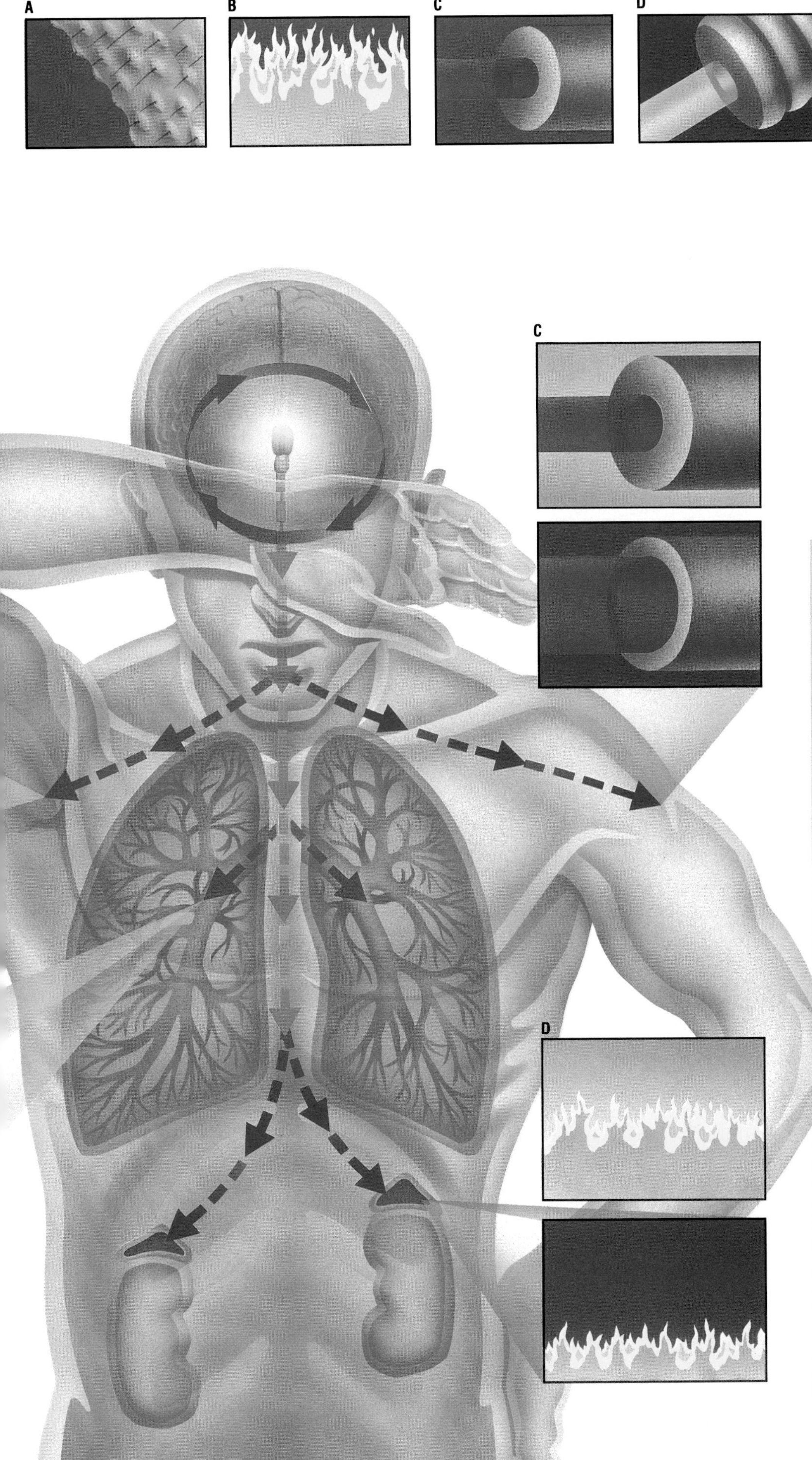

WARMING UP. When body temperature falls, the hypothalamus seeks ways to conserve heat. Goose bumps—holdovers from a time when humans were more hirsute—raise body hair off the skin to trap insulating air *(A, far left)*. While the adrenal medullas stoke the metabolic fires *(B)*, peripheral blood vessels *(C)* and bronchioles *(D)* constrict, reducing heat loss. Shivering *(near left)* generates heat by setting muscles in motion.

The Role of Fever

To fight infection, the hypothalamus often drives the body's temperature above the normal range—a condition commonly known as a fever. While its exact function remains something of a mystery, fever seems to serve a number of useful purposes.

Elevated temperatures may in fact destroy some invading viruses and bacteria. Fevers also appear to activate certain cells that produce the infection-fighting antibodies of the immune system.

When an infection sets in, the hypothalamus raises its temperature setpoint; it then directs the autonomic nervous system to activate the body-warming responses illustrated above. Once the infection subsides, the hypothalamus returns the setpoint to its normal range.

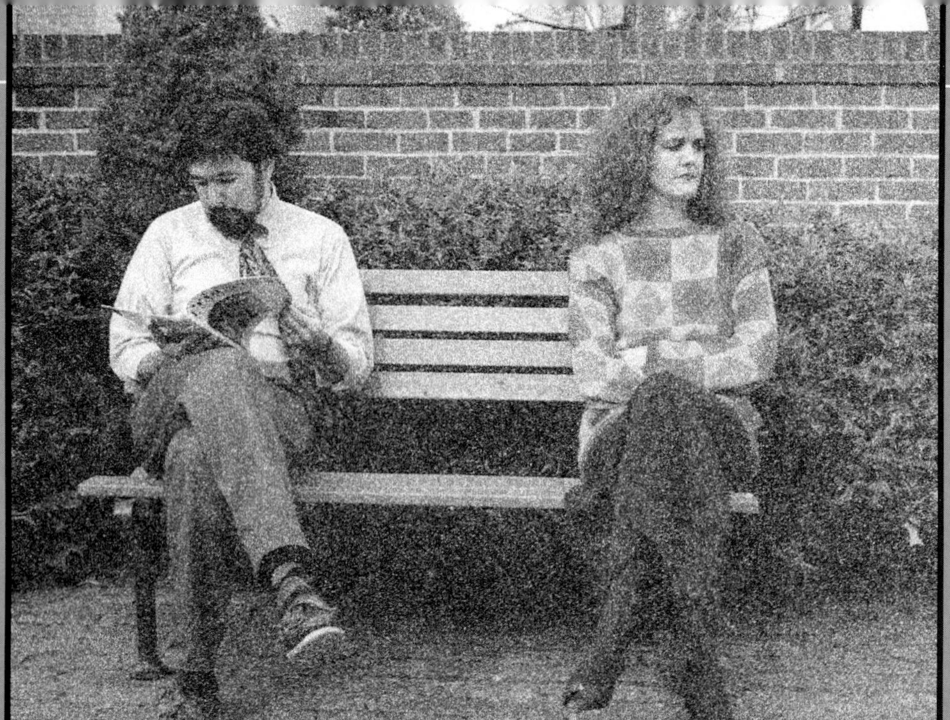

MALE SEX HORMONES. When the hypothalamus sends out GnRH *(orange arrow in panel 1, right),* the pituitary gland in males releases FSH and LH into the bloodstream. At the testes *(2),* these bind to seminiferous tubules, triggering the development of sperm cells and the release of hormones testosterone and inhibin, which are carried by the blood back to the brain. Their arrival *(3)* causes the hypothalamus to slow production of GnRH, which ultimately slows the release of sperm cells and the sex hormones *(4).* When the hypothalamus senses this hormone deficit, the cycle begins anew. Elsewhere in the body, testosterone *(red dots on figure, below)* contributes to sex drive and produces male secondary sex characteristics: facial, body, and pubic hair; robust bone and muscle growth; and a deep voice.

MEN, WOMEN, AND HORMONES

The regulation of sex hormones is perhaps the most vivid example of how the hypothalamus controls the endocrine system. For this task, the hypothalamus relies on a concept known as a feedback loop, in which the release of a particular hormone is determined by the amount already present in the blood. If the hypothalamus discovers that the concentration has dropped below a setpoint value, it alerts the pituitary gland, which in turn instructs whichever gland produces the hormone to produce more.

Normally, once the concentration climbs up to the setpoint level, the hypothalamus slows down the production of that chemical. But in rare, poorly understood instances—most notably during the female menstrual cycle—the hypothalamus raises the setpoint, allowing more hormone to be reieased.

The hypothalamus itself manufactures only one sex chemical, called gonadotropin-releasing hormone (GnRH). On arrival in the pituitary gland, this substance triggers the release of two others—luteinizing hormone (LH) and follicle-stimulating hormone (FSH)—in males and females alike. These pituitary messengers then travel to so-called target glands, where they prompt the release of sex-specific hormones.

In males, the target glands are the testes, which produce sperm cells and release the hormone testosterone. In females, the targets are the ovaries, which release eggs as part of the menstrual cycle. The ovaries also secrete hormones known as estrogens.

As with all other endocrine functions, the regulation of sex hormones is susceptible to disruption from the cortex and other higher centers in the brain. Stress, for example—brought on by illness or excessive physical activity—can affect a woman's menstrual cycle or a man's sperm count.

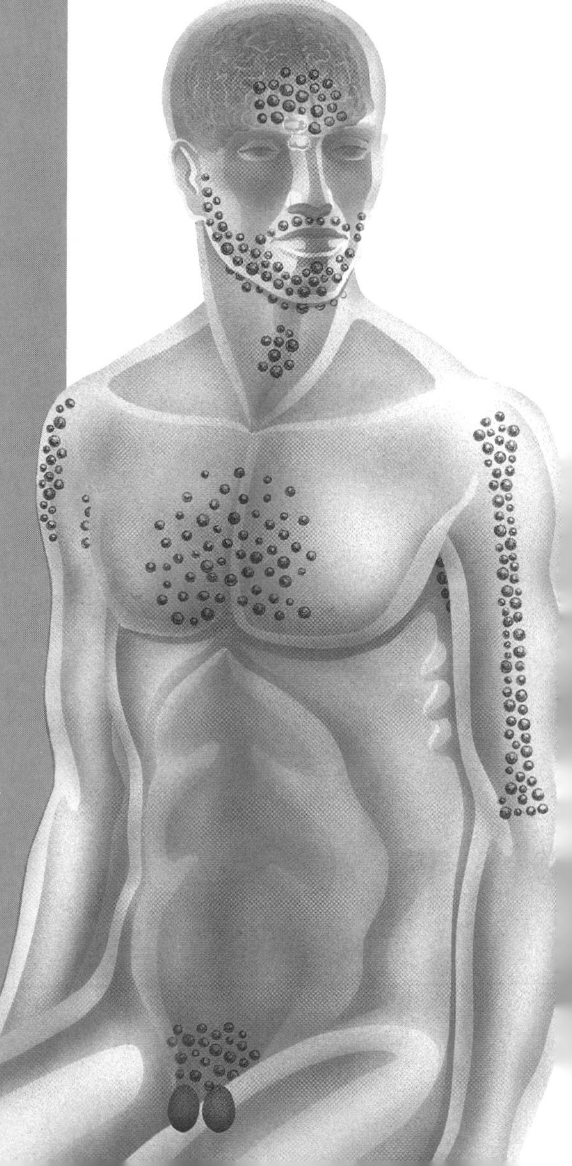

FEMALE SEX HORMONES. In women, sex hormones are responsible for the monthly menstrual cycle. At the start of the cycle, FSH and LH *(panel 1, left)* from the pituitary gland travel to the ovaries. There, they bind to a structure called a follicle, causing it to grow and triggering the production of estrogens *(2)*. These sex hormones then flow to the brain *(3)*, prompting the hypothalamus to raise its estrogen setpoint. The resulting hormonal surge, especially of LH, peaks with ovulation, when the follicle releases an egg *(4)*. Almost immediately, estrogen production drops sharply. In the female, estrogens *(purple dots on figure, below)* may contribute to sex drive in the brain and account for secondary sex characteristics: fat deposits in the breasts and hips; underarm and pubic hair; and a higher voice.

1

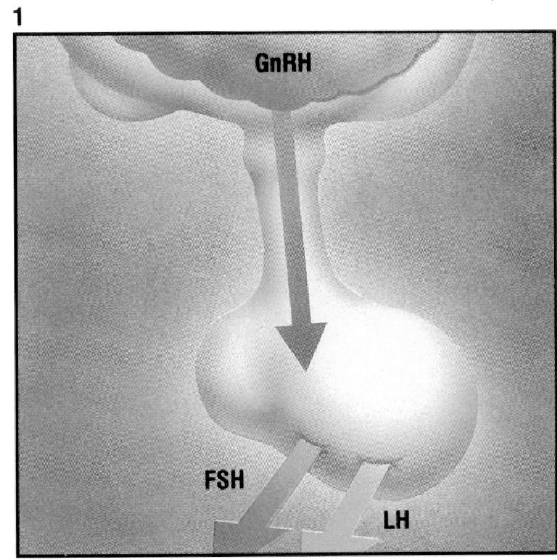

2

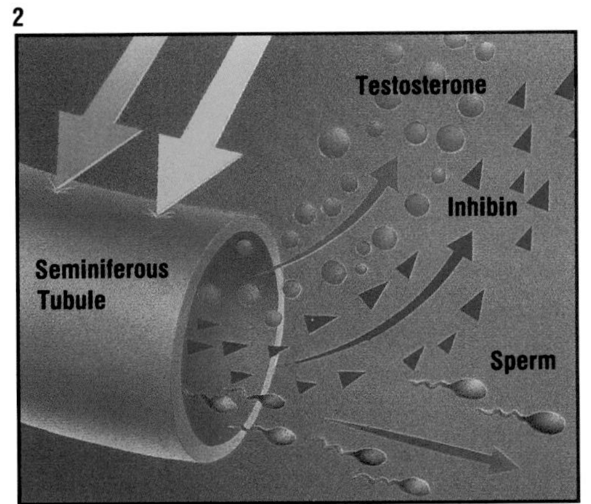

2

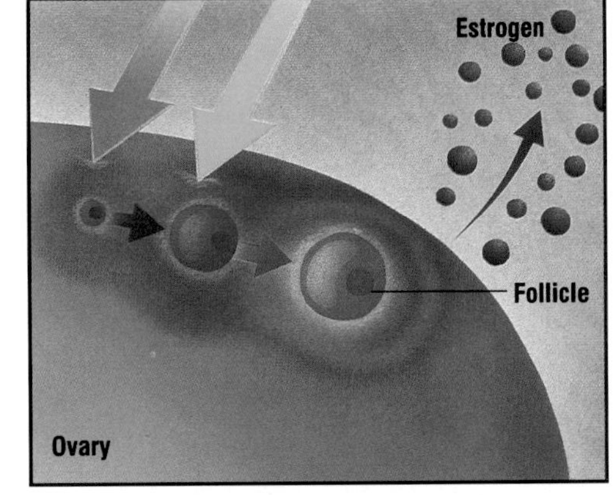

3

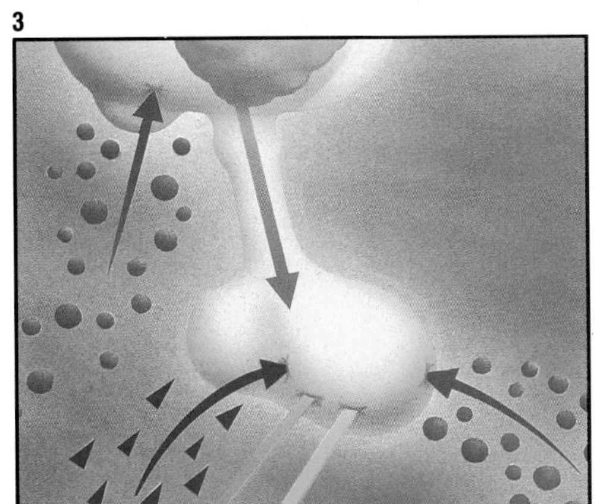

3

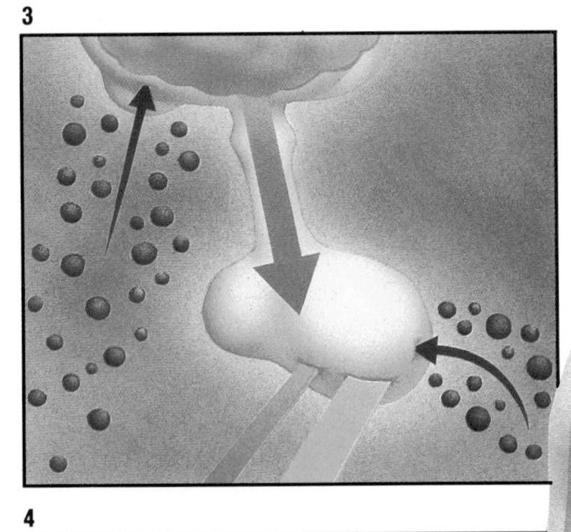

4

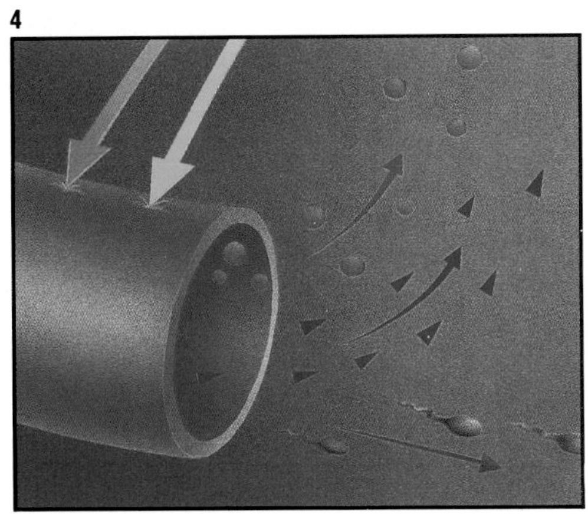

4

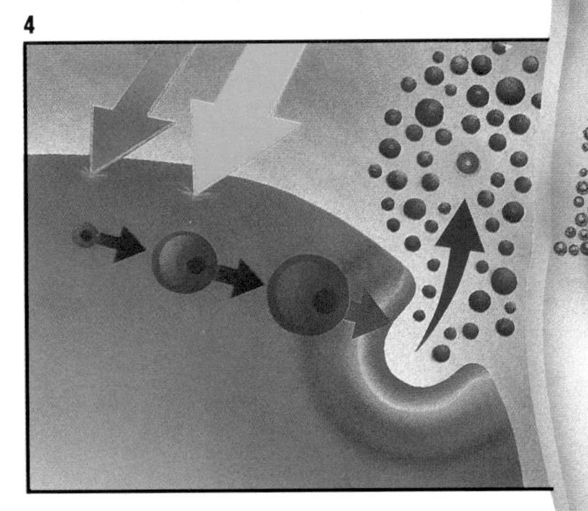

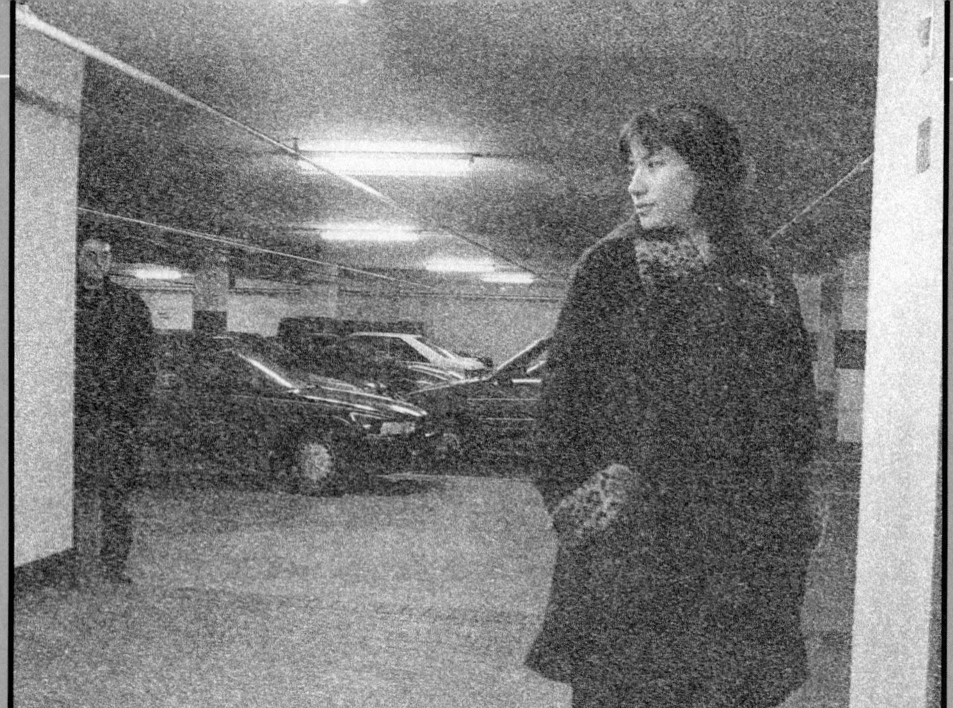

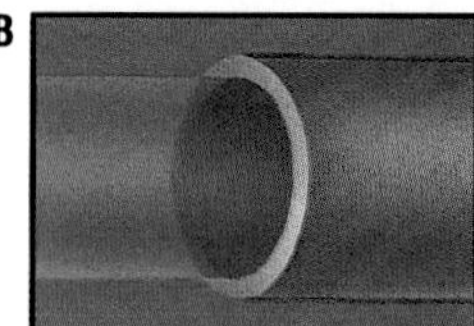

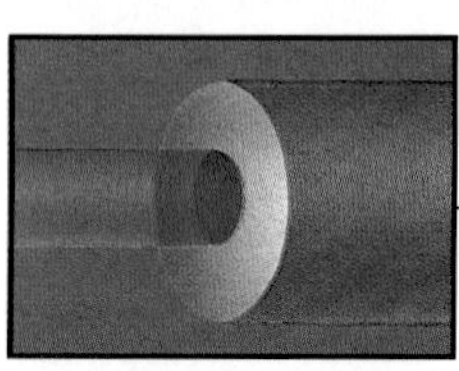

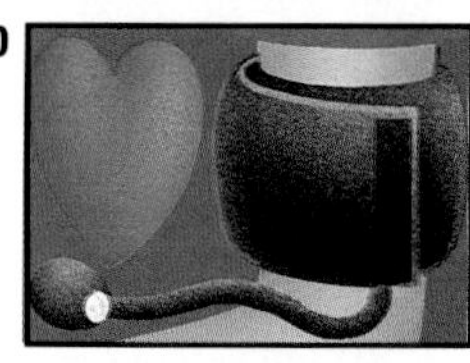

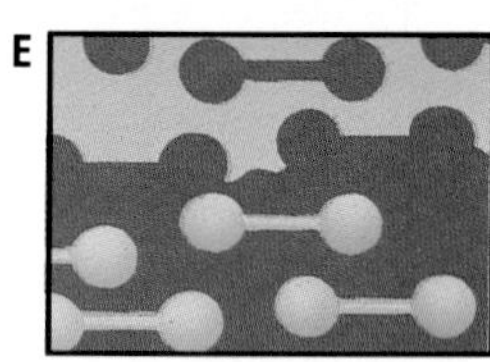

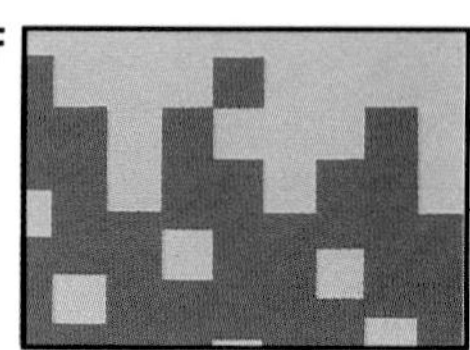

TO FIGHT OR TO FLEE?

Sudden fear—brought on, say, by a shadowy figure in a dimly lit parking garage—calls into play both the endocrine and autonomic nervous systems. Unless overridden by conscious effort, fear triggers a response in the body called the general adaptation syndrome, a series of involuntary actions orchestrated by the hypothalamus in ways that remain something of a mystery. According to conventional theory, illustrated at right, the cerebral cortex perceives the danger first, then signals the hypothalamus through the limbic system. However, some scientists believe that the hypothalamus, via its connections with that complex, can assess a frightening situation even before warning signals arrive from the cortex.

The first phase of the syndrome is the fight-or-flight response (*right, top*), a stream of impulses from the autonomic nervous system that alert the body within a matter of seconds to possible peril. During the second phase, called resistance (*right, bottom*), hormones of the endocrine system prepare the body for defending itself or fleeing. Although both phases begin almost simultaneously, hormones released during resistance can take a full minute to travel through the bloodstream to begin to influence their target organs.

Other stressful emotions, including anger, excitement, and anxiety, can activate the general adaptation syndrome—sometimes with serious consequences. Over time, elevated hormone levels can pose a severe health risk. Researchers have established, for example, that prolonged stress, such as the continuous anxiety some people feel at work, can raise levels of the hormone cortisol, boosting blood pressure and leading to hypertension. Stress also weakens the immune system, leaving the body more open to disease. In the long run, unrelenting stress can be far more hazardous than a temporary hair-raising scare.

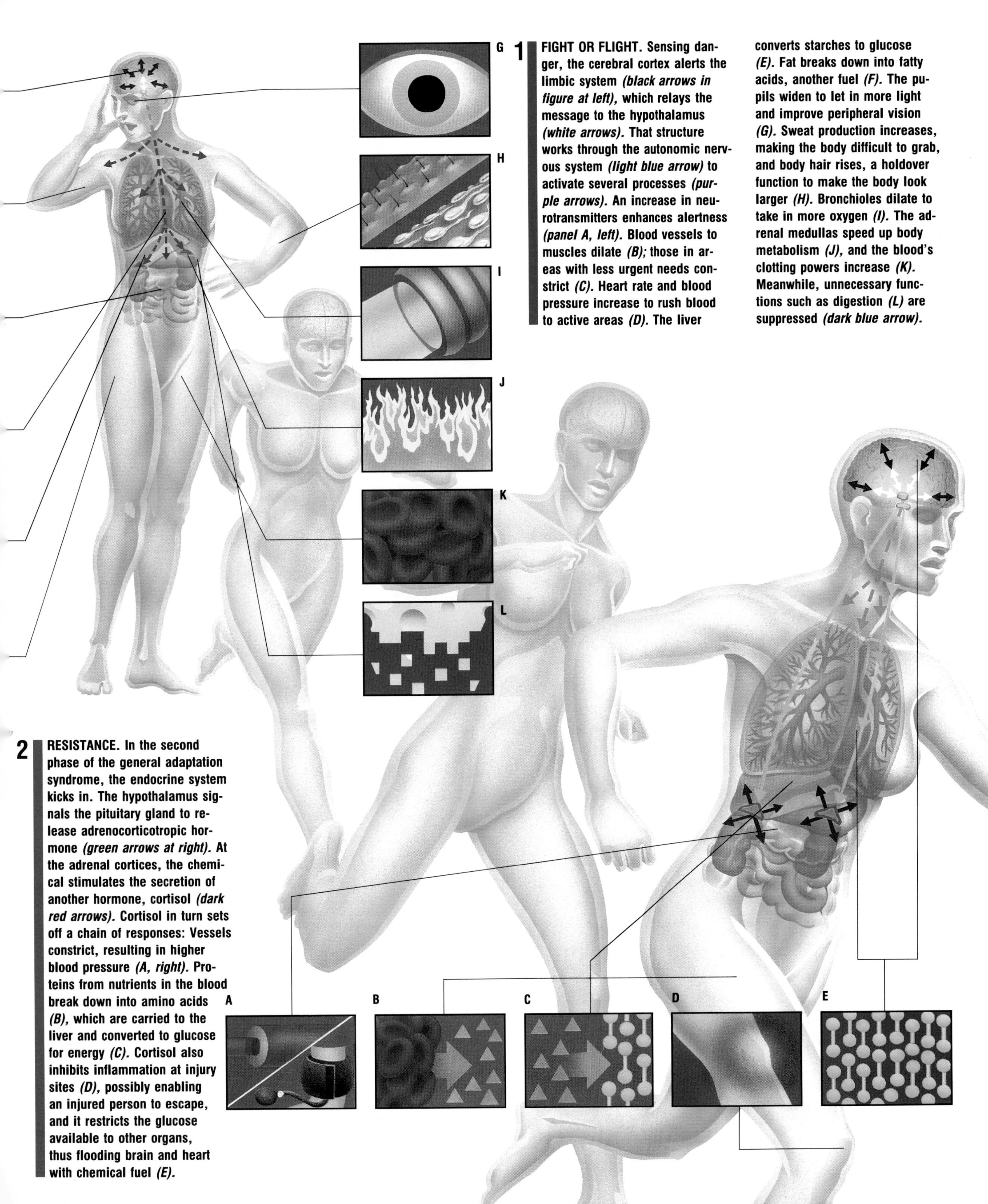

1 **FIGHT OR FLIGHT.** Sensing danger, the cerebral cortex alerts the limbic system *(black arrows in figure at left),* which relays the message to the hypothalamus *(white arrows).* That structure works through the autonomic nervous system *(light blue arrow)* to activate several processes *(purple arrows).* An increase in neurotransmitters enhances alertness *(panel A, left).* Blood vessels to muscles dilate *(B);* those in areas with less urgent needs constrict *(C).* Heart rate and blood pressure increase to rush blood to active areas *(D).* The liver converts starches to glucose *(E).* Fat breaks down into fatty acids, another fuel *(F).* The pupils widen to let in more light and improve peripheral vision *(G).* Sweat production increases, making the body difficult to grab, and body hair rises, a holdover function to make the body look larger *(H).* Bronchioles dilate to take in more oxygen *(I).* The adrenal medullas speed up body metabolism *(J),* and the blood's clotting powers increase *(K).* Meanwhile, unnecessary functions such as digestion *(L)* are suppressed *(dark blue arrow).*

2 **RESISTANCE.** In the second phase of the general adaptation syndrome, the endocrine system kicks in. The hypothalamus signals the pituitary gland to release adrenocorticotropic hormone *(green arrows at right).* At the adrenal cortices, the chemical stimulates the secretion of another hormone, cortisol *(dark red arrows).* Cortisol in turn sets off a chain of responses: Vessels constrict, resulting in higher blood pressure *(A, right).* Proteins from nutrients in the blood break down into amino acids *(B),* which are carried to the liver and converted to glucose for energy *(C).* Cortisol also inhibits inflammation at injury sites *(D),* possibly enabling an injured person to escape, and it restricts the glucose available to other organs, thus flooding brain and heart with chemical fuel *(E).*

4

Thought's Elusive Currents

Patricia S. Churchland lies in a small, brightly lit chamber at the University of Iowa Hospital in Iowa City, her head thrust into a massive device that rings her cranium like a high-tech metal doughnut. Churchland, who teaches philosophy at the University of California in San Diego, has been telling her philosopher colleagues for years that neuroscience holds a vital key to understanding the mind. Now, as if to underscore her point, she has volunteered to put her own brain on the line as a research subject.

A mask holds Churchland's head motionless in the doughnut's hole while a laser directs a threadlike crimson beam across her cheeks. The beam guides chief researcher Hanna Damasio as she positions the device—called a positron emission tomography (PET) scanner—around Churchland's brain. Once the scanner is in place, Damasio retreats to the control room, where she joins her husband and partner, Antonio Damasio, head of the hospital's neurology department.

"Ready!" announces a technician at the control terminal. On that signal, another researcher emerges from a room down the hall and rushes into the PET chamber carrying a sealed beaker. This is no time for delay. The beaker holds a radioactive form of water created mo-

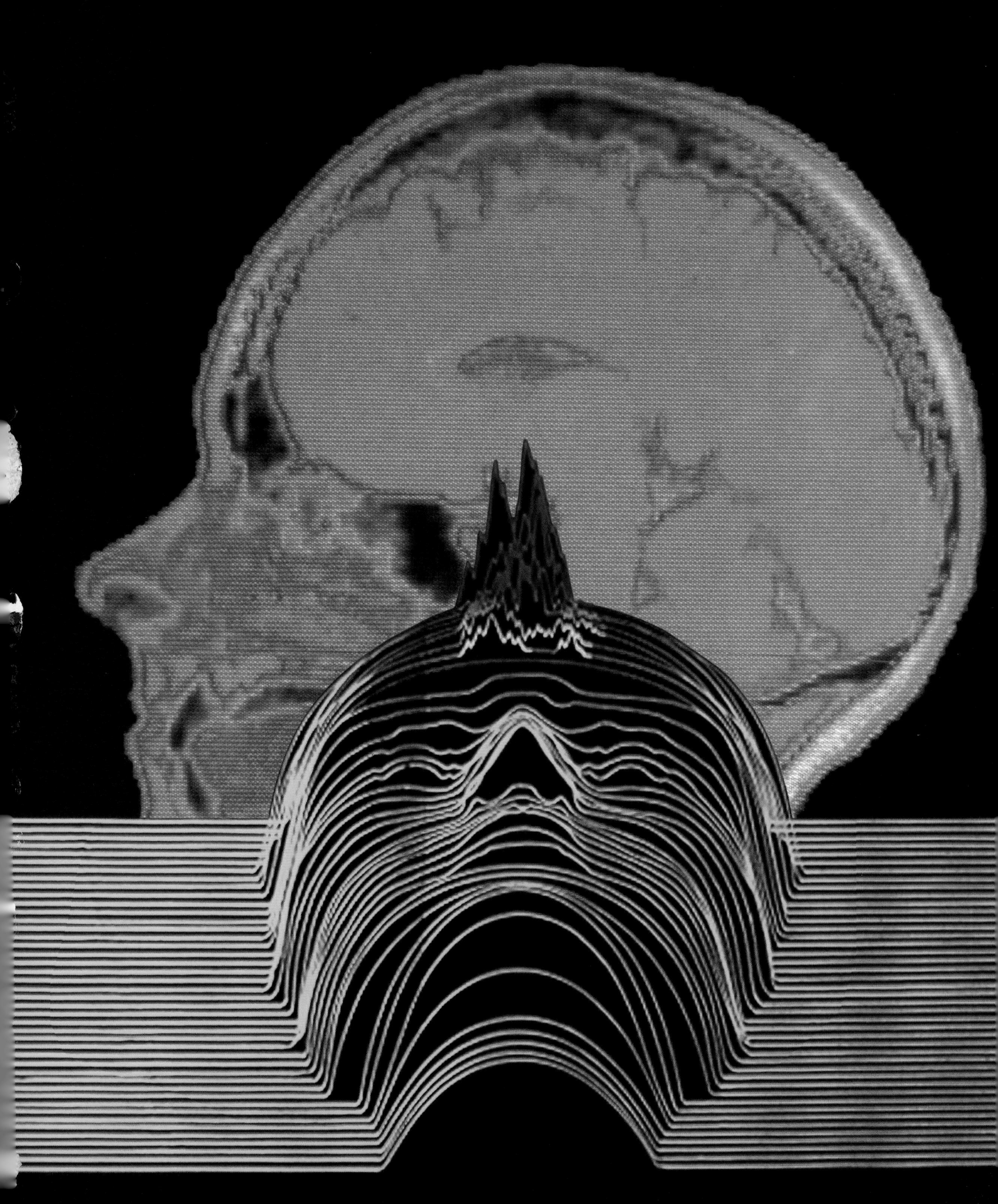

At the United Nations, multilingual individuals instantaneously translate the proceedings into a host of languages, from English and Arabic to Mandarin and French. The feat, which the most skillful translators seem to perform without conscious effort, exemplifies the vast powers of the cortex—hub of higher functions such as memory, thought, and language.

ments before on the hospital's cyclotron. Almost immediately after it is produced, the radioactive material begins to decay, which means that before too long this costly sample will become absolutely useless. Hanna Damasio switches on an intercom and begins reading names from a list, asking Churchland to visualize the person as she hears each name.

"Injection!" calls the technician, and in moments the water—containing a radioactive dosage smaller than that of a dental x-ray—begins pumping through a catheter directly into Churchland's arteries. The treated liquid spreads through her bloodstream and wends its way to her brain. As she continues to form mental pictures of people on Damasio's list, the blood concentrates in her brain's most active regions, forming radioactive "hot spots" that can be picked up by the scanner.

Within 40 seconds the solution has worn off, shutting the window into Churchland's brain. The PET images pop up on a computer screen five minutes later—15 ovals the size of poker chips, flecked with aqua, yellow, tangerine, and red against a blue background. Antonio Damasio excitedly points to glowing spots in two of the ovals. "What are those?" he exclaims. Hanna Damasio gently reminds him that much computer processing remains to be done before the meaning of these images becomes clear. Still, at a moment like this, even a seasoned professional finds it hard to stay calm.

The Damasios, who met and married while attending medical school in their native Portugal, are old hands at PET scans by now, having performed hundreds of them over the past decade. Yet for them, these brightly colored images are still the stuff of awe and magic. By recording the ebb and flow of the marked blood in Patricia Churchland's brain as she works on a mental task, the PET scanner has recorded the shifting currents of thought itself, producing, in effect, a kind of slow-motion picture of cognition—a graphic exploration of the workings of the mind.

Brain researchers such as the Damasios are feeling much like explorers these days. Their old maps of the brain were riddled with myths, misconceptions, blanks, and errors, just as maps of the world in the days before Columbus and Magellan were hopelessly flawed. Today, scientists are using PET scans, magnetic resonance imaging (MRI), and other advanced tools to redraw their old atlases, replacing mysterious isles and terra incognita with detailed renderings of charted lands. And nowhere have they been more successful than in their efforts to plot the outer layer of the brain, the cerebral cortex.

Only an eighth-inch thick (*cortex* is Latin for "bark"), this wrinkled, convoluted rind of neurons is an evolutionary newcomer. It began to develop extensively first among mammals and has reached its greatest development in humans. Indeed, scientists today view the cortex as the source of humankind's loftiest abilities. It is the home of language, the exclusively human mode of communication, and is responsible for conscious thought and decisions. The cortex, in a sense, is the brain's high-command center, the part of our anatomy that largely dictates personality and most defines the essence of the human self.

Neuroscientists probing the cortex enter a realm of astonishing complexity. Although at first glance, cortical tissue looks like a random tangle of neurons, one piece indistinguishable from any other, in reality, the cortex is organized into perhaps hundreds of neuron clusters, or networks, each specialized for a precise function. There are networks for touch and networks for muscle control, networks for understanding and for producing language. At least one network deals entirely with recognizing human faces.

The sheer quantity of networks, in fact, leaves neuroscientists to grapple

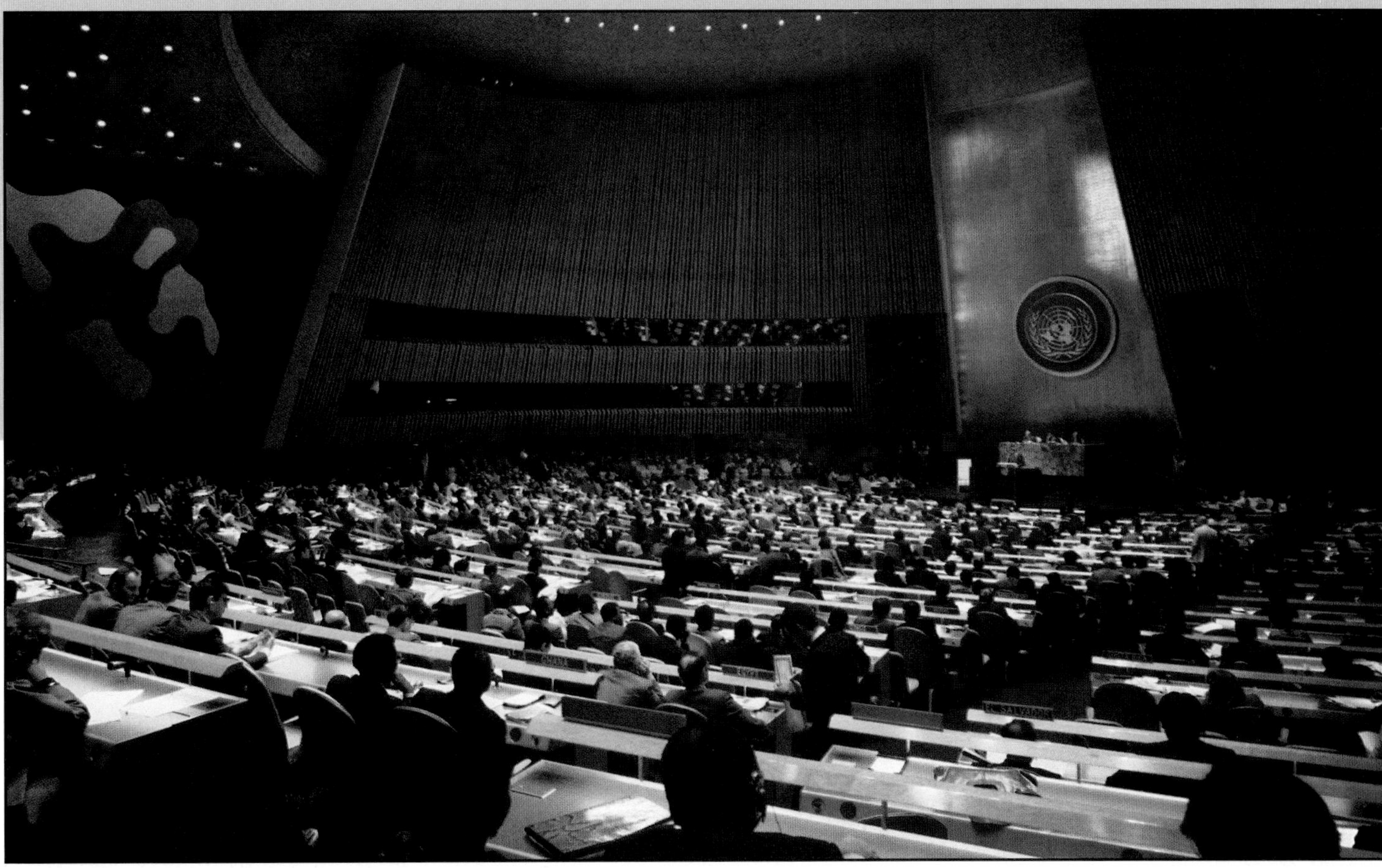

with a major mystery: How does the brain coordinate all the pieces? The simple act of playing middle C on a piano, for instance, floods the brain with a smorgasbord of stimuli. Some neurons detect the edge of the key, others its whiteness. Still others respond to the vibrations and the pressure on the fingertip. And yet, what emerges in the mind of the listener is not cacophony but simply the sound of middle C. The same sort of rapid synthesis occurs when we see a familiar face, grasp a doorknob, or bite into a raspberry. Somehow, the brain takes these isolated atoms of experience and forges them into an unfragmented whole.

Perhaps even more confounding, of course, is the deeper issue of how all these components come together to form the ineffable thing that philosopher Daniel Dennett and cognitive scientist Douglas Hofstadter have called "the mind's I"—our subjective sensation of awareness and self-awareness. Indeed, consciousness arguably represents the essence of humanity. But just what *is* it, and where does it reside in the brain?

Serious attempts to find the answer are of quite recent vintage. Scientists once tended to shy away from the issue, arguing that consciousness was too elusive to study experimentally, that the whole subject was best left to philosophers and theologians. Now that PET scans and other new techniques have actually begun to show thoughts in action, though, neuroscientists are shedding those old inhibitions and boldly searching for answers deep in the intangible mind.

Perhaps the greatest obstacle to explaining consciousness is the preconceived notion that it is one thing: the self. Yet if the brain is made up of many discrete components, consciousness—whatever it is—is not likely to be localized in just one of them. Somehow, it must arise from the organization and collective behavior of *all* the parts.

A giant step toward discerning that organization came half a century ago at McGill University in Montreal, where Nova Scotia-born psychologist Donald O. Hebb spent a long career laying the foundations for much of modern neuroscience. Hebb got his first taste of research back in 1928, when, as an aspiring novelist, he signed up for McGill's graduate program in psychology as a quick way to

Functional Landmarks in the Cortex

Early in the history of brain research, scientists learned that the structure of cells in the cortex varies from one area to another (*pages* 102-103). Shortly after the turn of the 20th century, researchers had already divided this crinkly landscape into more than 50 distinct regions. But figuring out each region's purpose proved more difficult. Not until the 1950s did neurosurgeons, starting with Wilder Penfield at the Montreal Neurological Institute, begin to fit together the cortical puzzle. Penfield found he could tease out the function of points on the cortex by mild electrical stimulation. Because the brain has no sensory receptors and cannot feel pain, he was able to perform the procedure on conscious patients who could describe sensations stirred by the electrode. Penfield discovered a correspondence between certain spots on the cortex and parts of the body: Excite the proper place in the brain, and the patient feels, say, a poke in the right big toe.

Over the years, scientist-explorers have mapped out a kind of functional hierarchy of the cortex. As they have increasingly come to realize, however, no single part of the brain operates independently. The communication network is complex: Impulses from the eyes, ears, and body are received first by three primary areas—the visual, auditory, and sensory cortices, shown in red on the schematic map below. Next are the higher-order regions (*blue*)—the secondary visual, auditory, and sensory cortices. These regions, which also include the posterior parietal cortex, analyze the signals for more specific information; secondary visual cortices, for example, detect color, motion, and form. Then come the association cortices (*gray*)—the prefrontal, parietal-temporal-occipital, and limbic. Often regarded as the seat of thought and perception, these areas integrate the sensory details into a coherent picture. They also connect the sensory cortices to the premotor cortex (*light green*), the last stage of mental processing before the motor cortex (*dark green*) instructs the muscles to act.

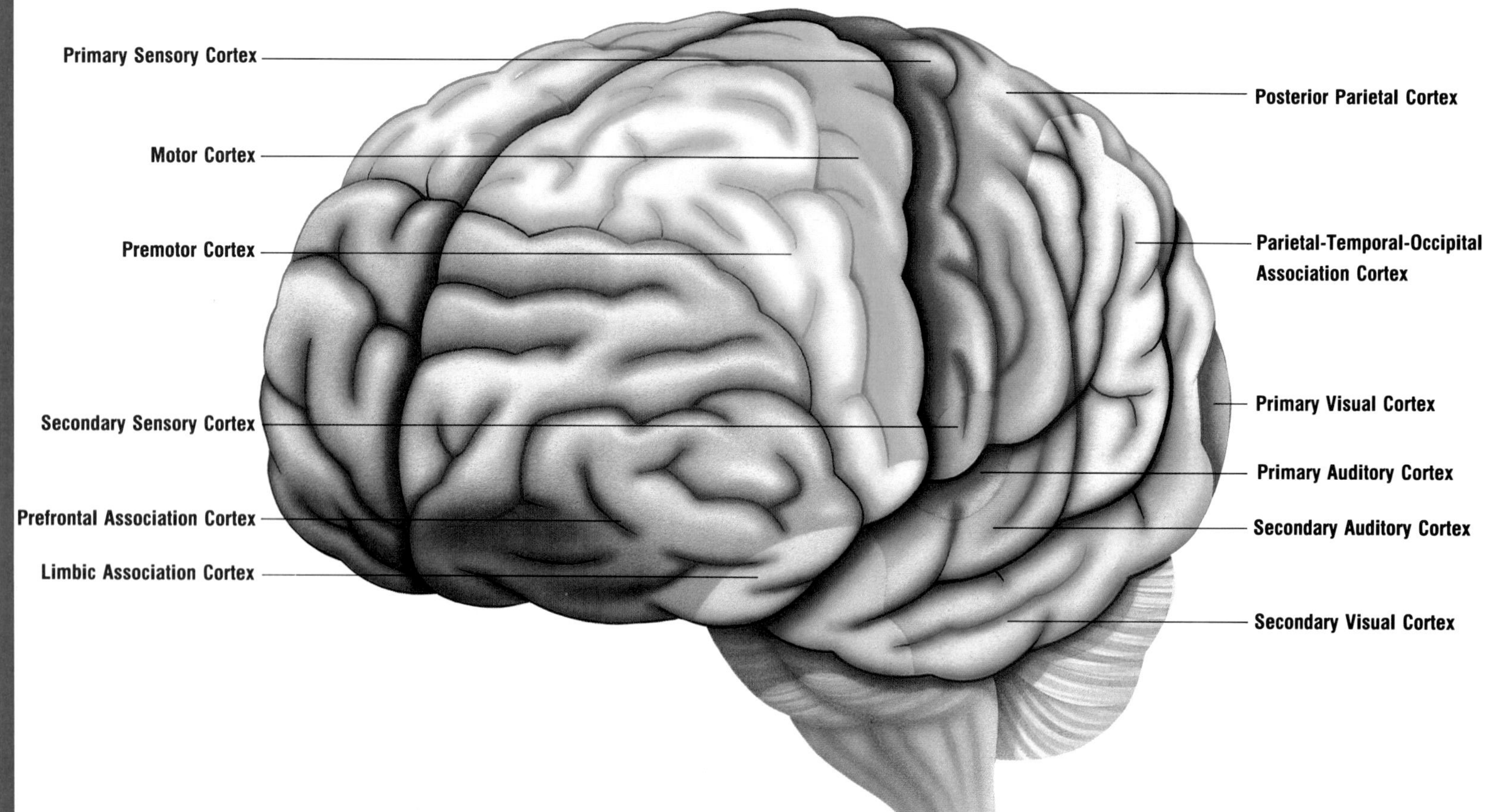

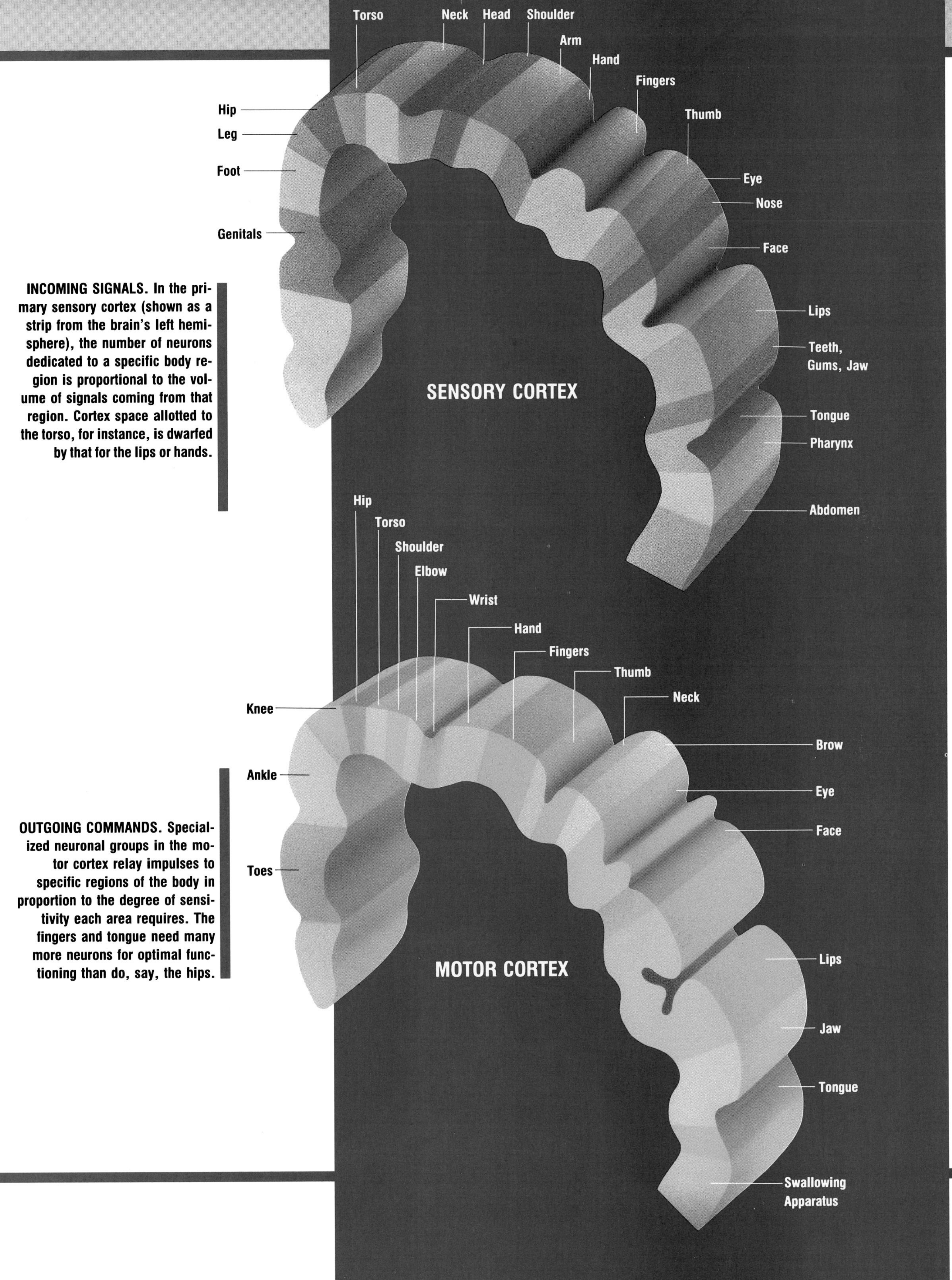

INCOMING SIGNALS. In the primary sensory cortex (shown as a strip from the brain's left hemisphere), the number of neurons dedicated to a specific body region is proportional to the volume of signals coming from that region. Cortex space allotted to the torso, for instance, is dwarfed by that for the lips or hands.

OUTGOING COMMANDS. Specialized neuronal groups in the motor cortex relay impulses to specific regions of the body in proportion to the degree of sensitivity each area requires. The fingers and tongue need many more neurons for optimal functioning than do, say, the hips.

learn about the psychoanalytic theories of Sigmund Freud. Fortunately for science, his passion for literature was soon overtaken by an even greater desire to understand human memory, a quest he was to pursue until his death in 1985.

Early in Hebb's career, most psychologists considered such a quest hopelessly naive. The field was dominated by "behaviorists" such as Harvard's B. F. Skinner, who declared that the inner world of the mind was utterly beyond the reach of scientific experiments. Whether the subjects are animals or humans, Skinner and company said, the only things actually measurable are input and output—that is, stimuli of various sorts and the brain's responses to those stimuli. Mental concepts such as "ideas," "thoughts," and "attitudes" were deemed unobservable, untestable, and unscientific. Humans and animals alike are simply "behaving machines," these researchers asserted. And what goes on inside the machine is unknowable.

Hebb was unconvinced. He vividly remembered the time he had been in charge of a colony of experimental apes, which loved to play and tease one another. They were hilarious to watch. But to Hebb, even funnier than the animals' antics were the verbal gyrations of his behaviorist colleagues as they tried to explain such goings-on in stimulus-response terms without any reference to what was happening in the apes' heads. No, Hebb reasoned, the mind was neither unobservable nor "unscientific."

The more he thought about it, the more he began to believe that learning and memory must involve changes in the brain's neural circuitry—real changes that could, in principle, be measured. "All the theories I knew made the brain out to be completely controlled by the things that were going on around it, by the sensory events that the brain was exposed to," Hebb later told author and neurologist Richard Restak. "But it occurred to me about 1945 that the brain might be functioning independently of the messages it is getting from the outside."

In time, Hebb came up with the idea that brain activity is actually the work of a number of separate, interactive systems—"little groups of cells influencing each other." These cell assemblies, as he called them, make it possible for activity to occur in the brain without any external stimulation. "For instance," he said, "if I sit quietly, with no noise and no visual stimulation—perhaps with my eyes closed—I still may have an intensely active brain with no messages from the outside coming at all. To this extent, the brain is not programmed by the environment, but instead is programming itself."

Hebb's concept of cell assemblies formed the basis of his 1949 book, *The Organization of Behavior*. He started from the well-established fact that nerve impulses coursing through the brain pass from one cell to the next by crossing the synaptic gap between them. To Hebb, it seemed reasonable to suspect that each passage would somehow strengthen the connection, so that the next impulse would find the crossing easier. He did not know precisely how this strengthening occurred, but he was convinced it did and that it was the brain's fundamental mechanism for learning.

If the synapses do change in some way with use, Hebb argued, each stream of sensory information from the eyes and ears, and each barrage of motor commands heading to the muscles, leaves its trace. In this way, the brain accumulates experience. More than that, he theorized, neurons that are active at any given moment begin to reinforce one another, each increasing the firing rate of the next.

Eventually, this reinforcement process organizes the neurons into specific circuits—cell assemblies—each an internal representation of the stimulus and each capable of resonating on its own. One assembly, for example, might record the image of an apple, while another represents the name attached to the object. Over time, the brain acquires knowledge and develops skills by establishing, then linking, vast numbers of cell assemblies. As Hebb explained, "The development of a child while he is in the stage before learning to speak will consist of the development of cell assemblies for hearing, vision, smell, taste, and skin contact. Each cell assembly corresponds to a particular kind of experience that the child may run into."

Hebb's book was enormously influential, posing many of the questions that have continued to dominate neuroscience. Experiments to prove the existence of cell assemblies and to determine precisely what kind of synaptic changes occur when memories are established are extraordinarily difficult even today. But researchers continue to accumulate indirect evidence that the organization of the brain follows Hebb's basic model—that synapses do change with use and that cell assemblies, or something very much like them, form the building blocks of thought. Moreover, scientists have found strong indications that this organization remains somewhat flexible, especially early in life.

Long before a baby is born, the overall organization of its brain is laid down by genetic instructions in its DNA, which provide general rules for wiring up the circuits during embryonic development. But even a newborn's brain contains billions of neurons and a near-infinite number of possible connections among them. A DNA molecule simply does not contain enough information to specify a wiring diagram of that complexity. (According to one scientist's estimate, a sperm cell that held that much DNA would have to be the size of a golf ball.) So instead, the brain seems to spend its time during embryonic development and childhood growing connections, many times more than it will actually need. Later, as it adjusts to its environment, the brain prunes the connections it does not need.

Such self-modification, or plasticity, of the brain manifests itself in many ways. One of the most striking perhaps is that certain types of development must occur within specific critical periods—or not at all. After hatching, for instance, a duckling or gosling will follow the first moving object it sees (usually its mother), a behavior called imprinting. The first 12 to 24 hours represent the most sensitive period, after which the bird's susceptibility to imprinting falls off rapidly. The die is cast, so to speak, within about 32 hours.

Similar critical periods also occur in young mammals. In 1963 David Hubel and Torsten Wiesel, then at Harvard University, showed that the visual system of a cat develops rapidly, starting when the animal first opens its eyes, at age 10 to 14 days. By age four weeks, when most of its neural connections are made, the kitten can judge distances and begins to move around confidently. Without visual input during this critical period, however, the animal's fast-growing neural connections cannot organize themselves properly. Hubel and Wiesel showed that if the kitten receives visual input from only one eye during the first month of development, the creature will never achieve binocular vision. The favored eye will become dominant, and the other eye, though perfectly healthy, will become effectively blind.

Hubel and Wiesel's work on the visual system eventually won the pair a Nobel Prize. But it also led immediately to another intriguing question: If the brain can organize itself from experiences early in life, can it *re*organize itself later on?

The answer seems to be a qualified

The Not-So-Simple Act of Making Up One's Mind

Every waking moment, the brain is bombarded by sensory inputs that demand a decision—even if no more than whether to pay attention to a sight, a sound, or a sensation. For instance, when an office worker hears her telephone ring, interrupting her conversation with a colleague, she must decide whether to pick up the receiver or let her answering machine take the call. Instantly, her brain begins weighing a flood of incoming signals. Her ears report how many times the phone has rung and the pause indicating that her visitor might be about to finish his sentence. Her eyes take in his expression—annoyed or accepting?—and the location of the phone relative to her hand. The muscles in her body relay information about the position of her hand.

The cortex receives these impulses in separate processing regions: the primary visual, auditory, and sensory cortices (shown in red on the brain map, right). Neural pathways connect these regions to the higher-order areas (*blue*), which subject the sensory bits to greater scrutiny. For example, is the hand close enough to grab the receiver before the phone rings again? These higher-order regions, in turn, relay signals to the largest components in the cortical architecture, the association areas (*gray*). Once called silent areas because they did not respond in obvious ways to electric stimulation, the association cortices are now believed to function as sensory clearinghouses, integrating the information from the disparate senses. Here, memories and emotions mix with sights, sounds, and body sensations to help the brain develop a course of action. Taking cues from the association areas, the premotor cortex (*light green*) formulates movement patterns and relays orders to the motor cortex (*dark green*) for execution.

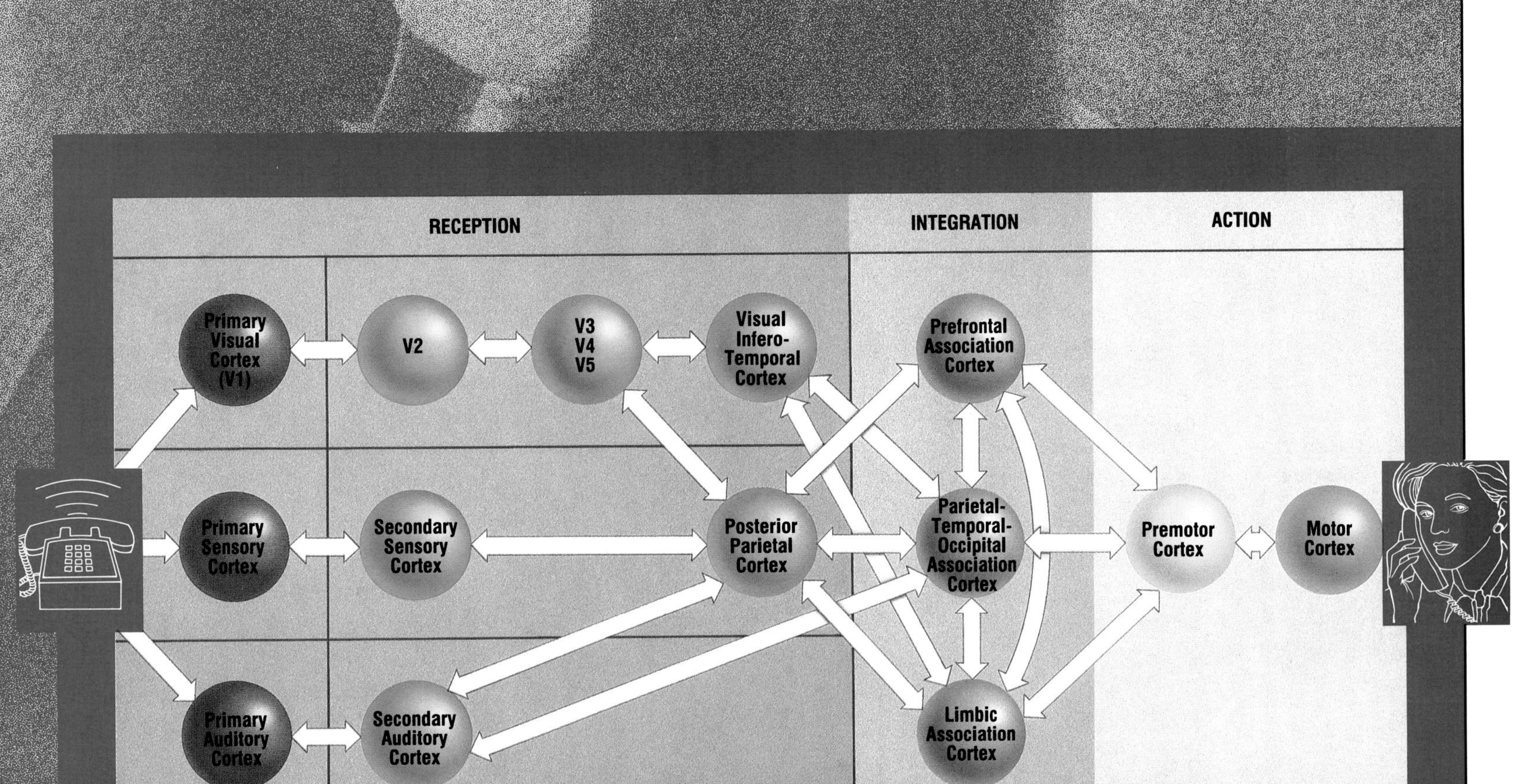

PATHWAYS TO ACTION. Sensory impulses set off by a ringing telephone go first to the brain's primary visual, auditory, and sensory cortices, represented above as red spheres. A two-way communication network *(arrows)* connects these primary sections with other parts of the cortex, most directly the higher-order areas *(blue spheres).* These specialized receiving centers pass interpretations of the input to the association areas *(gray spheres).* The prefrontal association cortex plays a key role in planning actions; the parietal-temporal-occipital, in bringing together sensory responses; and the limbic, in storing emotions and memories. Association areas feed into the premotor cortex *(light green sphere),* which prompts the motor cortex *(dark green sphere)* to activate the muscles.

The Multilayered Cortex

Hardly thicker than an orange peel, the cortex actually includes up to six distinct layers, constructed of two basic cell types: triangular-bodied pyramidal cells and their nonpyramidal counterparts *(right).* The size and distribution of these cells vary with each layer's function and location *(pages 96-97).* The impulse-receiving dendrites of pyramidal cells can extend to several layers, and their axons, used for transmitting signals, connect with distant parts of the brain and nervous system. But the dendrites and axons of nonpyramidal cells extend for only a few layers and never beyond the cortex.

Impulses from the eyes, ears, and body (shown as a red arrow on the diagram at right) enter the sensory cortices at layer IV, whose nonpyramidal cells bristle with dendrites. They then flow up to layers II and III, where pyramidal cells relay the signals *(dark blue arrows)* to layer IV of the association cortices. After ascending once again to levels II and III, the messages proceed to level III of the motor cortex—primarily an output area with little or no receiving layer of nonpyramidal cells. Some data feed back to previous stages by way of a secondary network *(light blue arrows).* Finally, large pyramidal cells in layer V translate the impulses into motor instructions.

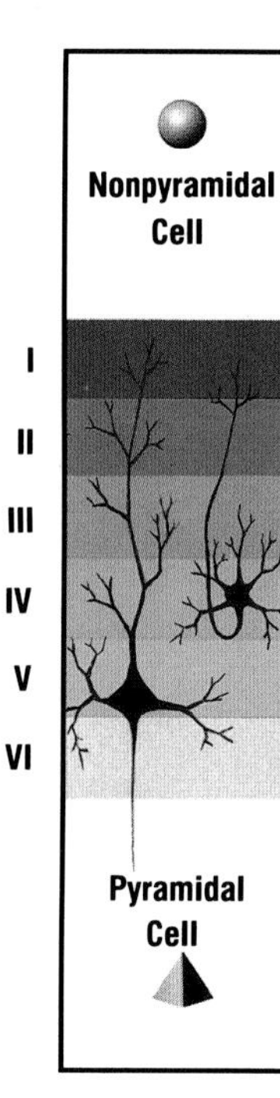

yes. Certainly children have an easier time of it than do adults, generally speaking. Language development, for instance, occurs during a critical period, starting about four months after a child's birth and continuing at least until the age of two and often for several years thereafter. Youngsters this age not only learn very quickly how to talk, but they easily pick up a second (or third or fourth) language and speak it without an accent. Children with no exposure to language at this time may never learn to talk at all.

Significantly, this critical interval coincides with a period of extremely rapid growth in the cerebral cortex. Before about age eight, a child can suffer major damage to the language centers on the left side of the brain and still make an excellent, even perfect, recovery. The brain is still so plastic that the right hemisphere, the supposedly nonlinguistic side, can take up the slack. Afterward, though, the rapid proliferation of nerve endings stops. Consequently, adults have a much harder time learning a new language—and when they do, they almost never manage to speak it without their native accent.

But as it turns out, even the adult brain's blueprint is not drawn in indelible ink. Starting in the mid-1980s, neuroscientists began to uncover compelling evidence that neural connections in the adult brain not only can reorganize themselves, but can do so with surprising alacrity. One of the most intriguing hints came from a troop of primates known as the Silver Spring monkeys. In the late 1970s, neuroscientist Edward Taub, who at the time worked at the Institute for Behavioral Research in Silver Spring, Maryland, wanted to learn how people might rehabilitate limbs that had been paralyzed by nerve damage. To do that, he needed to work with nonhuman subjects. So he took a dozen or so monkeys, most of them macaques, and surgically destroyed the point where sensory nerves from their arms entered their spinal columns, thereby causing paralysis.

In 1981, before the experiment had gone very far, the monkeys were confiscated by police during a raid initiated by animal-rights activists. Some of the animals lived for more than a decade after that, unaware of the long-running legal battle over who would have custody of them. In the meantime, they ended up making an unexpected contribution to science.

Mortimer Mishkin, Timothy Pons, and their colleagues at the National Institute of Mental Health in nearby Bethesda examined two of the monkeys in 1987, hoping to learn how the sensory maps—essentially neuronal atlases of the entire body (*pages 96-97*)—in the animals' brains had changed to accommodate the damage. What they found was a phenomenal degree of reorganization. The region of the monkeys' cortices that previously would have responded to sensations from the crippled arm and hand now responded to a gentle touch—on the face.

The discovery was astonishing. Although the regions corresponding to the face and the hand lie very near one another on the cortex, they are

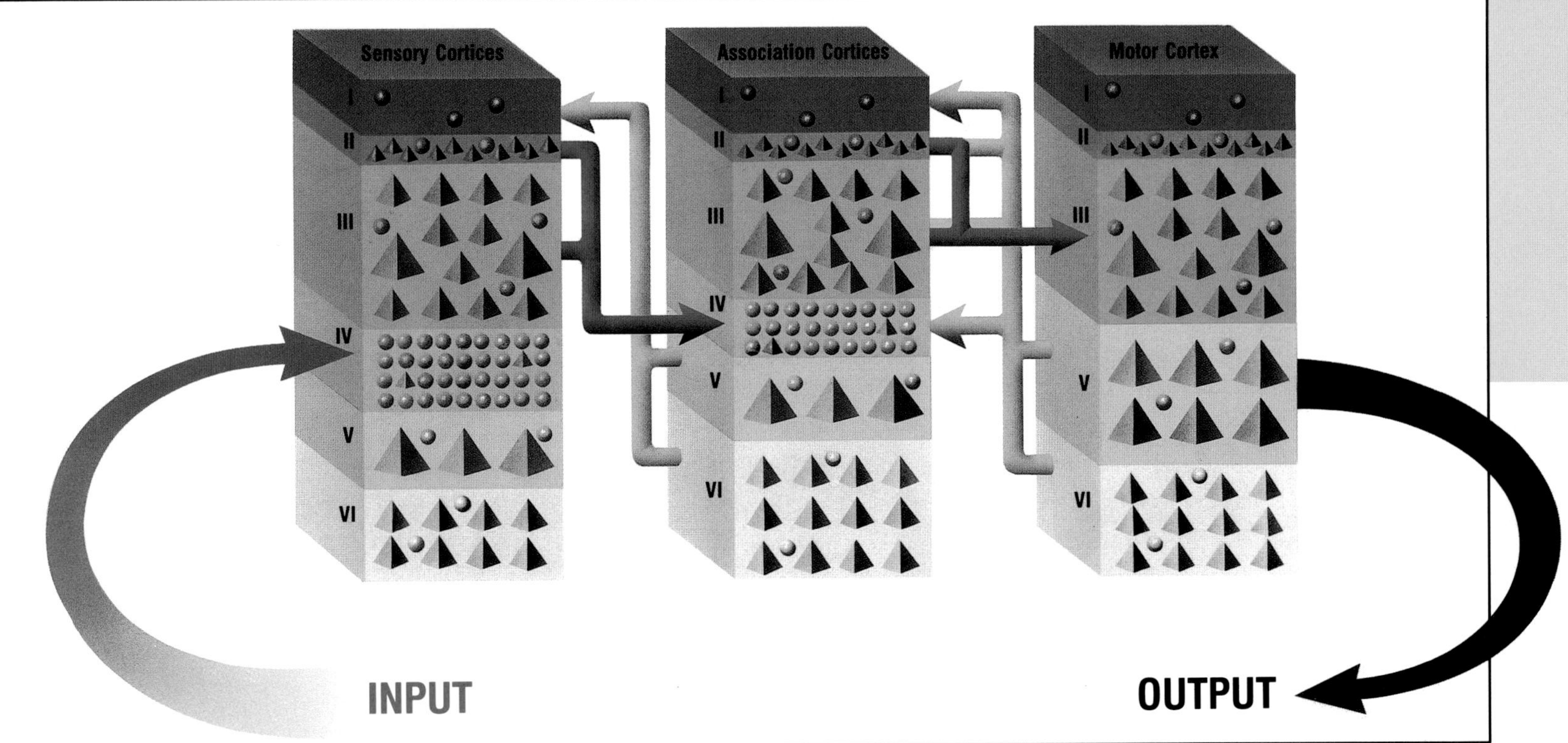

roughly a centimeter apart—light-years distant at the cellular level. It seemed as though the monkeys' brains had responded to the paralysis by putting out new connections on a colossal scale, a finding that, if true, would undermine the notion that nerve-cell connections proliferate at this rate only in childhood.

It was not long before evidence of another possible explanation began to emerge. Across the country, at the University of California in San Diego, neuroscientist V. S. Ramachandran was working with human subjects who had recently lost an arm. He discovered that many of these people, including one man whose arm had been severed only a month before, felt sensations from their missing hands when he stroked their faces with a cotton swab. Clearly, the subjects' brains had undergone map reorganizations similar to those of the Silver Spring monkeys. But Ramachandran believed that one month is far too short a time to grow new nerve connections; as far as he was concerned, another hypothesis was called for.

Ramachandran's findings were soon bolstered by an independent series of experiments with even more dramatic results. In April 1990 researchers Charles Gilbert at Rockefeller University and Jon Kaas at Vanderbilt University reported that, when they destroyed a point on a cat's retina, the part of the visual cortex that once had received signals from the damaged area began to expand its receptive field to take in information from surrounding areas of the retina—all within a matter of minutes.

Such "filling-in," contended Ramachandran, can occur only if another web of connections—a safety net, as it were—stands ready to provide backup assistance. Indeed, recent research has turned up evidence of just such a neural support network. Found first in the visual cortex and later in other parts of the cortex, these so-called horizontal connections link neurons of the cortex over distances as great as six to eight millimeters. Some neuroscientists think of these connections as auxiliary communication lines, always ready to take over if the main cables go down.

Scientists know that filling-in occurs throughout much of the brain, though many of the details of the process, as well as its exact purpose, remain something of a mystery. Obviously, filling-in allows for partial recovery from brain damage. But neuroscientist Michael Merzenich of the University of California in San Francisco has suggested that this activity represents

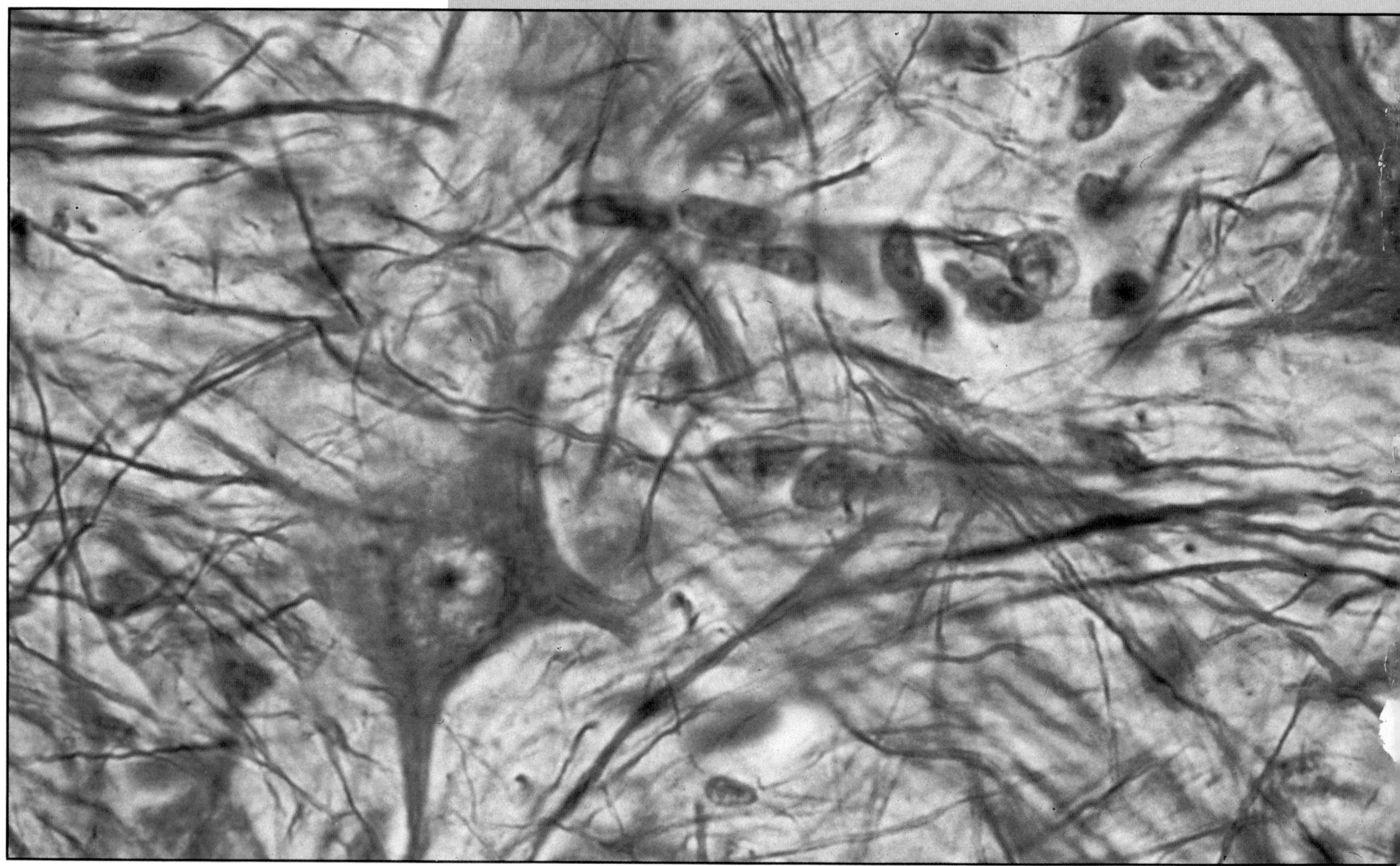

only part of a much bigger process: the continuous give-and-take among neurons in the brain.

In Merzenich's view, the brain constantly adjusts its organization to accommodate ever-changing demands. Some neuronal connections become stronger while others weaken, allowing parts of the brain once believed to be hard-wired to adapt instead. In a recent experiment, Merzenich and his colleagues used small vibrators to stimulate the middle fingers of research monkeys, which had been trained to respond to changing vibrational frequencies. Meanwhile, through electrodes implanted in each animal's brain, the researchers monitored neurons along the sensory map. They found that as a monkey improved at distinguishing one frequency from another, the region of the map corresponding to the middle finger expanded. Other researchers have since discovered that a similar expansion occurs in blind humans who use a single finger to read Braille. Presumably, the same thing happens with anyone who develops a particular skill, be it touch-typing 100 words a minute, running patterns on a football field, or being able to distinguish the subtle differences in taste between one red wine and another.

As these and other experiments suggest, the brain is capable of reorganizing itself to operate most efficiently—whatever the demand. Yet notions such as cell assemblies, plasticity, and filling-in, however intriguing, seem only to pick at the edges of the central knot. Consciousness—the subjective "I" that remembers learning to swim at age six (perhaps with the help of Hebb's cell assemblies) and anticipates a vacation next month—remains hidden from view.

Still, scientists in recent decades have made enormous strides in their

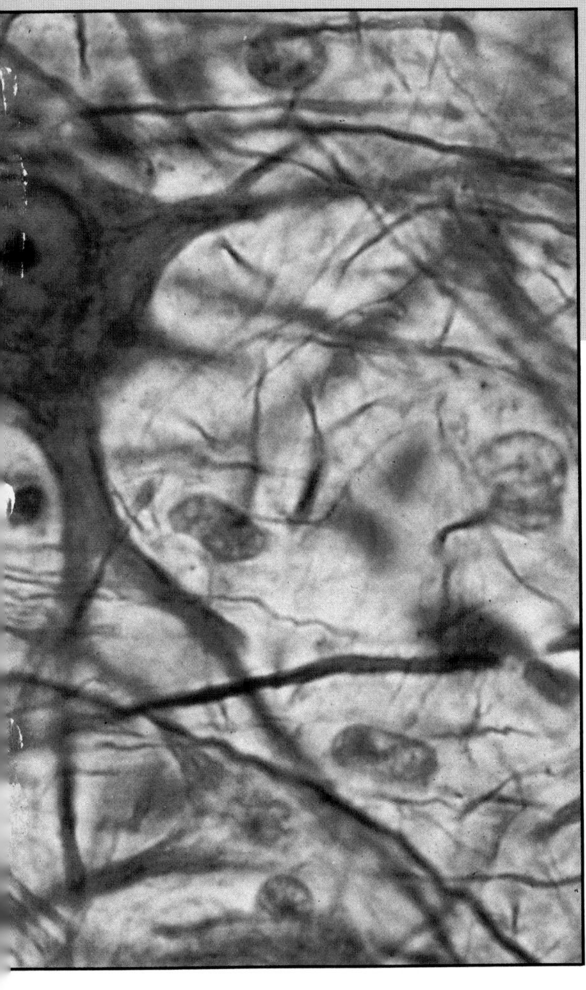

Under a microscope, a slice of cortical tissue reveals a dizzying mass of neurons *(stained orange in the photograph at left)* and their myriad connections—the avenues of knowledge. New challenges, such as learning a game, spark scattered activity across large parts of the cortex. As the game becomes more familiar, however, linkages between certain neurons appear to strengthen, allowing signals to move along more efficiently.

efforts to understand the cognitive aspects of the brain. Many brain researchers believe that with the advent of PET, MRI, and other sophisticated imaging techniques, the most exciting phase of this exploration has only just begun.

PET was one of the earliest techniques to come along, and its contribution has been profound. Although it was actually developed in the early 1970s, the concept dates back as far as 1928, when doctors in Boston first demonstrated that blood will flow to the most active parts of the brain. The story began with a man who checked into a hospital with failing vision and another, more bizarre complaint: Every time he opened his eyes, he heard a *shwih shwih* sound, like wind rustling through leaves. When he closed his eyes, the swishing stopped.

Exploratory surgery revealed that the man had an abnormally large cluster of blood vessels in the back of his brain. Removal was too risky, the doctors decided, but their probing left the patient with only muscle and scalp covering the visual cortex and the aberrant blood vessels.

The result, if unfortunate for the patient, was a windfall for medical science, for it gave the doctors a unique opportunity to confirm long-standing presumptions about blood flow. By holding a stethoscope to the back of the patient's head while he read a newspaper, they could hear the *shwih shwih* sound for themselves. As they had suspected, the noise was the rush of the man's blood surging through the stimulated visual cortex.

The great advance of the PET scan was to make this increased blood flow visible, by tracking the progress of radioactive compounds introduced into the bloodstream. At first, the images appeared rather fuzzy, since blood does not concentrate with pinpoint precision. A clearer picture emerged in the early 1980s, when advances in technology and software allowed researchers to superimpose a PET scan over a high-resolution MRI scan of the same brain. MRI, which charts the interior of the body by recording the response of atomic nuclei to magnetic fields, can produce detailed and highly accurate structural maps of the brain.

These combination guides to the brain's activity have galvanized brain research as well as increased the value of what can be learned from brain-damaged patients. Instead of simply guessing where the damage occurred (or waiting for an autopsy when the patient dies), researchers can now use MRI and PET scans to chart the lesion precisely and to demonstrate experimentally exactly how the damage affects thought processes.

By the 1990s, at least 40 centers in the United States were using PET for diagnosis and research, including the laboratory at Washington University School of Medicine in St. Louis where neurologist Marcus Raichle and his colleagues study how the brain processes language. In their first PET-scan experiments, Raichle's team started small, asking their subjects to read, silently, single words flashing on a computer screen at the rate of one per second. With each word, the subjects' visual cortex—the part of the brain that actually registers images—lit up just as expected. So did dime-

Vision Centers in the Brain

In a game of soccer, keeping track of the action is no small feat for the eyes and brain. The moving ball produces an ever-changing image on the retina, yet the brain recognizes these streaks and spinning blobs as one object—the ball. Meanwhile, the brain also monitors the position of the players, their movements, and the color of their jerseys. To make all of this possible, the eyes and brain join in an elaborate ballet of interpretation: The eyes, stimulated by events on the field, relay impulses to specialized regions of the occipital lobe, which sort and evaluate them as to form, motion, and color.

Research in the past 20 years has shed new light on the complex workings of vision. Led by neurobiologist Semir Zeki at the University of London, scientists have mapped out the traffic patterns for visual input and identified the higher-order cortical regions that collaborate to bring the world into view.

Signals from the retina travel first to V1 (*blue on illustration, opposite*), the primary visual cortex. This region, along with nearby V2 (*green*), serves as a general sorting, routing, and integrating center for visual information. The other three vision cortices are specialists, simultaneously scrutinizing the data for particular attributes. The cells of V3 (*yellow*) detect form—the outlines and borders of things—and motion. Region V4 (*orange*) analyzes color and form, while V5 (*black*) recognizes only motion. On the opposite page, four panels show how the soccer scene at right is processed in the visual apparatus—first by the retina, then by each specialized section of the cortex. (For simplicity, the cerebellum is not pictured.)

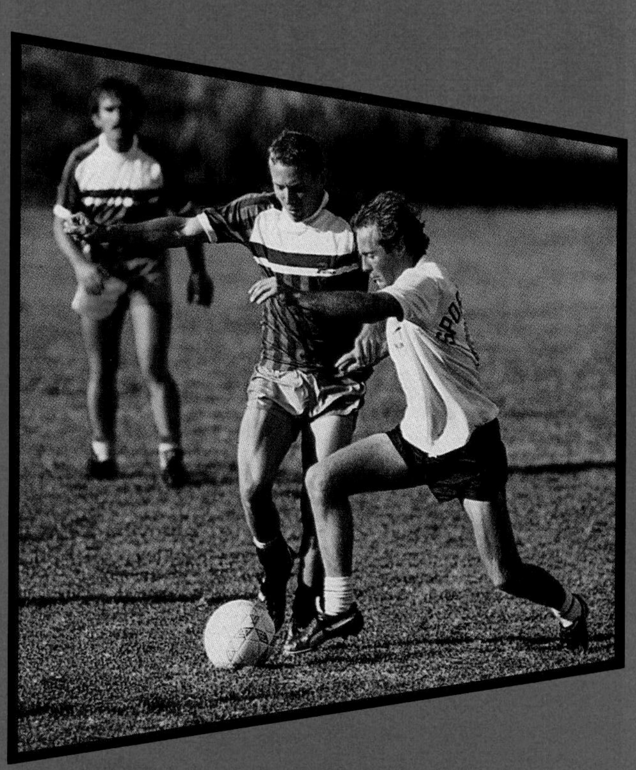

Crossed Wires, Clear Pictures

The eye divides the world into two fan-shaped visual fields, which cast images on opposite halves of the retina. Converted into electrical impulses, the visual input travels through nerve pathways to processing centers in the brain—but with a twist: Each cerebral hemisphere perceives only those images in the opposing visual field.

At a junction called the optic chiasm, signals from the inside half of one retina cross over to the other hemisphere; those from the outside half stay the course. The impulses continue along the optic nerve to a structure called the lateral geniculate nucleus, which forwards them to the primary visual cortex.

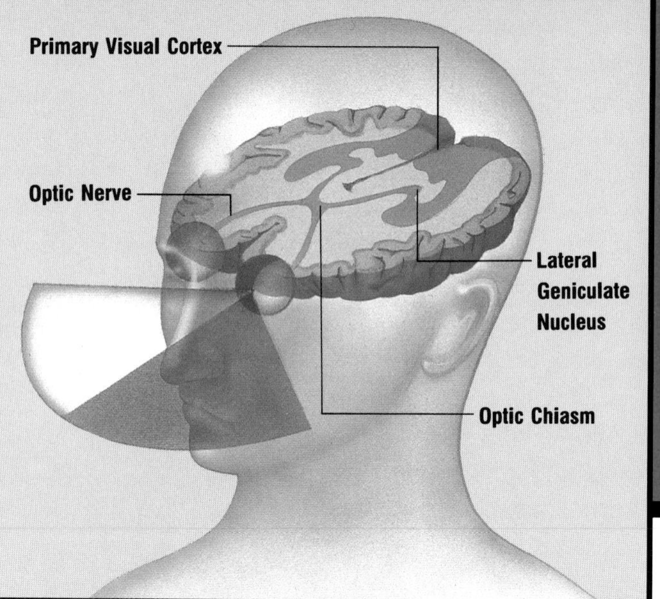

SHAPE AND MOVEMENT. From the retina, signals travel to cortical regions V1 *(blue)* and V2 *(green)*, where they are sorted and routed to V3 *(yellow)*. This higher-order processing area recognizes only movement and forms *(right)*.

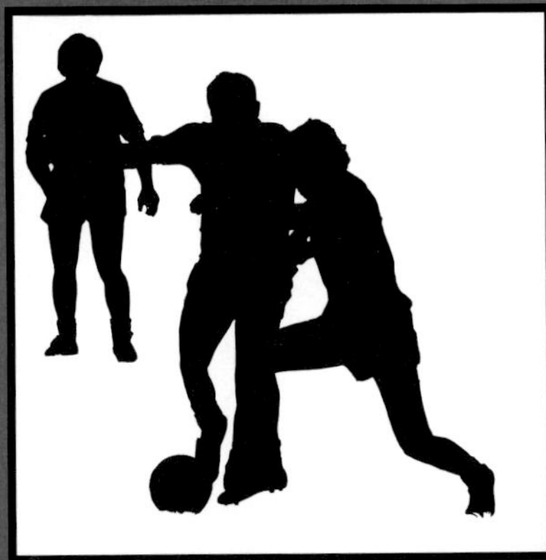

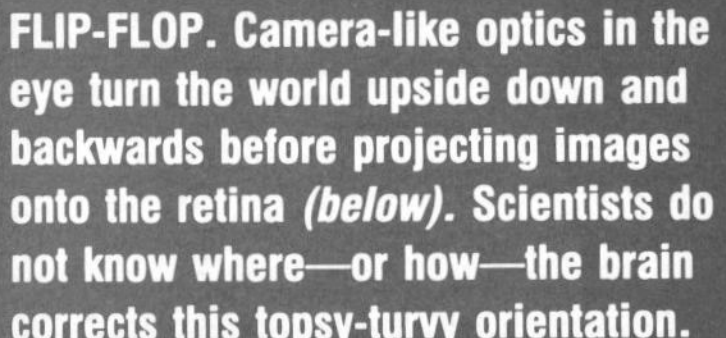

FLIP-FLOP. Camera-like optics in the eye turn the world upside down and backwards before projecting images onto the retina *(below)*. Scientists do not know where—or how—the brain corrects this topsy-turvy orientation.

COLOR AND FORM. Situated near V3 on the underside of the brain's occipital lobe, higher-order region V4 *(orange)* scours the messages for information regarding color and, to some extent, form *(below)*. Injuries to this area can destroy the ability to perceive—or even remember—different hues.

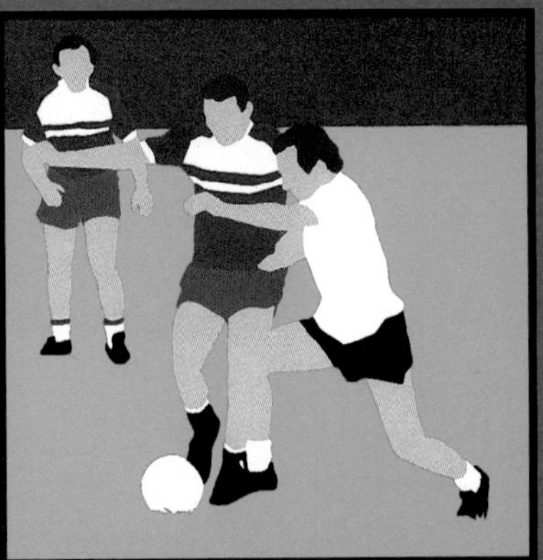

V3
V2
V1
V4

MOVEMENT. Region V5 *(red)*, located on the outer part of the occipital lobe, tracks movement by constantly comparing updated maps of the visual data with previous versions. In V5's interpretation of the soccer scene, one player is effectively invisible because he is not moving. For patients with damage to this higher-order region of the cortex, objects at rest are visible but seem to vanish when they move.

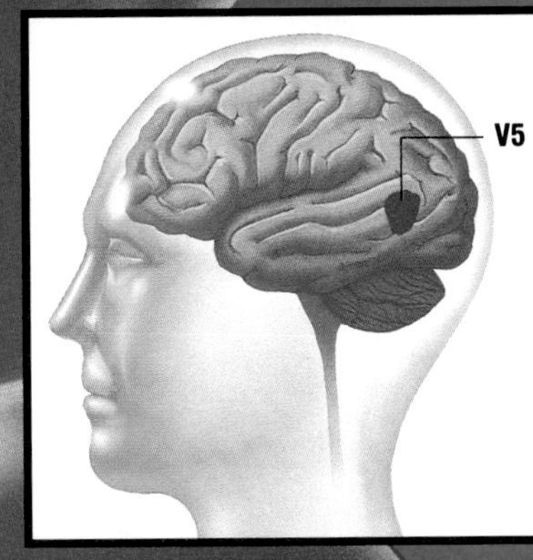

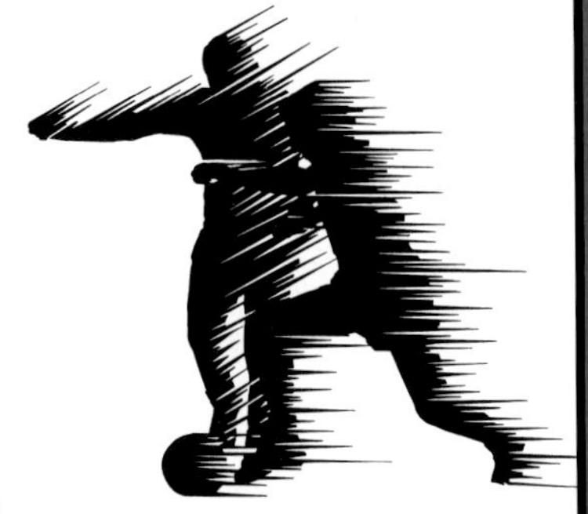

size clusters of neurons on the left-hand side of the brain, in the language centers, which were presumed to be busy recognizing the meanings of the words.

Surprisingly, however, the same semantic areas also lit up when the computer showed nonwords—*tweal* and *cade*, for example—that nonetheless obeyed spelling rules for English. It seemed that the brain was scrambling to make sense of nonsense constructions that looked like they ought to mean something. In contrast, when the volunteers were shown unpronounceable strings such as *nlpfz*, the semantic areas stayed dark. Clearly, the scientists reasoned, as the subjects had learned the rules of English spelling, their brains had developed special zones to analyze strings of letters that obey those rules.

In 1991, working with Larry Squire of the University of California in San Diego, Raichle found another surprise during a series of PET-scan experiments. The researchers showed a group of subjects a word, then asked them to recall whether it had been included on a previous list. Predictably, the scan showed hot spots in the hippocampus, which was known to be involved in the formation of long-term memories. But an area also lit up unexpectedly in the frontal lobe. This region, as it turned out, was least active in those subjects who remembered the most words. Evidently, the more efficiently the brain retrieves things from memory, the easier the task.

The findings of Raichle and Squire fit in neatly with those of many other PET researchers. In 1992, for example, Richard Haier of the Brain Imaging Center at the University of California in Irvine had volunteers play a complex computer game while he monitored their brain activity with a PET scan. Haier found that the people used considerable mental energy—that is, their brains were extremely active—while learning the game. After several weeks of practice, however, the activity was considerably reduced, even though their scores had improved 700 percent. Furthermore, the greatest reductions occurred in volunteers with the highest scores on standardized tests of abstract reasoning. Paradoxical as it may seem, says Haier, "It's possible that the brain learns over time what neural circuits *not* to use to perform a task, eventually relying only on certain important circuits." Moreover, the experiments would appear to indicate that intelligence—that elusive and controversial quantity known as IQ—has a real basis in physiological efficiency.

Without question, PET scans have helped usher in a new era of brain exploration. Still, for all its power, the technology has some severe disadvantages. The machines themselves are big, complicated, and expensive. The radioactive compounds that subjects must take into their bodies have to be produced by an equally expensive cyclotron. And at best, a PET scan will produce a fresh image of the brain only once every few seconds, a comparatively sluggish rate that makes the "motion picture" of the thought process look jerky. The ideal brain scanner, by contrast, would be cheap, easy, and fast.

In 1990 Alan Gevins, director of EEG Systems Laboratory, a private brain research center in San Francisco, announced a potentially important step in that direction. Called the Mental Activity Network Scanner, or MANSCAN, Gevins's device can record up to 250 brain images per second using a high-tech update of the classic technique of electroencephalography, or EEG.

Conventional EEG has been used for decades to monitor brain waves, the electrical signals emanating from the surface of the cortex. With early EEG machines, electrodes glued to the scalp produced a single, undulating line on a strip chart, allowing researchers and clinicians to track the fast, low-amplitude beta waves that

TRACES OF THOUGHT. The two brain-scan images below, each a hybrid of EEG and MRI data taken from five people, show differences in cortical activity between subjects who are simply waiting for a number to flash on a blank screen *(top)* and those who must remember two numbers while waiting for a third to appear *(bottom)*. The increased quantity and greater thickness of lines in the bottom image suggest intensified communication among different areas of the cortex. Researchers believe that this computer-generated sketch of neural processing represents the first glimpse of the widely dispersed brain activity that is involved with the everyday process of keeping something in mind.

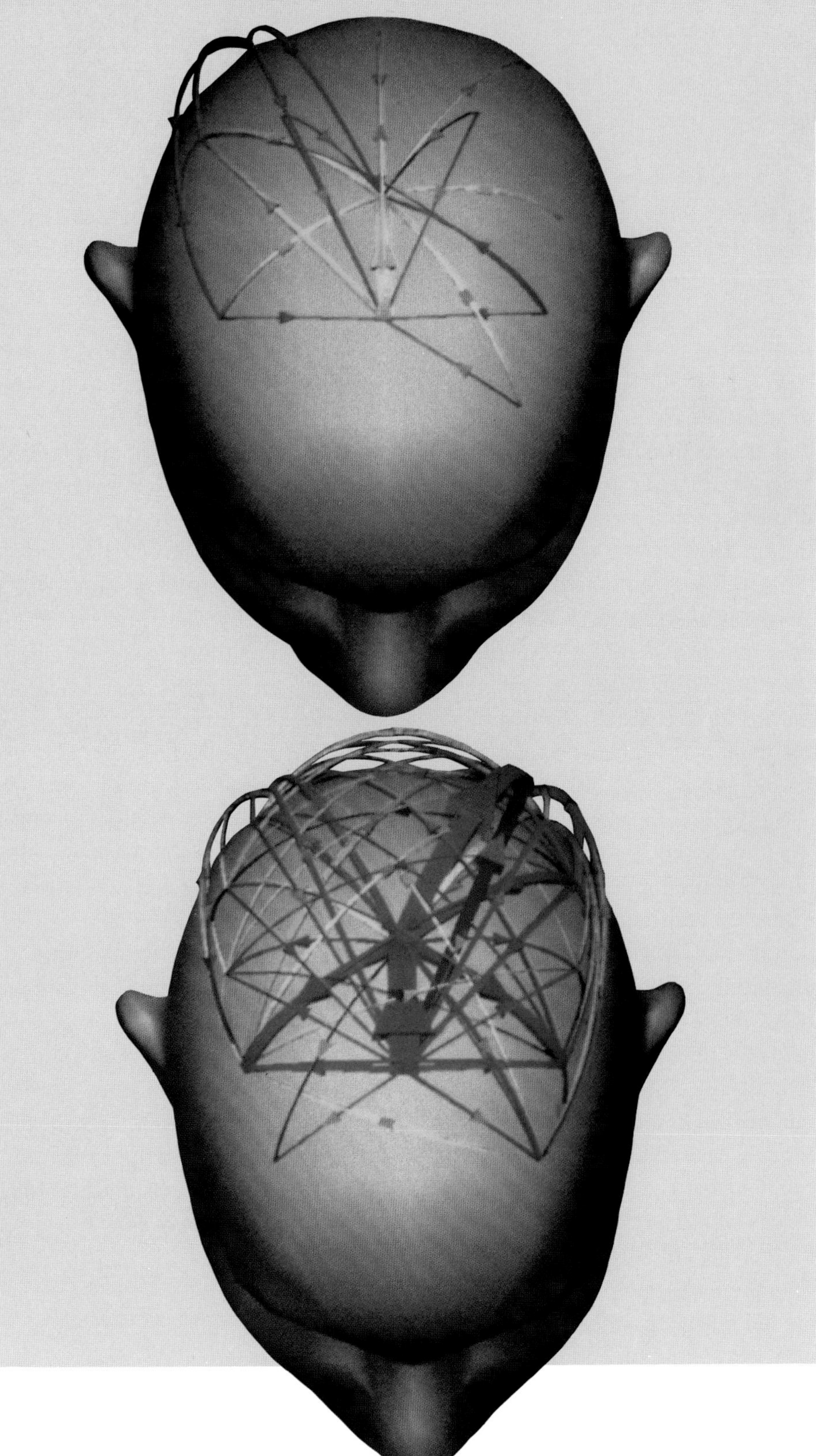

correspond to alertness as well as the slower, larger alpha waves that indicate relaxation.

In the 1960s and 1970s, with the advent of high-speed computers that could analyze the signals in more subtle detail, EEG researchers devoted a great deal of effort to understanding what these wiggly lines could reveal about the brain's response to a specific event. They pored over the strip charts like fortunetellers reading palms, hoping to glean clues from each peak, valley, and plateau.

Most of these attempts at divination ended in frustration. Conventional EEG machines took their input from fewer than 20 electrodes and produced only a small number of brain-wave traces at best, making it difficult for researchers to pinpoint a signal's origin. But in a MANSCAN experiment, the subject wears a soft helmet studded with 124 electrodes. Computers track the shifting centers of electrical activity, then plot the locations of those centers on a high-resolution, three-dimensional MRI map of the subject's brain. The result is a series of images that shows the ebb and flow of brain activity.

In one experiment, Gevins and his

colleagues used MANSCAN to monitor U.S. Air Force test pilots performing a battery of demanding mental tasks over a 10- to 14-hour period. Seated in front of computer screens, the pilots were shown a sequence of two numbers between one and nine and then asked to hold them in their minds while the screen went blank. The appearance of a third number a few seconds later was a signal for the pilots to push a pressure-sensitive button; the higher the first number in the sequence, the greater the pressure they were to exert. The scientists, meanwhile, tracked this mental activity with MANSCAN, which displayed the "cross talk" among different neuronal groups as colorful bolts streaking across the cortex.

The bolts were what Gevins calls shadows of thought—visible indications that the brain was busily reshaping and redefining its perception of the world based on experience (the numbers the pilots had been shown) and expectations (the numbers to come). Several hours before the pilots' ability to correlate number value with button pressure actually deteriorated, the scientists could detect signs of fatigue. The intensity of the bolts weakened and their configuration changed.

As the experiment suggests, higher mental functions—those that take the most concentration and energy—begin to falter long before lower functions, such as the ability to process visual information or control a motor response. To Gevins, the results also reveal a great deal about how we think. "Our brains are not mere stimulus-response devices," he says. "Rather, our brains seem to devote a very large portion of their activity to continuously forming, maintaining, and revising detailed simulations, or models, of what we imagine our self- and world-states to be." If Gevins is right, thought itself may simply be the process by which the brain builds and rebuilds these ever-changing models, creating the framework for how we perceive the world from one moment to the next.

As researchers slowly fill gaps in their understanding of the brain, one of their most striking and consistent findings is the division of labor between the right and left cerebral hemispheres. The most obvious proof of this is handedness: Roughly 90 percent of the human population is right-handed, which means—given that each side of the brain controls the opposite side of the body—that the left hemisphere is almost always dominant in terms of motor-skill superiority. (Right-handers are also usually right-footed and right-eyed.) Less than 10 percent of the population is right-brain dominant, meaning they favor their left hands, and an even smaller minority is ambidextrous, using both hands with equal skill.

Why the brain should prefer one hemisphere over the other has long confounded the experts. Monkeys and apes, our closest biological relatives, seem to show some tendency toward handedness, although the evidence is far from clear. Almost all other animals use either limb with equal ease. Many scientists have speculated that the uniquely human tendency toward right-handedness somehow sprang from the uniquely human capability for language. It may be no accident that the same side of the brain that controls language in most people (the left) also controls the dominant right hand. Perhaps spoken language began with hand signals. After all, newborns usually show no evidence of favoring one hand over the other. The distinction appears to set in after age two or three—at roughly the same time children begin to master language.

Whatever the reason, hemisphere specialization goes far beyond handedness or language. For evidence of the extent to which the halves of the brain allocate the work load, researchers turn to one of the most radical and bizarre operations in all of neurosurgery: the splitting of the brain. Doctors in the 1930s first tried the procedure as a last-ditch attempt to help people suffering from severe epilepsy, an electrical storm of nerve impulses raging from one side of the brain to the other. At its worst, epilepsy can produce violent convulsions and unconsciousness.

These pioneering surgeons found that they could give their patients enormous relief by reaching down into the fissure between the brain's hemispheres and severing the corpus callosum, the thick cable of nerve fibers connecting the two. By cutting off this communication, the operation short-circuited the epileptic attacks.

What most amazed the doctors, though, was that these split-brain operations seemed to have no obvious ill effects on the patients. Once they had recovered from surgery, the patients could not only walk, run, bicycle, and swim as well as ever, they could also read, write, and speak quite normally. The corpus callosum, it appeared, had no real function in the brain, giving rise to a popular joke in medical schools of the 1940s. Question: "What is the purpose of the corpus callosum?" Answer: "It transmits epileptic seizures from one side of the brain to the other."

As it happens, of course, the corpus callosum is far from a negligible structure. Researchers around the beginning of the 20th century had reported curious symptoms in people who had suffered damage to it. In 1908, for example, German neurologist Kurt Goldstein noted the strange case of one such woman, whose left hand would travel up to her neck and attempt to strangle her unless she sat on it. Another patient sometimes found himself pulling his trousers down with one hand while pulling them up with the other—or shaking his wife violently with one hand while using the other to protect her.

No one could explain the behavior, and the picture remained cloudy until the 1950s, when Roger Sperry, a neurophysiologist at the California Institute of Technology, and neurosurgeon Joseph E. Bogen of the University of Southern California perfected and tested the split-brain operation on animals. After they started using the procedure more widely on humans in 1961—again, only in patients with severe epilepsy—Sperry and his coworkers continued with experiments through 1969 to determine what the halves of the brain can know and do.

These experiments, which won Sperry the 1981 Nobel Prize in medicine, revealed that the impression of mental unity in split-brain patients is an illusion, created only because the two sides of the brain share the same body, the same eyes and ears, and the same experiences in the everyday world. "Everything we have seen so far indicates that the surgery has left these people with two separate minds, that is, two separate spheres of consciousness," Sperry wrote in 1966. "What is experienced in the right hemisphere seems to lie entirely outside the realm of experience of the left hemisphere."

In carefully designed experiments, Sperry's group demonstrated this independence of experience time and again. For example, they asked split-brain volunteers in one study to gaze at a spot in the middle of a screen while pictures flashed before them at the rate of 1⁄10 of a second, too quickly for their eyes to shift from one side to the other.

These were no ordinary pictures. Each was a composite, two half-images joined in the middle. One, for example, depicted half of an old man's face on the right and half of a child's face on the left—yet the volunteers saw nothing unusual about the image. Asked to say aloud what they had seen, they replied, "an old man." Since the left side of their brains, the hemisphere that houses the speech centers, could receive information only about the old-man half of the image, that was all they *could* say. But when the researchers showed the volunteers a group of undoctored pictures and asked them to point to the one they had seen on the screen, the subjects usually chose the image of the child. This time, the nonverbal right hemisphere took control.

Sperry knew, however, that the split-brain operation did not separate the halves of the brain completely. Even though the corpus callosum had been cut, other connections still held fast deeper in the brainstem. Indeed, Sperry found that somehow emotions could make the leap where facts could not. As one split-brain volunteer, a young woman, watched geometric shapes flash on the screen, Sperry suddenly projected a nude picture where it could be perceived only by her right brain. The volunteer blushed and giggled nervously. When asked why, she answered, "Oh, Dr. Sperry . . . that funny machine." But she could not explain any more than that: Her left brain was not aware of the facts of the matter, only of her embarrassment.

Skeptics argued that these experiments revealed nothing about the normal brain. After all, they said, split-brain patients suffered from

One Brain, Two Minds

In 1970 Caltech neurophysiologist Roger Sperry used half-and-half images similar to the one below to demonstrate that the brain's two hemispheres perceive the same world in curiously different ways. He split photographs of two perfectly normal faces down the middle and recombined them to create a composite. Then, using a special device, he flashed the image before the eyes of patients whose left and right cerebral hemispheres had been surgically disconnected as treatment for severe epilepsy. The image was presented to one eye for only 1/10 of a second, far too quickly for the eye to scan from side to side. Because of the twisting path visual impulses follow to the brain (*pages* 106-107), the right half of the image was visible only to the left hemisphere, and the left half only to the right hemisphere.

When the subjects were asked to say aloud what they had seen, they usually mentioned the image viewed by the left hemisphere, home of the language centers. But shown a stack of original, uncut images and asked to point to the face that had flashed before them, they almost always chose the one detected by the brain's nonverbal right half. As Sperry noted, the subjects consistently selected with greater confidence and accuracy when pointing, an indication that the right hemisphere is more adept at recognizing forms such as faces.

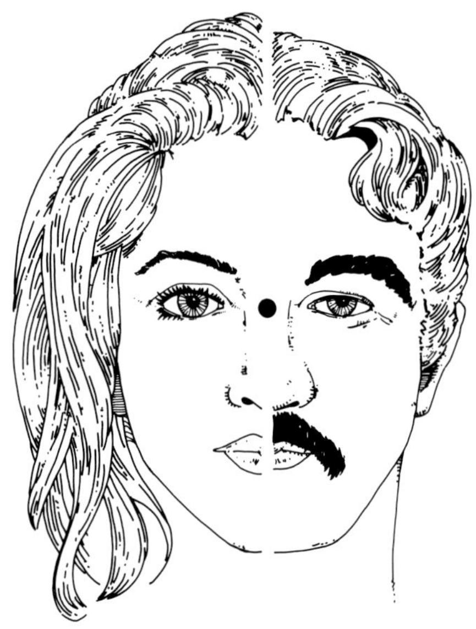

severe epilepsy and may have had other brain abnormalities as well. Perhaps the bizarre disconnection Sperry had found was simply a side effect of his patients' illness and nothing more.

Over the years, however, Sperry's split-brain findings have been confirmed many times in normal people. By carefully injecting an anesthetic such as sodium amytal into the arteries supplying blood to the brain, researchers can put one hemisphere to sleep while the other continues to function normally—with some intriguing results. When volunteers receive an injection in the left hemisphere while they are singing a song, for example, they can still carry the tune, but they suddenly forget the lyrics: Their language areas have ceased to function. With an injection on the right side, they can remember the lyrics, but they lose all sense of melody and rhythm.

Taken as a whole, split-brain studies seem to confirm what many scientists had already suspected: The left hemisphere not only contains the centers for speech and understanding language, it also seems to be specialized for orderly, analytical thinking in general. This is the side that would be particularly active in someone who was solving, say, a complicated arithmetic problem. For reasons not completely understood, even in left-handed people—who might be expected to have their language center in the dominant right hemisphere—the verbal, analytical part of the brain most often lies on the left.

The right hemisphere, meanwhile, might be characterized as the intuitive side of the brain. It shows little verbal ability, although it can process simple words. It can also perform simple arithmetic, but unlike the literal left, which proceeds step by step, the right brain appears to solve problems through leaps of insight and intuition. The right hemisphere is the part of the brain that responds to musical rhythm and melody. It also appreciates humor, metaphor, and connected themes, making it better equipped than the left hemisphere to grasp the point of a story. Indeed, people with right-brain damage can have trouble getting the punch line of a joke: They simply do not understand why it is funny. Instead of laughing, they tend to analyze the story and criticize small details. Researchers also have found that the right hemisphere excels at recognizing shapes and their relationships to one another. People with right-brain damage sometimes cannot dress themselves, cannot orient themselves spatially, and often cannot recognize familiar faces.

Not surprisingly, such conclusions have captured the imagination of scientists and laypeople alike. The romanticized tugs of war between heart and mind, emotion and reason, conscious and subconscious all seem to have found a physical embodiment in the brain's two hemispheres. However, the public fascination with the distinction has also led to exaggerated claims that make many scientists extremely uncomfortable.

The right brain–left brain fad really blossomed in 1970, with the publication of *The Psychology of Consciousness* by psychologist and science popularizer Robert Ornstein. According to Ornstein, Western culture in general and Western schools in particular have put a near-exclusive emphasis on the logical, mathematical, language-based skills of the brain's left hemisphere while letting the more intuitive skills of the right brain go to waste. Although these left-brain modes of thought form the foundation of the West's technological, rational culture, he said, Western men and women have been using only half their mental capacity. By contrast, right-brain abilities are far more developed in the intuitive, mystical cultures of the East. In the book's aftermath, many adherents took the debate much further than had Ornstein himself. The resulting wave of enthusiasm included everything from mail-order pop-psychology tapes urging listeners to awaken the latent creativity of their right hemispheres to social theorists equating the left hemisphere with all the evils of modern society.

Most responsible scientists dismiss such either-or dichotomies as simply wrongheaded. For one thing, tests on split-brain patients reveal considerable variation in each hemisphere's specialty. Language does not always dwell exclusively in the left hemisphere, for instance, and spatial ability does not always concentrate entirely in the right. More significant, brain scans show activity in both hemispheres all the time.

Long before MANSCAN, Alan Gevins and his colleagues found that even the simplest mental tasks generated a pattern of brain waves that spread rapidly over the cortex. "When you're reading or writing, it isn't as if the left half of your brain is turned on and the right half is turned off," says Gevins. "There are many areas on both sides of the brain involved in the process of comprehending and expressing language."

Many scientists agree that every situation requires both sets of skills. Indeed, together the halves of the brain wield far more power than either could by itself. When we read a story, for example, our left hemisphere translates the written words and figures out the meanings of complex sentences. At the same time, our right brain appreciates the humor and the emotional content, fitting new events and characters into the general story framework and comparing the tale with past experiences.

Elkhonon Goldberg and Louis Costa, cognitive neuroscientists at the Medical College of Pennsylvania and the University of Victoria in British Columbia, respectively, suggest that the right brain is not so much a center for artistry as a jack-of-all-trades: It tackles new problems by trying one solution after another until it finds one that works. The left hemisphere, in their view, functions as a specialist, able to solve familiar problems quickly by using well-tested methods. PET-scan studies appear to support this theory, showing activity in the right brain while the subject learns new tasks. After the tasks have become familiar, the left brain seems to take over. The way we listen to music provides an example. Most people recognize melodies with their right brains; to them, the *Nutcracker Suite* may be simply an enjoyable, familiar musical work. But professional musicians—who are likely to recall compositions in terms of structure, chord progression, and harmony—use their left.

The interplay between the two hemispheres provides valuable clues, but researchers still cannot explain how the brain's specialized components give rise to the vaporous force we call consciousness—the mind capable of a single, coherent perception of the world and of purposeful, coordinated behavior. Perhaps no one has attacked the problem more doggedly and systematically than Antonio and Hanna Damasio. The couple, working together at the University of Iowa Hospital, have spent more than 15 years assembling the records of some 1,500 brain-injured patients, the most extensive compendium of its kind in the history of brain science.

This immense body of experience with brain damage has led Antonio Damasio, in particular, to challenge the prevailing view of how brain function is organized and to offer an alternative. According to conventional wisdom, the brain's structure follows a kind of hierarchy: "Low-level" sensory neurons select relevant details from swarms of real-world stimuli and relay summaries up to "high-level" neurons, which refine these snippets of data and splice them together. The information arrives at the hierarchy's

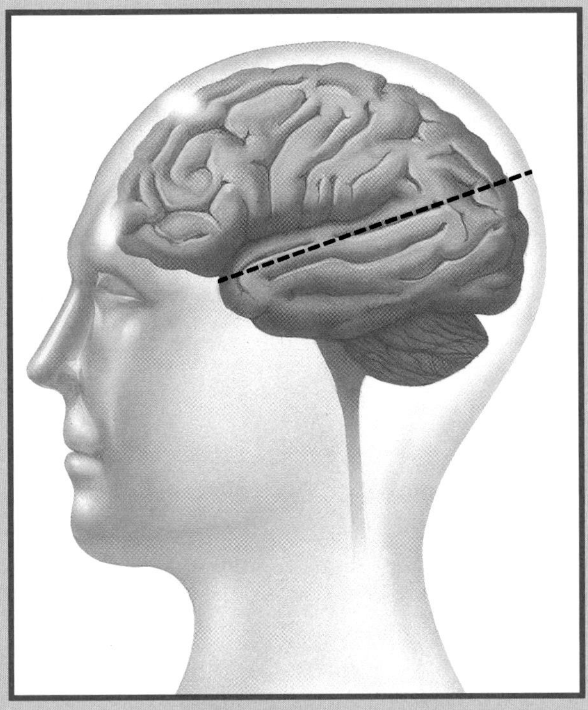

Getting to Know the Asymmetrical Brain

In the latter part of the 19th century, French surgeon Paul Broca and German neurologist Carl Wernicke pinpointed areas in the left hemisphere of the cerebral cortex that seemed to be responsible for specific language functions—Broca's area for producing speech, Wernicke's for understanding the sounds of language. Although most scientists accepted Broca's declaration, in 1861, that "Nous parlons avec l'hemisphere gauche!" ("We speak with the left hemisphere!"), this functional specialization was long assumed not to be reflected anatomically, in differences between the brain's two hemispheres; outwardly, at least, the brain appears to be essentially bilateral and symmetrical.

As shown in the schematized drawings here and on the following two pages, however, the right and left hemispheres differ substantially in the amount of area associated with language. In addition, scientists have found in recent decades that emotion-based, or affective, functions—once thought to be the purview of the whole brain—are also localized, this time in the right hemisphere. The counterpart in the right hemisphere to Wernicke's area, for example, enables us to understand the emotional content of language—whether a tale is happy or sad. Similarly, the counterpart to Broca's area allows us to express our own emotion in speech or writing.

A diagonal incision through the cerebral cortex *(above),* from the occipital lobe to the tip of the temporal lobe, reveals the asymmetrical nature of the brain's two hemispheres *(below).* In the left hemisphere, the region called the temporal plane *(blue),* which houses Wernicke's area, the site involved in recognizing sounds as words, is significantly larger than its counterpart in the right hemisphere *(red),* which is part of the area responsible for recognizing emotional content.

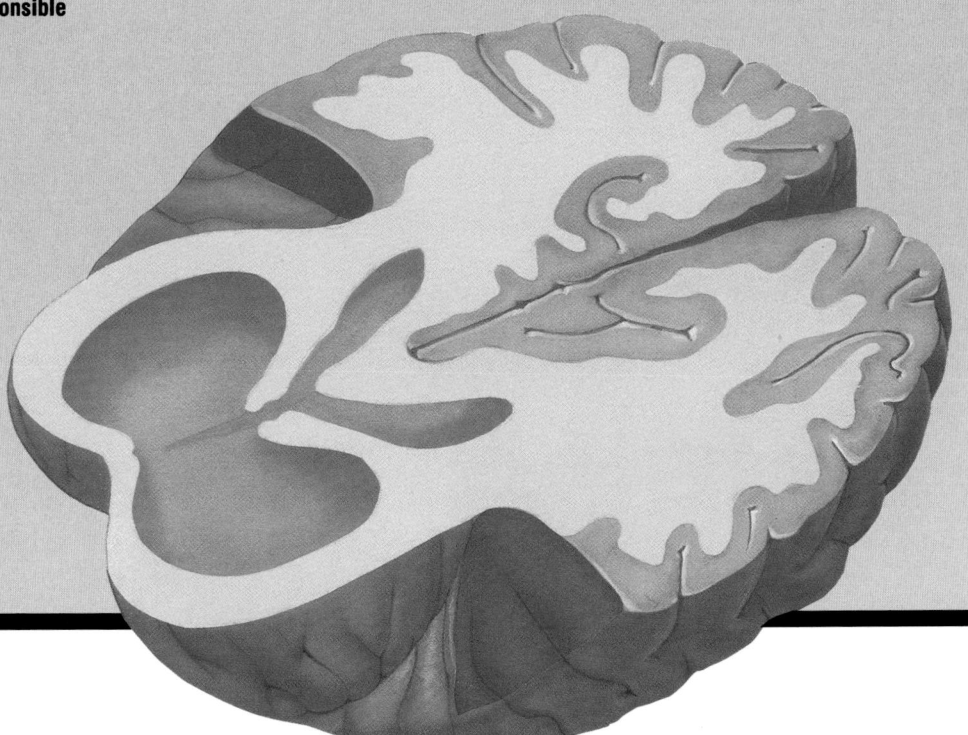

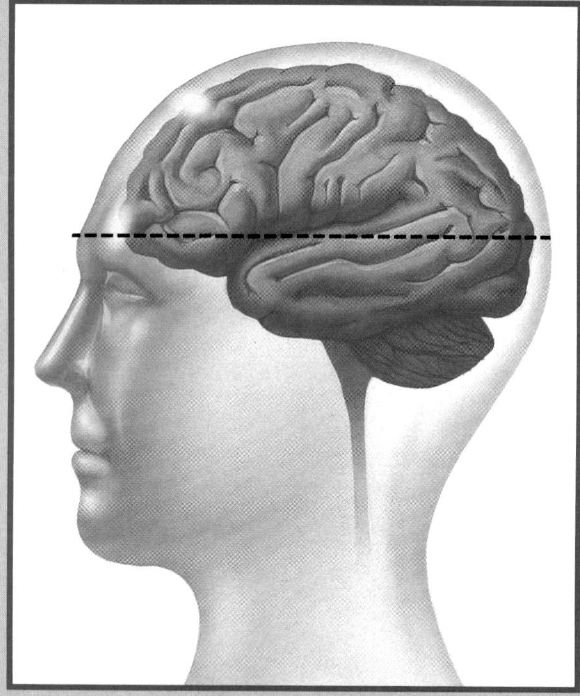

READING A WORD. A horizontal incision *(above)* uncovers regions responsible for language, according to a model *(below)* based on early studies. When a subject sees an object, information moves from the retina to the lateral geniculate nucleus *(1)*, which relays it to the primary visual cortex *(2)* and the higher-order visual area *(3)*. Other sense impressions join in at the parietal-temporal-occipital association cortex *(4)*. Then, this model postulated, the word is associated with meaning in Wernicke's area *(5)*, the memory for word articulation comes into play in Broca's area *(6)*, and pronunciation occurs via instructions from the facial area of the motor cortex *(7)*.

The Traces of Language

Until recently, nearly everything scientists knew about where in the brain different language functions reside came from studies of patients with various forms of aphasia, or language loss. Researchers analyzed the patients' difficulties with expressing and comprehending language, and then later conducted postmortem examinations of the brains of such patients to locate the lesions that might have caused the aphasia. Although the method was somewhat hit-or-miss, scientists could deduce, for instance, that a lesion in the neuronal pathway between Wernicke's area and Broca's area was the likely cause of a condition in which the patient is unable to use words correctly and—despite understanding what he hears and reads—cannot repeat even simple phrases.

With the refinement in the 1980s of noninvasive brain-imaging techniques such as PET and MRI scans (*opposite*), researchers have been able to watch the brain's language processes in action. By monitoring radioactive compounds introduced into the bloodstream, scientists can track the increased blood flow that indicates heightened activity in specific regions of the brain. Such techniques have enabled scientists not only to discover functional regions not found with the old methods but also to greatly refine their understanding of how the brain operates.

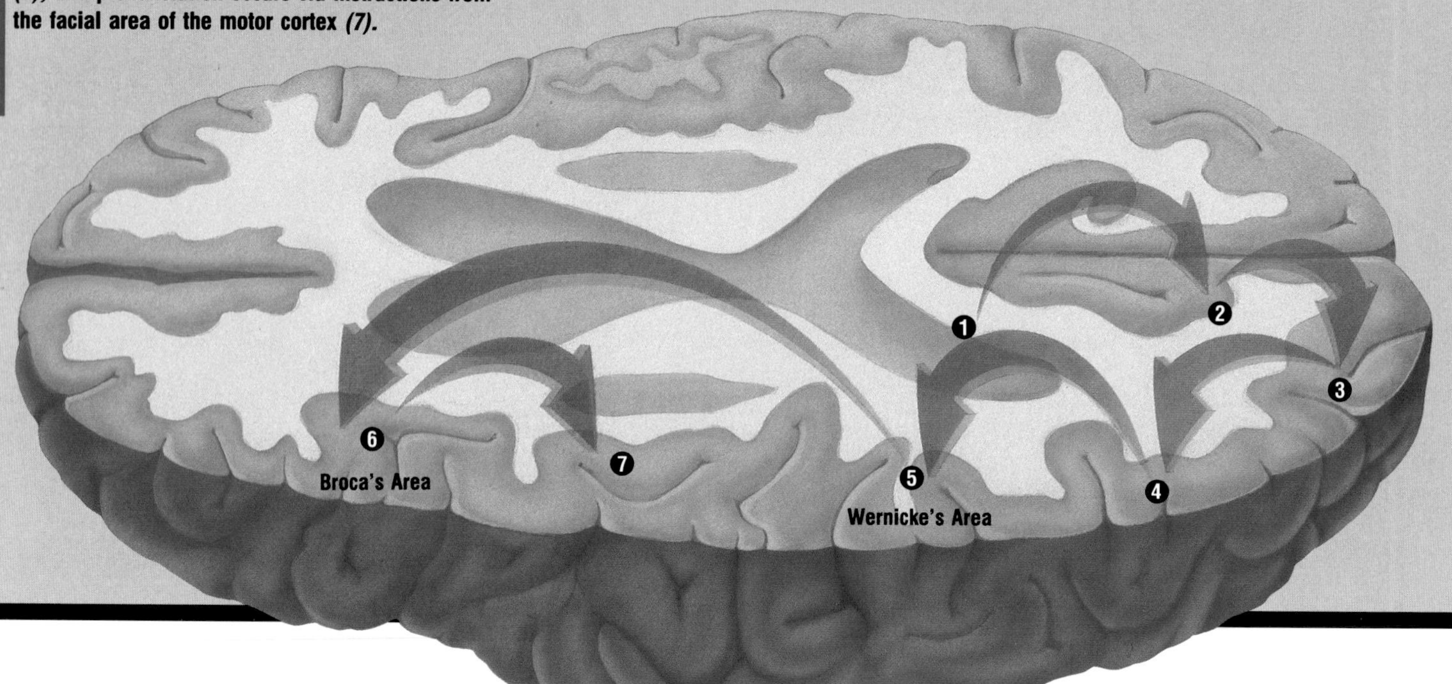

Superimposed over an MRI blueprint of neural structure is a composite of three PET images *(yellow and red dots),* each depicting a separate test of brain activity in the left hemisphere. Thinking about a word's meaning activates a region in the frontal lobe *(A),* speaking engages a region in the motor cortex *(B),* and silent reading activates part of the visual cortex *(C).* Images such as these show that the pathways of language are more complex than predicted by earlier models *(opposite).* Scans suggest, for example, that spoken language is identified as such in Wernicke's area, but that meaning is a function of several areas, including the frontal lobe, working together.

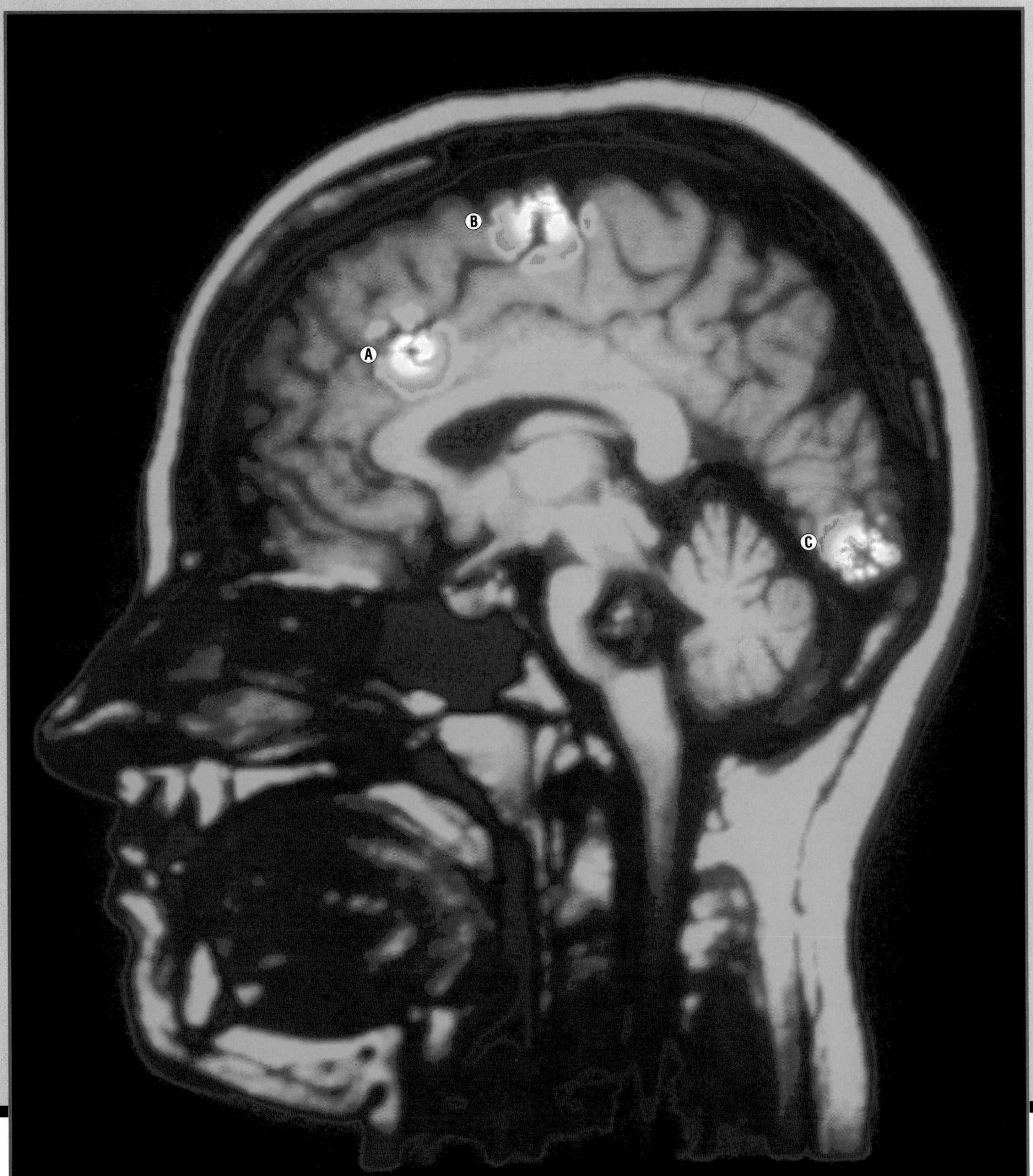

To the brain, language is language, whether expressed in spoken words or hand signals *(below)*. Generally, gestures and spatial perception are the province of the brain's right hemisphere. But studies with deaf subjects reveal that sign language is processed in the same specialized areas of the left hemisphere as spoken language.

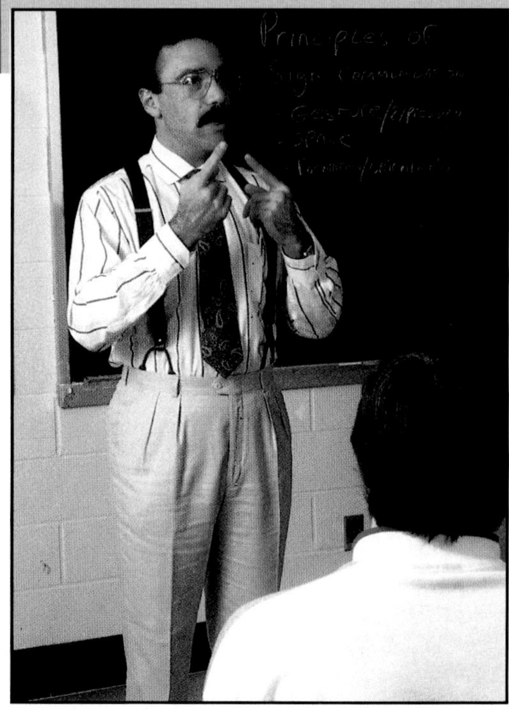

highest levels, which presumably correspond to the conscious mind, as a distilled version of the experience —something like the final cut of a motion picture.

The problem with this view, according to Damasio, is that, unlike images on film, the pictures produced by the brain are not fixed. Characters, plot, setting, dialogue—all are subject to infinite revision and substitution. Instead of Humphrey Bogart, why not cast Ronald Reagan in *Casablanca*, or even Danny DeVito? If the brain had to store every possible combination, real or imagined, it would have to be infinitely large. "People know this," says Damasio, "but they don't have a clear idea of how memory can be represented otherwise. We're trying to come up with a workable idea."

Damasio's first insight into how memory might be organized came in the late 1970s, when he examined a 65-year-old woman who had a curious disability: She could not recognize people's faces. The woman had suffered a stroke several months earlier and apparently had recovered. Her vision was normal, and her memory was sound. Yet she could not identify her husband's face, nor even her own. To her, a face was as meaningless as a word in a foreign language.

The woman's condition, called prosopagnosia, was unusual but not unknown. According to the conventional view of brain organization, her stroke had knocked out a region of the cerebral cortex that was specialized for one thing: recognizing faces. But when Damasio examined the woman more closely, he discovered that her difficulties with recognition involved more than faces. She could not distinguish her car from the one parked next to it, or her socks from her husband's. Damasio tested other prosopagnostics, with similar results. A dairy farmer could not tell one cow from another. A bird watcher had lost the ability to identify birds.

To Damasio, it was absurd to imagine special nerve networks for recognizing faces, socks, and cows—or, for that matter, that this region of the brain would store memories of individual objects at all. Instead, he began to think of it as a "convergence zone," an area where the brain brings together the myriad visual details that allow it to distinguish one object from others like it.

Going further, Damasio hypothesized that the brain contains not just one but a complex hierarchy of convergence zones. The prosopagnostics he studied had retained the lower zones that link up the small number of features that indicate a face is a face, for example, and not a birdbath. They had also retained the higher-level convergence zones that allowed them to connect diverse general characteristics such as gait, voice, and name. But they had lost the intermediate zones that allowed them to distinguish unique visual images, be they faces, birds, or automobiles.

The only thing actually stored in a convergence zone, according to Damasio's theory, is information about how to link knowledge fragments—the color of an eye, the curve of a cheekbone, the shape of a lip. The fragments remain scattered throughout the sensory cortex. In order to recognize an object or recall an image, the convergence zone has to summon together all the various fragments. In other words, instead of trying to store all possible images at the highest level, the brain attempts to reconstruct them by organizing fragments in different patterns, much as an artist can create infinite designs in mosaic from the same tiles. "There is no complete picture in any part of the brain," says Damasio. "You have to reconstruct it every time."

Somewhere in these convergence zones, presumably, lurks consciousness, the knowing mind. But Damasio, like most brain scientists, is extremely careful about what he claims in this area. Consciousness, as he knows full well, is a subtle and slippery notion.

As modern brain research has shown, "consciousness" refers to at least two distinct concepts, each arising from a different part of the brain. Consciousness as a state is the difference between being awake and being asleep or in a coma. Consciousness as a sense of self is the mysterious inner voice that gives form to thought, passes judgments, makes choices. And although philosophers and theologians have pondered this kind of consciousness for millennia, in many ways it still represents the ultimate imponderable. Many people would argue that it lies beyond the realm of science entirely.

Yet neuroscientists have known for a long time that thought, will, and judgment do have a reasonably precise location in the brain: the prefrontal cortex, which lies on the front of the frontal lobe, just behind the forehead. EEGs and other types of brain scans show that when a person or animal moves a limb, for example, the prefrontal cortex becomes active a fraction of a second before movement begins—a flicker that might represent the decision to move.

Furthermore, the prefrontal cortex contains a number of "gatekeeper" regions that greatly influence a person's ability to act. Patients with damage to the area known as the supplementary motor cortex, for example, are essentially creatures without a will. Their brains work perfectly well. They can talk to other people. They can understand the words they hear. But they have no volition. Ask them a question and they may answer the next day. Or they may just sit there, utterly inert.

The prefrontal cortex is likewise where the brain produces the so-called stream of consciousness, the set of thoughts the mind processes at any given time. More precisely, this area plays an important role in working memory, the mental blackboard where the brain briefly records its moment-to-moment awareness of the surrounding world, then combines it with knowledge and experience retrieved from long-term memory. Working memory is not a large blackboard. It can hold only five to 10 items at a time, for no more than 10 to 30 seconds each; new items drive out those already there.

Even so, Yale neuroscientist Patricia Goldman-Rakic has called working memory "perhaps the most significant achievement of human mental evolution." It is here that humans plan for the future and string together thoughts and ideas—to make a chess move, construct a sentence, drive a car, or simply daydream. Patients who have suffered damage to the prefrontal cortex can do very little of this sort of thinking. Although they may continue to score well on intelligence tests, they seem to be guided almost entirely by habit and reflex rather than by understanding events unfolding right in front of them.

Evidence indicates that most of consciousness dwells in the prefrontal cortex, but the mechanism of "awareness"—which scientists recognize as a separate state of alertness—is spread more widely throughout the brain.

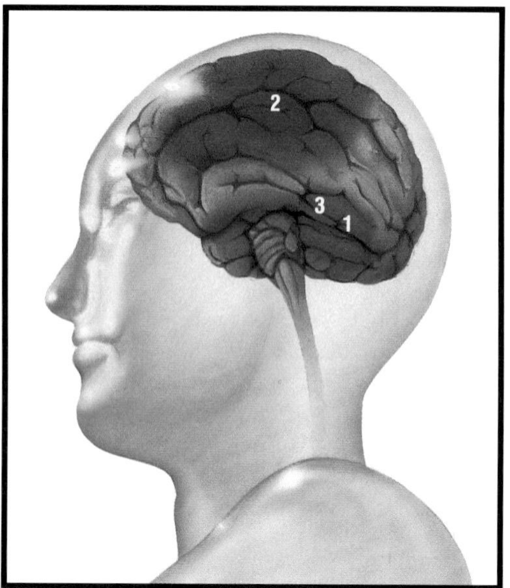

The ability to see and describe different hues is controlled largely by three regions in the cortex, as shown at left. In the back part of the lingual gyrus, a region *(1)* that includes the specialized higher-order visual area V4 *(pages 106-107)* oversees the initial perception of color. A section of the motor cortex involved in the production of spoken and written language *(2)* helps ensure correct pronunciation of all words. Part of the visual cortex *(3)* found in the front of the left lingual gyrus serves as mediator between areas 1 and 2, locating the appropriate word for a given color or, conversely, evoking a mental image to match a color term.

The Complex Task of Describing Color

Functioning normally, the brain can apprehend a color, turn it into a concept, then almost instantly match that concept with words or symbols. But according to University of Iowa neurologist Antonio Damasio, damage to certain regions of the cortex (*diagram, above*) can seriously impair these abilities. As shown here, three people with specific types of lesions have difficulty answering the simple question, "What color is the sky?" Their responses shed light on the function of each region and offer clues to the way the brain processes language.

To subject 1, the sky looks gray. Damage to a structure in the occipital lobe called the lingual gyrus—specifically, to the area that translates impulses from the eyes into color concepts—has stripped her mental palette of all pigment. Once able to see and imagine all colors, she now views everything in shades of black and white. Subject 2, by contrast, sees all colors normally. But because of a lesion in the part of the motor cortex that contains the machinery of language, he cannot properly form words. His brain perceives blue, but his tongue and lips mispronounce it "buh." Subject 3 recognizes all colors correctly and speaks without impediment. Yet damage to his mediation region, which lies largely in the forward part of the left lingual gyrus, makes him unable to link colors with the appropriate words. Thus, he sees a blue sky and calls it red.

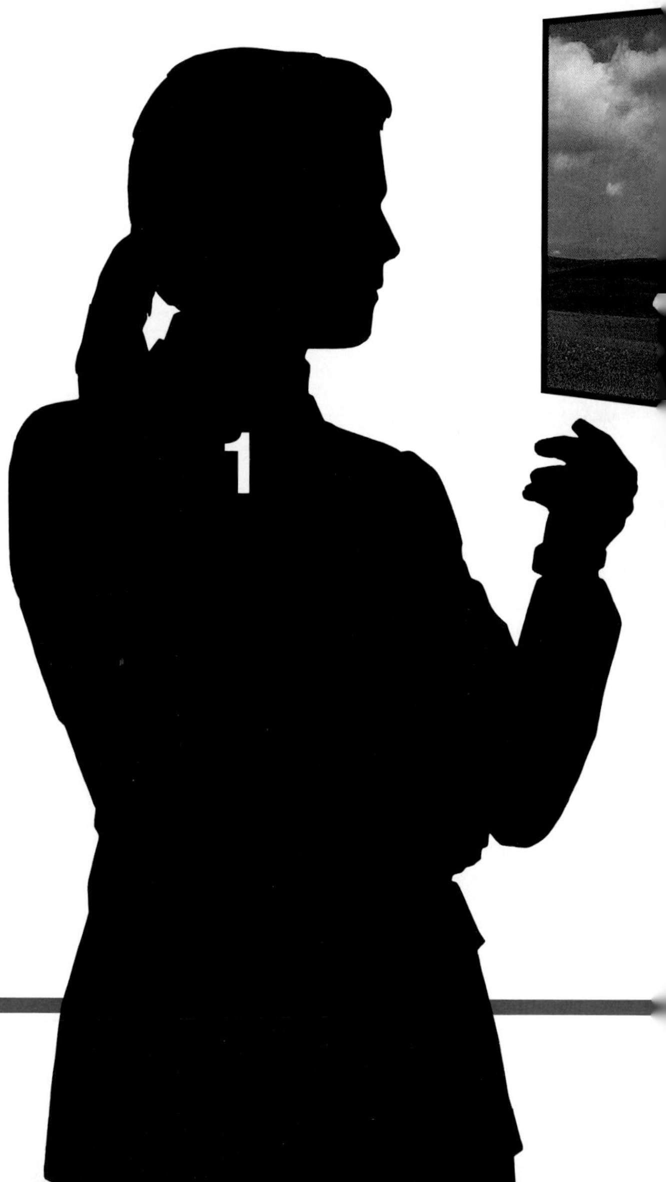

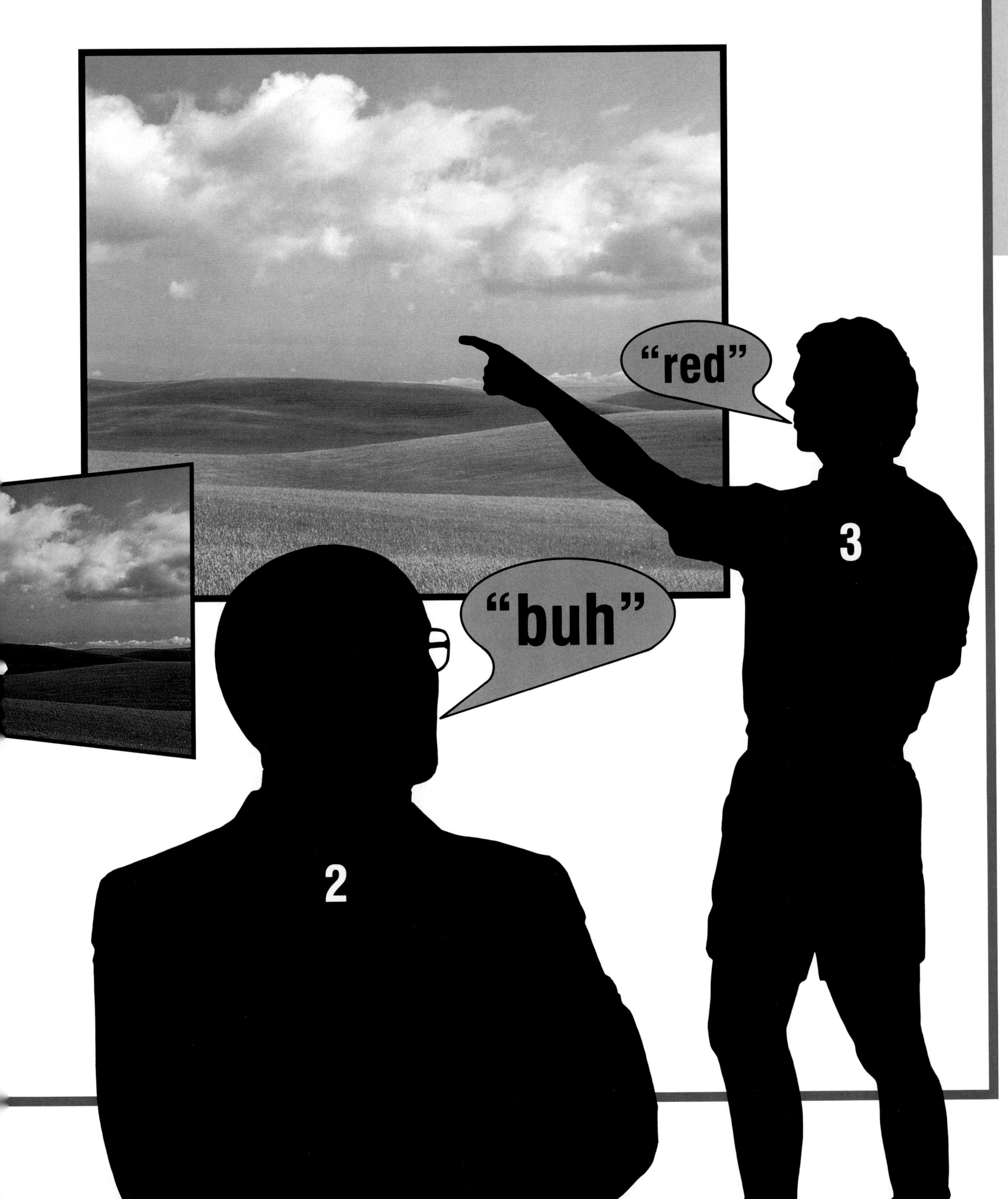
"red"
3
"buh"
2

Perhaps nothing illustrates the distinction between the two concepts more dramatically than the phenomenon called covert awareness. This bizarre ability to "know without knowing," in effect, was first described in 1917 by a neurologist who played a harmless trick on one of his patients, a woman who had suffered some brain damage and could not remember recent experiences. Once when they shook hands, he lightly pricked her finger with a concealed pin. Next time they met, she did not recognize him and had no memory of their previous encounter—yet she declined to shake hands. She did not know why, she said. She just had a feeling it might be "unpleasant."

Physicians and scientists turned up many similar cases over the years. But only in the mid-1970s did they begin to take a more systematic look at covert awareness. One notable example was the patient known as H. M. (*pages* 81-82), who could not form new memories. Extensive tests revealed that his ability to solve a puzzle steadily improved although he was unable to remember working on it. Later, in 1991, psychologist Melvyn Goodale and his colleagues at Western Ontario University in London, Ontario, tested a woman who had suffered carbon monoxide poisoning and had lost her ability to recognize objects and shapes. They found that she could not describe to them whether a pencil held in front of her was horizontal or vertical. And yet, she could reach out and grab the pencil without difficulty, as though her motor cortex was aware of information to which her conscious mind had no access.

In Iowa the Damasios have found many examples of covert awareness among their 1,500 brain-damage patients. Prosopagnostics, for example, cannot recognize faces. But when shown pictures of people they know, the patients' pulse rates increase, and they reveal other signs of recognition at some unconscious level. Equally intriguing is the Damasios' finding that brain damage can leave consciousness intact while blocking covert awareness—sometimes with odd and disturbing results.

In one recent case, a 35-year-old man they call E. V. R. suffered damage to a decision-making region in his prefrontal cortex during the removal of a brain tumor. Before the operation, E. V. R. had a successful career, a happy marriage, two children, and a blameless social life. Afterward, he passed every neuropsychological test. Yet within months he had forced himself into bankruptcy through questionable business deals. He divorced his wife and married a prostitute—who divorced him after six months—then married and divorced a third time. Since the surgery, E. V. R. has been unable to hold a job, and his uncharacteristic behavior continues.

The Damasios have studied four stroke patients who suffered damage to the same region of the frontal lobes as E. V. R., all of whom have undergone abrupt personality changes. In one experiment, the researchers hooked up E. V. R. and the four stroke patients to sensors that monitored, for example, pulse, perspiration, and blood pressure, factors controlled subconsciously by the autonomic nervous system. The Damasios then showed their subjects a series of slides depicting such grisly scenes as children being burned alive and people being cut into pieces—the kind of visceral jolt that would cause normal subjects to send the laboratory monitors off scale. But this group simply watched passively, showing no reaction at all. Afterward, however, when asked to discuss the scenes, the subjects used words such as "shock" and "disgust" in describing what they had seen.

To the Damasios, the patients have lost immediate access to their "gut feelings" of good and bad, pleasure and pain—to the area where the brain stores memories of reward and punishment. In everyday life, the

Damasios suggest, this memory repository serves as a form of covert awareness that guides our decisions more than we realize; lack of such guidance is presumably what led E. V. R. to make a mess of his life. The puzzling thing, of course, is that E. V. R. and his fellow unfortunates evidently could tap the memories during discussion of the slides, presumably by routing them through their undamaged verbal channels.

Scientists who investigate covert awareness hope it will someday explain a number of other puzzling memory quirks, such as déjà vu—that eerie feeling of familiarity without recognition—and posthypnotic states, in which patients can repeat things learned under hypnosis without recalling how they learned them. Meanwhile, efforts to locate and explain consciousness continue in diverse scientific fields.

One of the most radical approaches has been taken by the Massachusetts Institute of Technology's Marvin Minsky, a pioneer in the field of artificial intelligence and author of the 1987 book *Society of Mind*. "I think consciousness is an illusion," he says.

Minsky suggests the mind consists of a huge number of simple neural processors, which he calls agents. Individually, these agents have no brain power; their strength lies in their ability to join forces with other agents by way of myriad connections. Larger groups of agents, called agencies, pursue common goals in a machine-like way. In other words, no one is in charge. Knowledge of any sort does not reside in a particular spot in the brain; rather, it is spread out across an intricate web of connections. If a person knows how to ride a bicycle, for example, it is because numerous little processes needed for bike riding—vision, balance, and so on—have learned to exploit one another. Although Minsky's "agencies" are reminiscent of Donald Hebb's "cell assemblies," Minsky believes that agencies are the end of the story. "The brain is just hundreds of different machines connected to each other by bundles of nerve fibers," he says. "There isn't any 'you.' "

Not everyone goes that far, but many scientists suspect that Minsky is right in one sense. With so many neural subsystems operating in parallel, the mind is much more like an uneasy coalition than an all-powerful executive ego. As split-brain researcher Michael Gazzaniga, now at the University of California in Davis, has put it: "The mind is not a psychological entity but a sociological entity."

Our subjective sense of being a unified consciousness is, as Gazzaniga might put it, just slick public relations. A left-brain system he calls the interpreter watches what the body is actually doing and sensing—that is, the interplay of the competing neural subroutines—and then, after the fact, tries to make up a coherent story about why the body behaved as it did. This story is what creates a sense of mental unity, of self.

Roger Sperry's work with split-brain patients in the 1960s laid much of the groundwork for the interpreter theory, suggesting that the left hemisphere manufactures some sort of rationale for behavior initiated by the right. But perhaps the most compelling evidence has come from a series of experiments that Gazzaniga conducted at Cornell University beginning in 1975 with Joseph LeDoux, one of his students at the time. Their chief subject was a 15-year-old split-brain patient known as P. S., who had undergone the operation as treatment for severe epilepsy.

In one key experiment, LeDoux and Gazzaniga projected pairs of pictures on a screen in front of P. S. in such a way that his right brain could perceive only one image and his left brain the other. Then the scientists

Computer Glimpses into Chaos

With their tracings of voltage shifts beneath the scalp, EEGs (*right, top*) are far from lucid windows on the mind, supplying only an approximate notion of brain activity. But a new branch of science called chaos theory is turning those cryptic squiggles into distinctive patterns, the very shape of thought.

Through a range of advanced mathematical techniques, chaos theory reveals underlying order in wildly complicated phenomena, from the workings of the weather to the turbulence of boiling water. Its approach is a kind of geometric magic: The functioning of any given system is represented as movements of a single abstract point within an imaginary space made up of many dimensions—the minimum number required to describe the system as a whole. The movements, calculated by computer, sketch an image that theorists evocatively call a "strange attractor," a reference to a complex system's attraction to particular states—its deep order.

The two attractors at right were created by Paul Rapp of the Medical College of Pennsylvania, a pioneer in applying chaos theory to neuroscience. Derived from two EEGs with similar patterns of peaks and valleys, they are very different—proof of the technique's power of finding structure in confusion.

lined up a number of small pictures and asked P. S. to use both hands to point to images that related to those he had seen on the screen. This he could do quite easily. When a snow scene appeared to his right brain and a chicken claw to his left, he dutifully pointed with each hand to pictures of a snow shovel and a chicken.

The surprise came when LeDoux and Gazzaniga asked, "What did you see?" Using the language centers of his left brain, P. S. replied, "I saw a claw and I picked the chicken, and you have to clean out the chicken shed with a shovel." His left brain had no idea why his left hand (controlled by his right brain) had pointed to the shovel; it had not seen the snow scene and had no way of learning about it. And yet, in its response, the left brain attempted to explain—or interpret—the actions of the right.

The young man gave similar responses in trial after trial. When the scientists flashed the written command "laugh" to his right hemisphere, for example, P. S. did indeed laugh. But when asked why, his left brain replied, "You guys come up and test us every month. What a way to make a living!" When the command "walk" was flashed to his right hemisphere, P. S. stood up to leave. "I'm going in the house to get a Coke," he told the researchers.

These and similar experiments led LeDoux and Gazzaniga to the interpreter theory of consciousness. "The emerging picture is that our cognitive system is not a unified network with a single purpose and train of thought," they later wrote. "A more accurate metaphor is that our sense of subjective awareness arises out of our dominant left hemisphere's unrelenting need to explain actions taken from any one of a multitude of mental systems that dwell within us."

At first glance, Gazzaniga's interpreter theory of consciousness seems to have little to do with Antonio Damasio's convergence-zone theory of perception and coordination. Yet the two theories go together quite well if, in fact, the convergence process is what actually produces the interpretation. This is essentially the theory that Tufts University philosopher Daniel Dennett put forward in 1991.

Dennett, among the handful of philosophers who pay serious attention to neuroscience, compares the various functional networks of the brain to a "Pandemonium of Homunculi": a riotous swarm of imps who clamor and compete for attention. (In medieval lore, a homunculus was a tiny human being supposedly conjured in an alchemist's test tube.) In the brain, each of these "imps" concentrates on a particular aspect of perception. One might analyze shape, for instance,

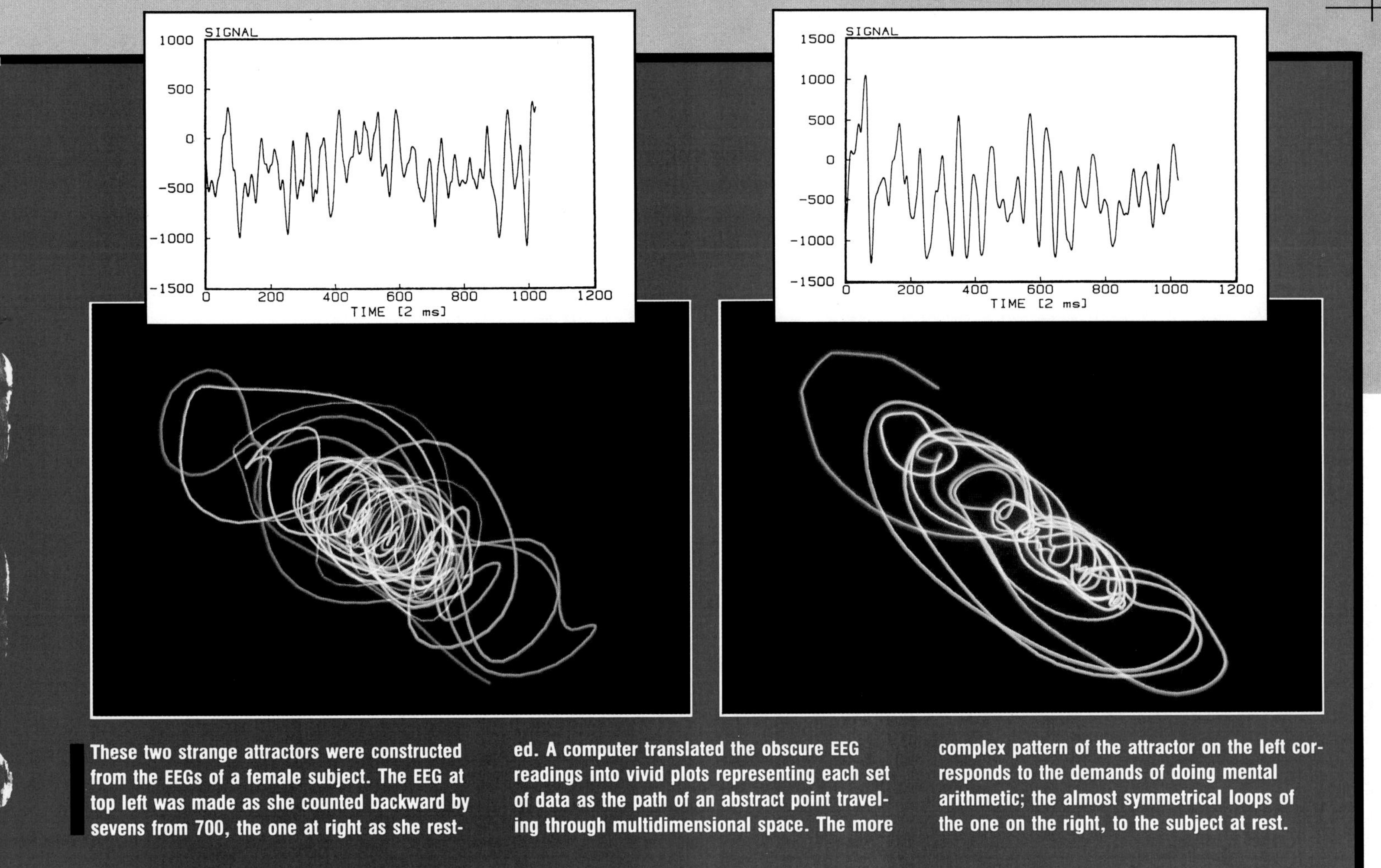

These two strange attractors were constructed from the EEGs of a female subject. The EEG at top left was made as she counted backward by sevens from 700, the one at right as she rested. A computer translated the obscure EEG readings into vivid plots representing each set of data as the path of an abstract point traveling through multidimensional space. The more complex pattern of the attractor on the left corresponds to the demands of doing mental arithmetic; the almost symmetrical loops of the one on the right, to the subject at rest.

while another deals with language or motion. As they perform their individual duties, says Dennett, they also communicate among themselves about the meaning of incoming data.

Like teams of indefatigable scribes, these imp networks form coalitions that produce collated, revised, and enhanced drafts of the interpretation. "Information entering the nervous system is under continuous 'editorial revision,' " Dennett says, "so that at any point in time there are multiple 'drafts' of narrative fragments at various stages of editing in various places in the brain."

As the multiple drafts come together—possibly in Damasio-style convergence zones—they sometimes coalesce, sometimes conflict. But ultimately, after a great deal of editing, the mind experiences this evolving interpretation of events as a sort of silent narrative, one coherent stream of consciousness that produces what appear to be consecutive thoughts.

Still another theory of consciousness—the synchronization model—also happens to work well with convergence zones and evolving interpretations. It may also solve a major problem with all such theories: explaining how the brain's many networks actually communicate. In neural terms, the brain is an incredibly noisy place, with signals running in every direction. For two brain networks to communicate amid this neural din is like trying to hold a quiet conversation at a rock concert.

The first hints of how the brain succeeds in doing just that came to light in 1986, when neuroscientists Charles Gray of the Salk Institute and Wolf Singer of the Max Planck Institute in Germany found that cooperating neurons do not actually communicate directly. Instead—as theorized by Donald Hebb nearly four decades earlier—they reinforce each other in a process Gray and Singer called "phase locking," in which the neurons synchronize their firing rate. The researchers inserted a number of electrodes into the brains of anesthetized cats or monkeys; then, as they beamed light onto an animal's retina, they watched signal patterns appear and begin to mesh. "These responses would start; they would coalesce; they would phase-lock in," says Gray. "That would last for a certain number of cycles, and then as the stimuli left the receptive fields or changed, the reaction changed."

These observations led quickly to the idea that synchronization is the brain's way of pulling things together. When the eyes focus on a bus, for example, separate populations of nerve cells—those responding to the color, shape, texture, motion, smell, and sound of the bus—all send out impulses at the same firing rate. That synchronization holds for a fraction of a second, during which time the network of perceptions coalesces to form the conscious perception of a bus.

Neither Gray nor Singer is eager to speculate about the broader implications of these findings. As Gray cheerfully admits, synchronized firings could be like the redness of blood: there, but not important. Redness is simply a by-product of the chemistry of hemoglobin, and the brain's oscillations may be just as meaningless. Other scientists, however, are not so shy. Antonio Damasio, for example, speculates that synchronization plays a key role in the operation of his hypothetical convergence zones. Maybe consciousness occurs when higher- and lower-level convergence zones fire simultaneously, causing the whole hierarchy effectively to light up like a hotel switchboard.

The possibility of coming to grips with the ineffable is exciting and compelling for many in the field. But there remains one significant hurdle. After all, this emphasis on the neuronal basis of the mind leaves out a fundamental part of our conscious selves—namely, feelings, or more precisely, what philosophers call the subjective state of being. Convergence zones, interpreters, and synchronization cannot yet explain what it feels like to perceive the color red or to taste a peach. Nor can those theories pinpoint the *you* that feels the pain of biting your tongue.

Some scientists and philosophers are convinced these questions will never be answered—that the human mind is simply not equipped to understand itself at the deepest level. "It's like monkeys trying to do physics," offers philosopher Colin McGinn of Rutgers University. "It's just not available to us." Moreover, many people seem to prefer that state of affairs. The attempt to explain human nature in terms of the functioning of cells in the brain is distasteful to them, an exercise that reduces the human spirit to something mechanical, less than human.

Cognitive neuroscientist Christof Koch of Caltech disagrees. In his view, the more scientists learn about the workings of the mind, the more magnificent and unknowable it becomes. Even if it turns out that "neurons are all there is," Koch argues, "I don't think this should take away any of the wonder. It certainly hasn't diminished my sense of admiration for how logic or speech or Beethoven comes out of these tiny things."

Perhaps, as Nobel Prize winner David Hubel suggests, the difficulty lies less in the magnitude of the task we have set ourselves—daunting though that task may be—than in the words we use when we talk about trying to "understand" the mind or the brain. "The problem comes when we ask about understanding," Hubel says, "because such a word carries with it the implication of a sudden revelation or dawning, the existence of a moment when we might be said to leave the darkness of the tunnel. It is not clear to me that there can be such a moment, or that we will know it when it comes."

UNDERSTANDING THE ACT OF PERCEPTION

One of the reasons communication is often so difficult—and eyewitnesses so often unreliable—is that we each carry around a lifetime's worth of memories and experiences that color our perceptions of reality. What we see and hear at any given moment is deeply influenced by what we have seen or heard or felt in the past. Say, for example, that a vacationer has just returned, painfully sunburned, from Hawaii. As he walks past a church, he sees the title of Sunday's sermon: "Relief for the Sunburned Soul." On second glance, the words turn out to be "Sin-burdened Soul." Later, he is stunned when the waiter at a restaurant asks, "How was Hawaii?" The question was actually, "How is the wine?" Both times, the things that were literally "on his mind" determined what the vacationer saw and heard.

These memory-based expectations are highly dynamic. As some investigators theorize, our brains seem to spend a lot of time mentally revising who we are, what the world is, and thus what we expect to perceive. As illustrated on the following pages, perceptions are not only shaped by short- and long-term memories, they also interact with those memories and with new sensory information to adjust the frameworks for future perceptions.

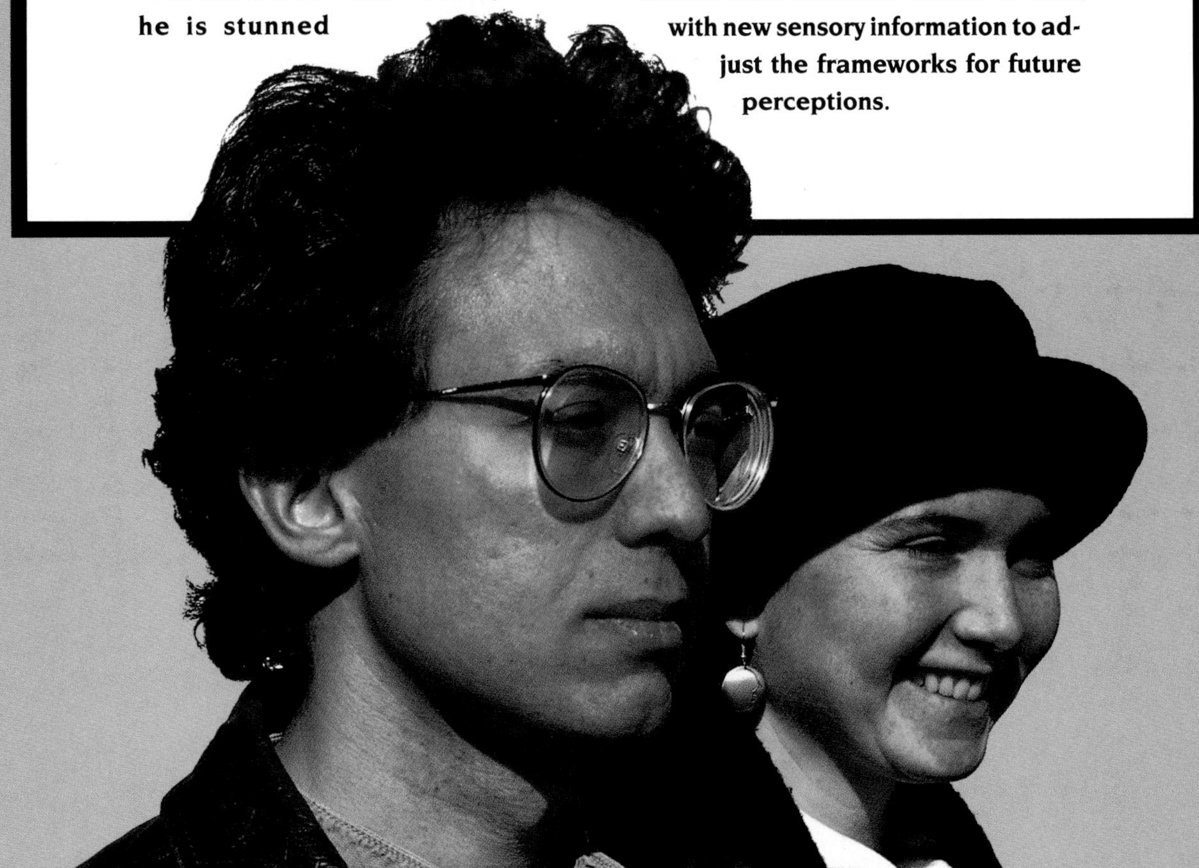

TWO PEOPLE AND TWO VIEWS OF THE WORLD

Scientists use the term "perceptual framework" to describe the memories—images, sounds, textures, smells, emotions—that shape our expectations. Although certain memories and associations may not be wholly applicable to the situation at hand, the mind draws on them to interpret reality. Moreover, since our memories are unique to each of us, so too are the lenses through which we view the world. In a sense, then, we each create our own reality—a notion that might smack of mysticism or science fiction but is receiving serious attention from brain researchers.

A given perceptual framework is both powerful and fleeting. Every in-

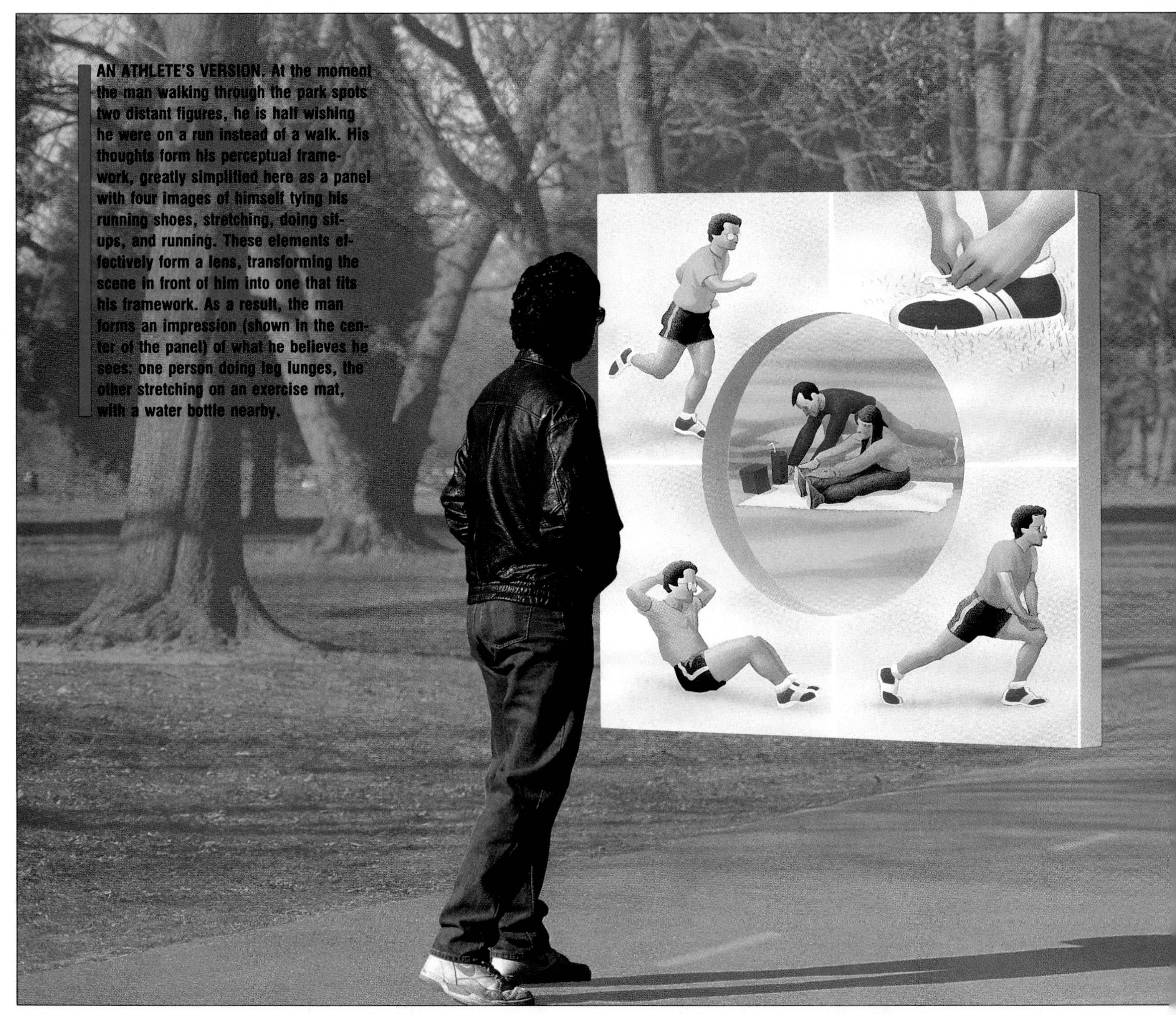

AN ATHLETE'S VERSION. At the moment the man walking through the park spots two distant figures, he is half wishing he were on a run instead of a walk. His thoughts form his perceptual framework, greatly simplified here as a panel with four images of himself tying his running shoes, stretching, doing sit-ups, and running. These elements effectively form a lens, transforming the scene in front of him into one that fits his framework. As a result, the man forms an impression (shown in the center of the panel) of what he believes he sees: one person doing leg lunges, the other stretching on an exercise mat, with a water bottle nearby.

stant a new sight, sound, sensation, or thought modifies the current version. Thus, not only will two people perceive the same thing differently, but one person will perceive the same thing differently at different times.

The scenario depicted below and on the following pages describes in highly simplified form the effects of separate perceptual frameworks on the experiences of two people who are strolling through a park, beginning with the moment they notice two figures in the distance. When someone shouts the word "dog," the new stimulus activates memories and associations (*overleaf*) that will alter the pair's existing frameworks.

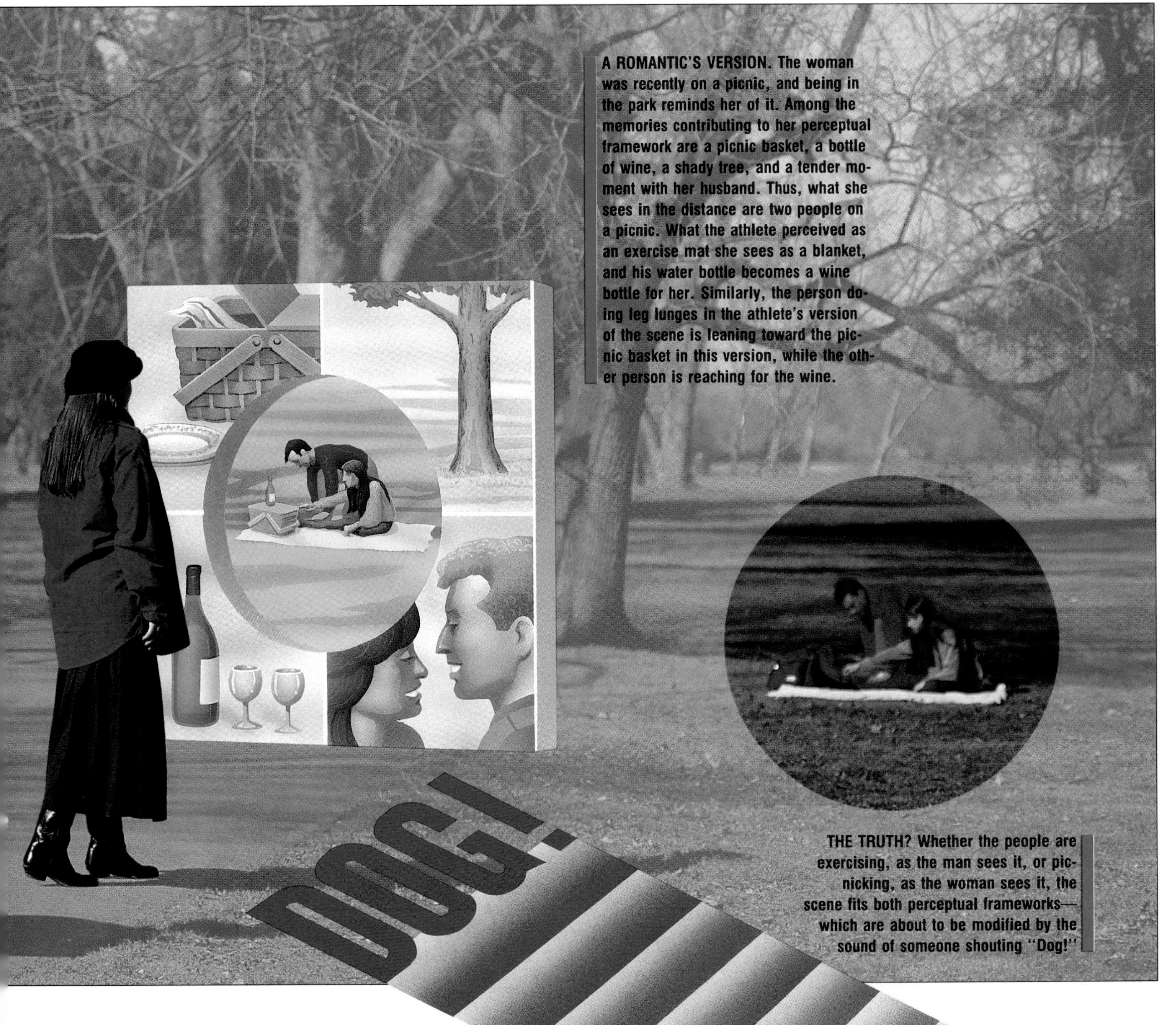

A ROMANTIC'S VERSION. The woman was recently on a picnic, and being in the park reminds her of it. Among the memories contributing to her perceptual framework are a picnic basket, a bottle of wine, a shady tree, and a tender moment with her husband. Thus, what she sees in the distance are two people on a picnic. What the athlete perceived as an exercise mat she sees as a blanket, and his water bottle becomes a wine bottle for her. Similarly, the person doing leg lunges in the athlete's version of the scene is leaning toward the picnic basket in this version, while the other person is reaching for the wine.

THE TRUTH? Whether the people are exercising, as the man sees it, or picnicking, as the woman sees it, the scene fits both perceptual frameworks—which are about to be modified by the sound of someone shouting "Dog!"

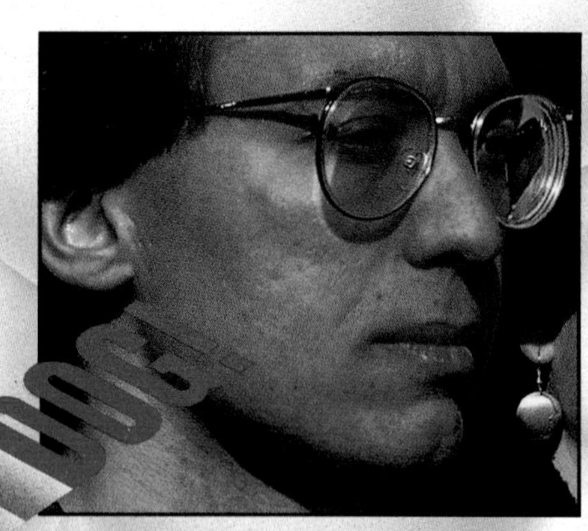

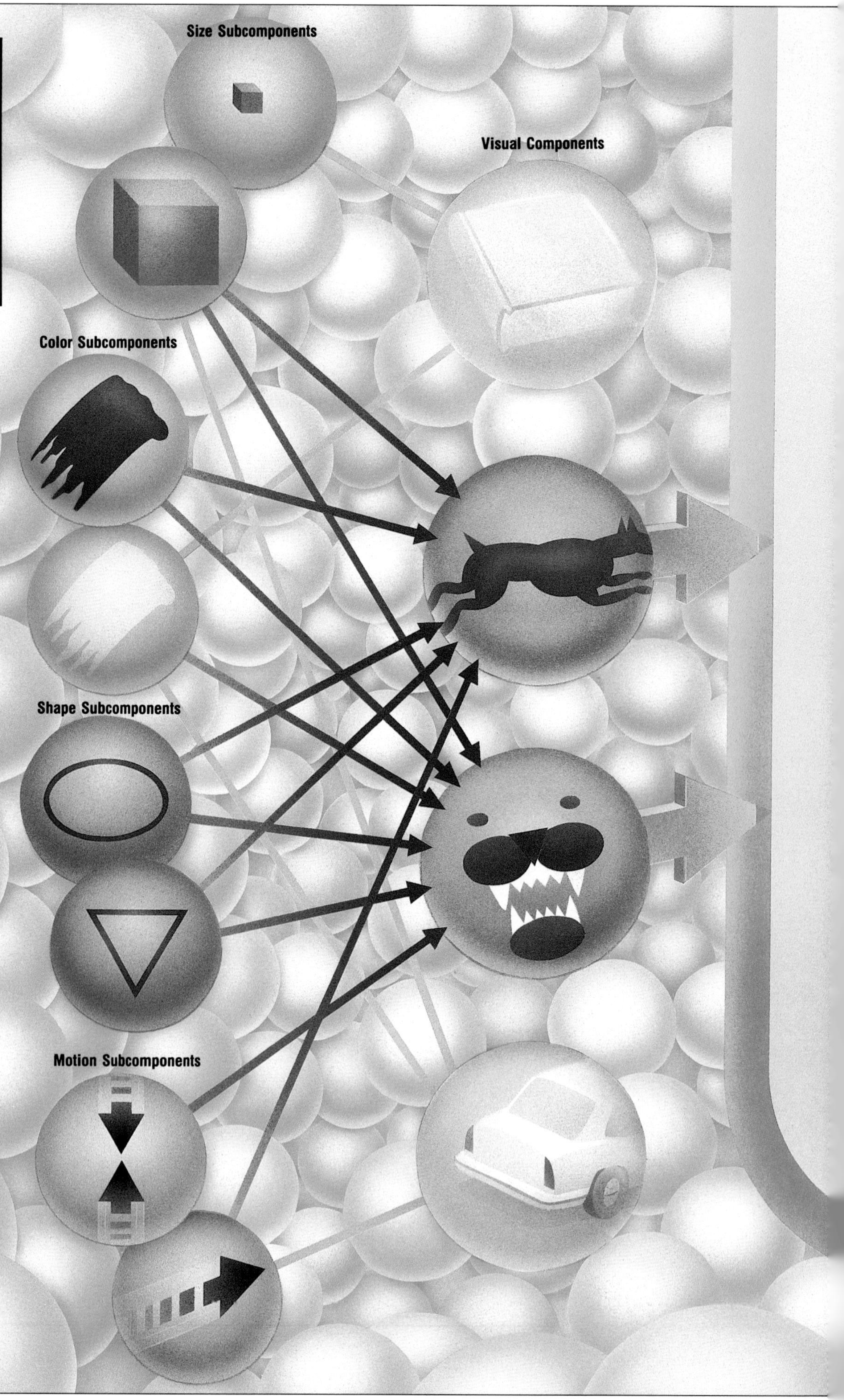

Size Subcomponents

Visual Components

Color Subcomponents

Shape Subcomponents

Motion Subcomponents

INTEGRATING THE PARTS OF MEMORY. According to one theory of memory, the brain reduces the concept of an object into many smaller subcomponents *(blue spheres)*. Any object has such visible features as size, shape, color, and motion (or lack thereof). It also has other sensory features such as smell, taste, and texture, as well as nonsensory verbal or emotional attributes. The theory suggests that, in the act of perception, each feature activates its own cluster of neurons—which are reactivated in the act of recall. Thus, the cluster for "roundness" could be triggered by stimuli as varied as a puppy's tummy or a full moon, and "forward motion" could be triggered by a charging bull or a speeding car.

In the example shown here, the word "dog!" excites a number of subcomponents in the brain of the man at the park that reflect his personal experience. He has been chased by dogs while running, for instance, and was once bitten. The word thus triggers visual subcomponents that tend to reflect his negative predisposition—large (body), triangles (teeth), white (teeth again), and up-and-down motion (snapping jaws)—as well as more neutral elements such as ovals (eyes) and brown (fur). The subcomponents (some of which might also be activated by, say, a book or a police car) come together to form larger dog-related assemblages (pink spheres). Along with related nonvisual elements *(far right)*, the visual components may be combined by an integration area or areas to conjure the mental image of a ferocious canine *(opposite)*.

BUILDING A CONCEPT FROM FRAGMENTS OF MEMORY

Any stimulus triggers a number of responses in the brain, but the nature of those responses—which areas are stimulated and to what degree—varies widely from one person to another, depending on individual experience. Hearing the word "dog," for instance, will induce one response in the listener if the word is shouted in a loud, angry voice, another if the speaker is a giggling child. Moreover, a given listener will respond one way if his experience with dogs has been largely pleasant and quite differently if he carries scars from a nasty encounter with a Doberman pinscher.

Whatever reactions are triggered, the process can be extraordinarily complex. Many researchers think that the brain does not store memories as coherent units but rather as discrete fragments, or subcomponents, that reside as patterns of interaction among small groups of neurons. The neuronal pattern that encodes the color white, for example, may well be evoked in recalling vanilla ice cream, a sheet of paper, or snow.

Although scientists think they have a fair understanding of how the brain might create visual subcomponents, they are less certain of the breakdown of input from other senses. More difficult still are abstract stimuli. How does the brain store the concept of "freedom," for example, or anger, or pity? In any event, how all the pieces of information come together remains a deep mystery. One theory, illustrated here, involves a hierarchy of widely distributed encoding areas. Another theory stresses temporal rather than spatial integration, suggesting that the various neuronal networks may synchronize their firing rates for a fraction of a second.

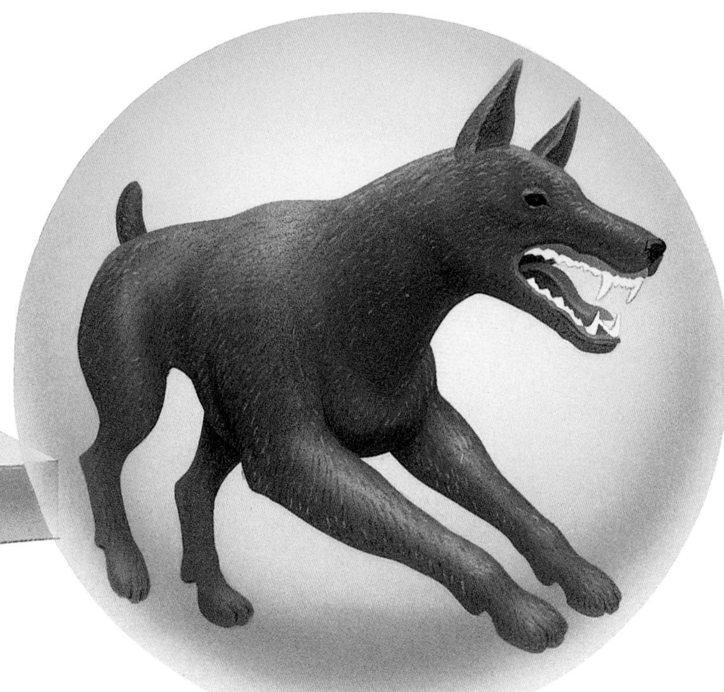

UPDATING THE FRAMEWORKS

Once a stimulus has been processed through the brain's assortment of neuronal clusters, it interacts with an individual's existing perceptual framework to produce a new framework. Depending on the particular memories and associations that are triggered by the stimulus, the revised version may turn out to be quite similar to the original one or drastically different from it. Because this revision—despite its phenomenal complexity—takes only a fraction of a second, it will instantly influence ongoing acts of perception. Indeed, we experience these revisions several hundred thousand times a day.

As the man and woman in this ex-

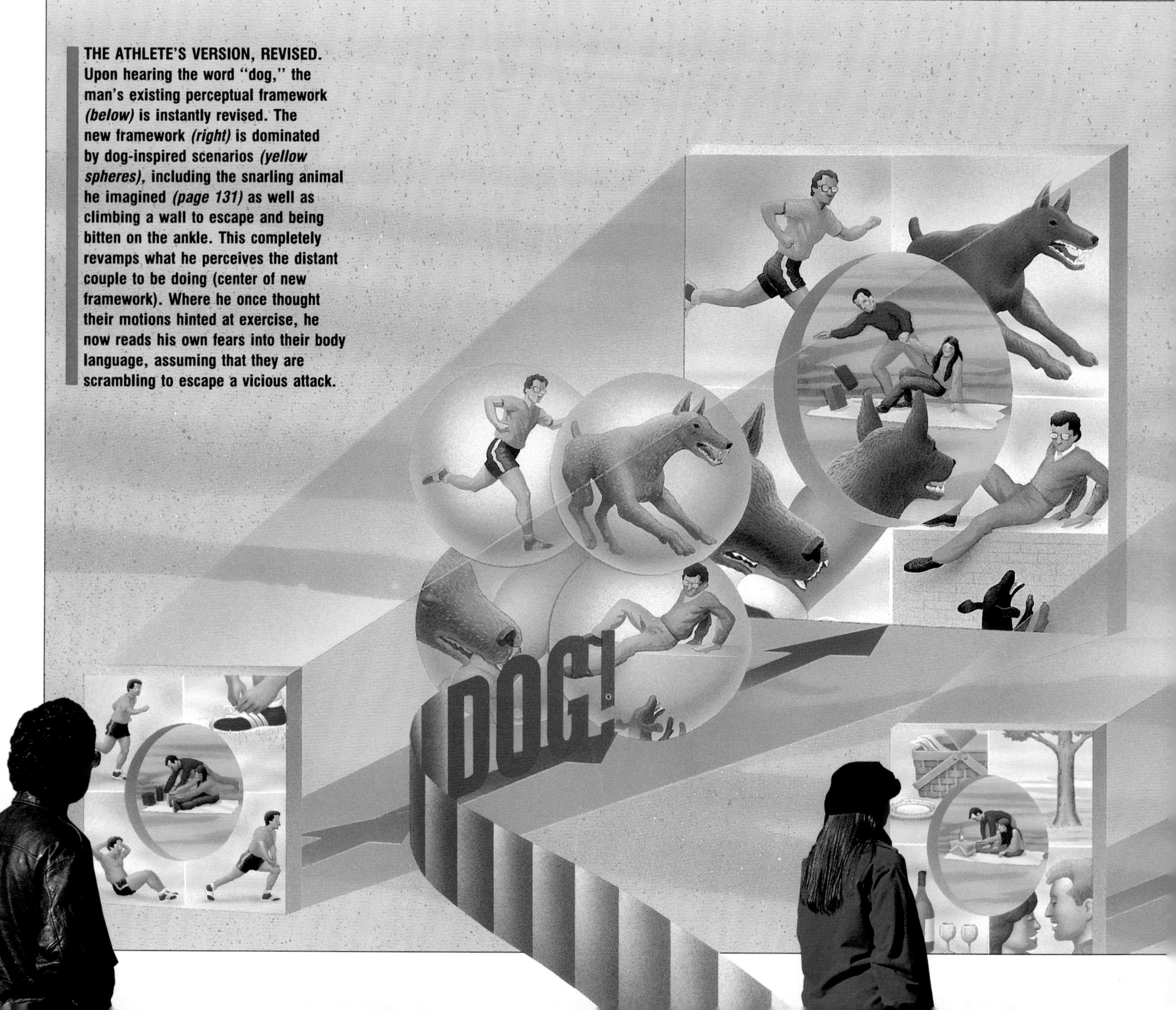

THE ATHLETE'S VERSION, REVISED. Upon hearing the word "dog," the man's existing perceptual framework *(below)* is instantly revised. The new framework *(right)* is dominated by dog-inspired scenarios *(yellow spheres),* including the snarling animal he imagined *(page 131)* as well as climbing a wall to escape and being bitten on the ankle. This completely revamps what he perceives the distant couple to be doing (center of new framework). Where he once thought their motions hinted at exercise, he now reads his own fears into their body language, assuming that they are scrambling to escape a vicious attack.

ample walk through the park, the activities of the distant pair may come into sharper focus, and the offstage dog may in fact enter the scene. As the perceptual frameworks of the strolling people adjust in response to new stimuli, the frameworks will to some degree grow more alike. But they will never be identical, because each of us interprets even small details differently—one of the profound truths of the human condition.

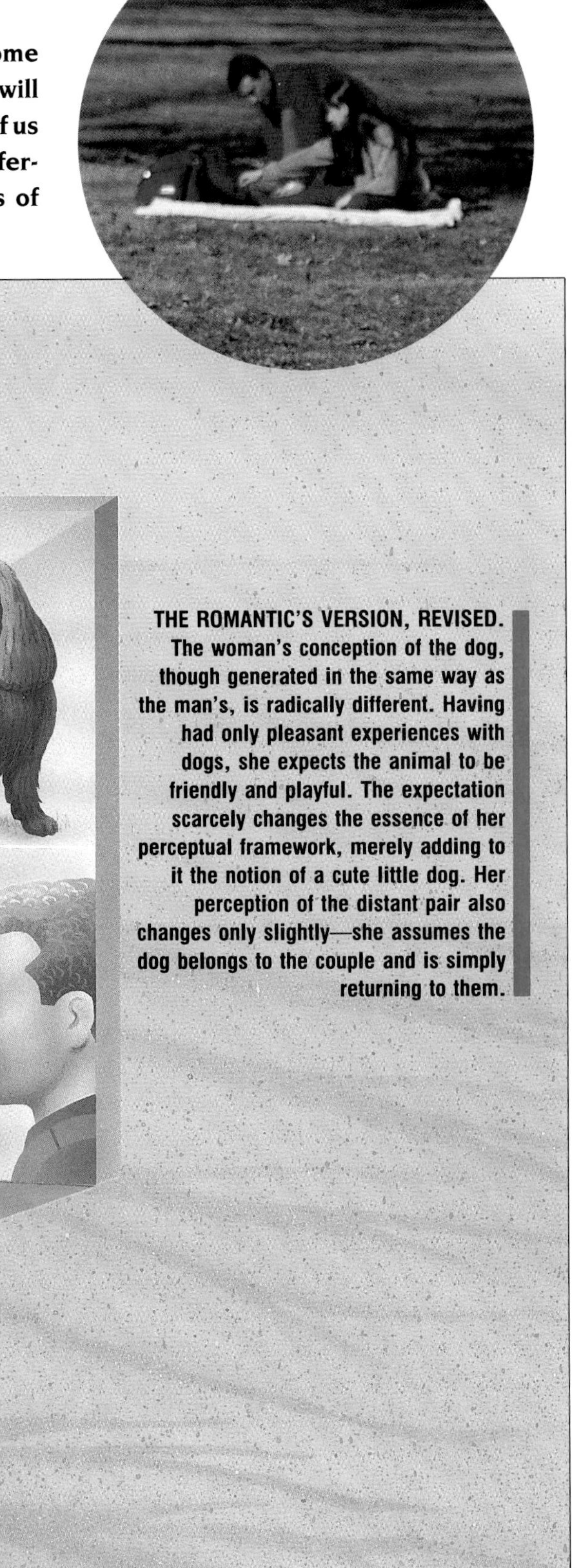

THE ROMANTIC'S VERSION, REVISED. The woman's conception of the dog, though generated in the same way as the man's, is radically different. Having had only pleasant experiences with dogs, she expects the animal to be friendly and playful. The expectation scarcely changes the essence of her perceptual framework, merely adding to it the notion of a cute little dog. Her perception of the distant pair also changes only slightly—she assumes the dog belongs to the couple and is simply returning to them.

GLOSSARY

Alzheimer's disease: an affliction that destroys areas of the limbic system and other parts of the brain, resulting in gradual loss of memory and the ability to think rationally; named for German neurologist Alois Alzheimer, who identified it in 1907.

Amygdala: a structure in the brain that helps generate emotions associated with thoughts or memories; from the Latin for "almond," a reference to its shape.

Aphasia: a condition, usually caused by injury to certain areas in the cerebral cortex, marked by loss of the ability to speak or understand written or spoken language.

Association areas: regions of the cerebral cortex that neither receive direct sensory input nor transmit direct motor signals but instead integrate sensory input with memories and plans for action.

Autonomic nervous system: the system of nerves that regulates involuntary bodily processes, such as blood pressure, heartbeat, breathing, or digestion.

Axon: the long fiber, extending as much as three feet from the cell body of a neuron, that transmits electrochemical impulses. Axons generally branch only near their tips.

Axon terminal: one of many structures at the branched end of an axon that convey electrochemical nerve impulses across the synaptic gap.

Basal ganglia: several clusters of neurons, located atop the brainstem within the two cerebral hemispheres, that play a role in memory and emotions and in coordinating movement.

Blood-brain barrier: the tight seal between cells that form the capillaries in the brain, isolating brain tissue from most harmful blood-borne substances.

Brainstem: the part of the brain that consists of the medulla, pons, and midbrain.

Broca's area: a region in the left frontal lobe of the cerebral cortex responsible for the physical aspects of producing speech; named for 19th-century French surgeon Paul Broca.

Cell assembly: according to one theory, a group of neurons that have exchanged impulses so often that the synapses between them have become easy to activate; the circuit thus forms an internal representation—or memory—of the stimulus.

Central nervous system: a component of the nervous system made up of the brain and spinal cord.

Cerebellum: a part of the brain, situated behind the brainstem and below the cerebrum, involved in coordinating complex movements.

Cerebral cortex: the outer, one-eighth-inch-thick covering of the cerebrum, divided into segments called lobes; the part of the brain most directly responsible for thought, memory, planning, and decision making.

Cerebrospinal fluid: a liquid that circulates throughout the brain and spinal cord; among other things, it supplies the brain with nutrients and hormones, and cushions it against shocks.

Cerebrum: the largest part of the brain, consisting of two hemispheres, overlain by the cerebral cortex; it is primarily responsible for voluntary movement and mental activity.

Computed tomography (CT): a method of combining x-rays taken from different angles to generate a three-dimensional picture of an internal part of the body.

Consciousness: on a physiological level, the state of being alert and aware of one's surroundings; on a psychological level, the state of being aware of one's own existence, thoughts, feelings, and so forth.

Corpus callosum: a thick band of neurons connecting the left and right cerebral hemispheres; from the Latin for "hard body."

Declarative memory: the conscious recollection of facts or experiences. *See* Procedural memory.

Dendrites: filaments that branch out from the body of a neuron to receive information transmitted by the axons of other neurons.

Dualism: a philosophical theory holding that the mind is a separate entity from the brain.

Electroencephalograph (EEG): a device that monitors the electric signals given off by neurons firing in the cerebral cortex.

Endocrine system: the network of endocrine glands in the body, as well as other organs that secrete hormones.

Endorphin: any of a class of molecules, produced naturally in the brain and in other tissues, that bind to the brain's opiate receptors; endorphins thus can act as painkillers and can induce a euphoric state of mind.

Epilepsy: a disorder of the nervous system marked by seizures resulting from the uncontrolled firing of neurons in the cerebral cortex.

Fever: an elevated body temperature brought about when the hypothalamus, in response to an infection, raises the body's temperature setpoint.

Fornix: a large bundle of nerve fibers that link each hippocampus to the mammillary bodies of the hypothalamus.

Frontal lobe: the portion of the cerebral cortex in each hemisphere that lies immediately behind the forehead; it is in these lobes that reasoning and decision making are carried out.

Functional localization: in neuroscience, the concept that different parts of the brain are responsible for performing different tasks.

General adaptation syndrome: a series of physical responses initiated by the hypothalamus in response to stress.

Gland: any of several organs within the body whose primary function is releasing various substances, especially hormones.

Gonads: the human sex glands; they consist of the testes in males and the ovaries in females.

Gray matter: any region of the central nervous system, such as the cerebral and cerebellar cortices, that is poor in myelin. *See* White matter.

Hippocampus: a seahorse-shaped structure, generally regarded as part of the limbic system, that is involved in the creation of emotions as well as in memory storage and retrieval.

Homeostasis: a condition of internal equilibrium, in which most of the body's proc-

esses function within limits set by the hypothalamus.
Hormones: chemicals released by glands and a few other organs that travel through the bloodstream and regulate the activities of specific tissues, organs, and other glands.
Hypothalamus: a small, olive-size structure, located just below the thalamus, that controls many of the body's autonomic functions.
Inhibitor neuron: a neuron whose firing suppresses the firing of other neurons.
Lateral geniculate nucleus: a region of the thalamus that relays visual information from the eye to other parts of the brain.
Limbic system: a group of structures within the brain, including the hippocampus and amygdala, thought to play a major role in emotions.
Locus ceruleus: a cluster of neurons in the brainstem that produces the neurotransmitter norepinephrine; from the Latin for "blue area," for the color of its cells.
Magnetic resonance imaging (MRI): a procedure that uses magnetic fields and radio waves to provide a highly detailed structural map of the brain.
Mammillary body: one of two structures in the hypothalamus that receives information from the hippocampus and sends information to other parts of the brain, such as the thalamus.
MANSCAN: for Mental Activity Network Scanner; a device that combines electroencephalograph readings with magnetic resonance imaging data to create a three-dimensional view of brain activity.
Materialism: A theory holding that the mind is not an entity on its own, but rather a by-product of the brain's activity. *See* Dualism.
Medulla: the lowest of the three segments of the brainstem, responsible for, among other things, the regulation of breathing and blood pressure.
Metabolism: the process by which the body's cells assimilate nutrients to produce energy.
Midbrain: the uppermost of the three segments of the brainstem, serving primarily as an intermediary between the rest of the brain and the spinal cord.
Motor cortex: a part of the cerebral cortex involved in movement; it receives instructions from the premotor cortex and then sends impulses to the appropriate muscle groups.
Motor neuron: a neuron that sends instructions from the brain to other parts of the body, especially muscles and glands.
Muscle memory: a type of procedural memory that stores the physical movements required to perform a task.
Myelin: a white fatty substance that insulates the axons of many neurons.
Nerve: one or many bundles of axons bound together that form the central and peripheral nervous systems.
Nerve impulse: an electrochemical signal that travels down the axon of a neuron.
Neurology: the study of the brain and nervous system and their disorders.
Neuron: a nerve cell, consisting of a central body from which extend a number of dendrites and a single axon; the human brain is made up of somewhere between 10 billion and 100 billion neurons.
Neurotransmitter: a chemical, synthesized by neurons, that carries information across the synaptic gap between neurons.
Occipital lobe: the rearmost section of the cerebral cortex in each hemisphere, responsible for processing vision and visual associations.
Olfactory bulb: a mass of neurons in the brain that relays information on smell from the nose to the amygdala and cerebral cortex.
Pain receptor: a sensory neuron that fires whenever tissue damage occurs.
Parietal lobe: the section in each hemisphere of the cerebral cortex, situated behind the frontal lobes, that deals with sensory and motor information.
Parietal-temporal-occipital association cortex: an area of the cerebral cortex that combines visual information with the sensory and emotional responses that accompany it.
Parkinsonism: an affliction whose symptoms appear in Parkinson's disease but also arise from external factors, such as drug abuse or repeated blows to the head, which severely damage cells in the substantia nigra.
Parkinson's disease: an affliction in which the substantia nigra stops producing the neurotransmitter dopamine; the symptoms include muscle weakness, tremors, and difficulty in speaking. It is named for English physician James Parkinson, who first described the disease early in the 19th century.
Perceptual framework: the memories and associations that deeply influence current perceptions.
Peripheral nervous system: the nerves that extend from the spinal cord throughout the rest of the body. It has two subcomponents: the autonomic nervous system, made up of the nerves that regulate involuntary functions like heartbeat; and the somatic nervous system, made up of the nerves that control voluntary functions, such as walking.
Pituitary gland: a structure located near the hypothalamus, which controls all other glands in the body through the release of hormones.
Plasticity: the ability of neurons or groups of neurons to acquire new functions.
Pons: the middle of the three segments of the brainstem. Its functions include linking the cerebral cortex to the cerebellum; from the Latin for "bridge."
Positron emission tomography (PET): a technique that traces emissions from a radioactive substance injected into a patient to produce a map of specific receptors in the brain.
Premotor cortex: an area of the cerebral cortex that formulates movement patterns and relays orders to the motor cortex.
Primary cortex: an area of the cerebral cortex that receives information regarding a specific sense and channels it to the appropriate areas of the brain for in-depth processing. There are primary cortices for hearing, vision, and bodily sensations.
Procedural memory: knowledge of a proc-

ess or procedure, such as how to ride a bicycle or solve a particular puzzle; this kind of memory is associated with the cerebellum and the basal ganglia.

Prosopagnosia: a disorder marked by the inability to recognize faces; it is caused by damage to the cerebral cortex.

Purkinje cell: a type of neuron, found in the cerebellum, capable of forming connections with as many as 150,000 other neurons; named for Czech physiologist Jan Purkinje, who described them in 1837.

Receptor: a large molecule on the surface of a neuron that is specially shaped to bind with a particular neurotransmitter.

Reticular formation: a network of neurons, extending from the spinal cord through the brainstem and into the cerebrum, that seems to affect virtually every aspect of nervous system function.

Secondary cortex: a part of the cerebral cortex responsible for the analysis of sensory information; it receives information from a corresponding primary cortex.

Sensory neuron: a neuron that sends a signal to the brain in response to an external stimulus, such as touch or heat.

Septum: a structure near the center of the brain that links the hippocampus and hypothalamus; believed to play a role in pleasurable emotions.

Setpoint: a standard value, set by the hypothalamus, for a particular bodily function, such as blood temperature.

Sham rage: a physical state induced in test animals through the stimulation of the hypothalamus and other parts of the brain; it involves outward manifestations of anger and aggressiveness without any emotional motivation.

Spinal cord: a thick cable of nerves and associated nerve cells, housed within the backbone, that relays impulses between the brain and the rest of the body; with the brain, part of the central nervous system.

Substantia nigra: a collection of neurons in the midbrain that produces the neurotransmitter dopamine; named for the cells' black color.

Synapse: a narrow gap, less than 1/1,000 of a millimeter across, between the axon terminal of the presynaptic, or sending, neuron and the dendrites or cell body of the postsynaptic, or receiving, neuron.

Synaptic vesicle: a structure, located in an axon terminal, that contains molecules of neurotransmitters.

Temporal lobe: the section of the cerebral cortex, on both sides of the brain, that is involved with, among other things, communication, hearing, and memory.

Thalamus: a structure within the brain that initially processes all sensory input except smell and routes it to the cerebral cortex.

Wernicke's area: a region in the left temporal lobe of the cerebral cortex, named after 19th-century German neurologist Carl Wernicke, responsible for recognizing the sounds of language.

White matter: bundles of nerve fibers within the central nervous system—white because their axons are coated with myelin—that link neurons in the spinal cord and in the cerebral and cerebellar cortices to other parts of the brain.

Working memory: memories that are temporarily stored in the cerebral cortex—and perhaps the hippocampus—for immediate use in decision making.

BIBLIOGRAPHY

BOOKS

Ackerman, Sandra. *Discovering the Brain.* Washington, D.C.: National Academy Press, 1992.

Adams, Raymond D., M.D., and Maurice Victor, M.D. *Principles of Neurology* (4th ed.). New York: McGraw-Hill, 1989.

Adelman, George (ed.). *Encyclopedia of Neuroscience* (Vols. I and II). Boston: Birkhäuser, 1987.

Altman, Harvey J. (ed.). *Alzheimer's Disease.* New York: Plenum Press, 1987.

Andreasen, Nancy C. *The Broken Brain.* New York: Harper & Row, 1984.

Atlas of the Body. New York: Rand McNally, 1980.

Bailey, Ronald H., and the Editors of Time-Life Books. *The Role of the Brain* (Human Behavior series). New York: Time-Life Books, 1975.

Beaumont, J. Graham (ed.). *Brain Power.* New York: Harper & Row, 1990.

Bevan, James. *Anatomy and Physiology.* New York: Simon and Schuster, 1978.

Bloom, Floyd E., and Arlyne Lazerson. *Brain, Mind, and Behavior* (2d ed.). New York: W. H. Freeman, 1985.

The Brain. New York: G. P. Putnam's Sons, 1982.

Changeux, Jean-Pierre. *Neuronal Man.* New York: Random House, 1985.

Coleman, P. D., and D. G. Flood. "Dendritic Proliferation in the Aging Brain as a Compensatory Repair Mechanism." In *Aging of the Brain and Alzheimer's Disease* (Vol. 70 of *Progress in Brain Research*). Edited by D. F. Swaab, et al. New York: Elsevier Science, 1986.

Diamond, Marian C., Arnold B. Scheibel, and Lawrence M. Elson. *The Human Brain Coloring Book.* New York: HarperCollins, 1985.

Fincher, Jack. *The Brain: Mystery of Matter and Mind* (The Human Body series). Washington, D.C.: U.S. News Books, 1981.

Frank, Joseph. *Dostoevsky: The Years of Ordeal.* Princeton, N.J.: Princeton University Press, 1983.

Gazzaniga, Michael S.:

Mind Matters. Boston: Houghton Mifflin, 1988.

The Social Brain. New York: Basic Books, 1985.

Gilling, Dick, and Robin Brightwell. *The Human Brain.* New York: Facts on File, 1982.

Grollman, Sigmund. *The Human Body: Its Structure and Physiology* (4th ed.). New York: Macmillan, 1978.

Hampden-Turner, Charles. *Maps of the Mind.* New York: Macmillan, 1981.

Hauser, Thomas. *Muhammad Ali: His Life and Times.* New York: Simon & Schuster, 1991.

Hooper, Judith, and Dick Teresi. *The Three-Pound Universe.* New York: Putnam, 1992.

Isaacson, Robert Lee. *The Limbic System.* New York: Plenum Press, 1974.

Jones, Edward G. "The Anatomy of Sensory Relay Functions in the Thalamus." In *Role of the Forebrain in Sensation and Behavior* (Vol. 87 of *Progress in Brain Research*). Edited by G. Holstege. New York: Elsevier Science, 1991.

Jubak, Jim. *In the Image of the Brain.* Boston: Little, Brown, 1992.

Julien, Robert M. *A Primer of Drug Action* (6th ed.). New York: W. H. Freeman, 1992.

Kandel, Eric R., James H. Schwartz, and Thomas M. Jessell (eds.). *Principles of Neural Science* (3d ed.). New York: Elsevier Science, 1991.

Kapit, Wynn, Robert I. Macey, and Esmail Meisami. *The Physiology Coloring Book.* New York: HarperCollins, 1987.

Kjetsaa, Geir. *Fjodor Dostojevskij—et dikterliv.* Oslo: Gyldendal Norsk Forlag, 1985.

Kolb, Bryan, and Ian Q. Whishaw. *Fundamentals of Human Neuropsychology* (3d ed.). New York: W. H. Freeman, 1990.

Kosslyn, Stephen Michael. *Wet Mind: The New Cognitive Neuroscience.* New York: Macmillan, 1992.

Kuffler, Stephen W. *From Neuron to Brain* (2d ed.). Sunderland, Mass.: Sinauer Associates, 1984.

LeDoux, Joseph E., and William Hirst (eds.). *Mind and Brain.* New York: Cambridge University Press, 1986.

Legg, Charles R. *Issues of Psychobiology.* New York: Routledge, 1989.

Liebman, Michael. *Neuroanatomy Made Easy and Understandable* (4th ed.). Gaithersburg, Md.: Aspen, 1991.

McGoon, Dwight C. *The Parkinson's Handbook.* New York: W. W. Norton, 1990.

Martin, John H. *Neuroanatomy.* New York: Elsevier Science, 1989.

Melzack, Ronald, and Patrick D. Wall. *The Challenge of Pain* (rev. ed.). New York: Basic Books, 1983.

Mind and Brain. New York: Cambridge University Press, 1986.

Netter, Frank H., M.D. *Nervous System* (Vol. 1 of *The CIBA Collection of Medical Illustrations*): *Anatomy and Physiology* (Part 1). Ed. by Alister Brass, M.D. West Caldwell, N.J.: CIBA Pharmaceutical, 1983.

Niedermeyer, Ernst, M.D. *The Epilepsies: Diagnosis and Management.* Baltimore: Urban & Schwarzenberg, 1990.

Nilsson, Lennart. *The Incredible Machine.* Washington, D.C.: National Geographic Society, 1986.

Ornstein, Robert, and David Sobel. *The Healing Brain.* New York: Simon and Schuster, 1987.

Ornstein, Robert, and Richard F. Thompson. *The Amazing Brain.* Boston: Houghton Mifflin, 1984.

Pandya, Deepak N., Benjamin Seltzer, and Helen Barbas. "Input-Output Organization of the Primate Cerebral Cortex." In *Comparative Primate Biology, Vol. 4: Neurosciences.* Edited by Horst D. Steklis and J. Erwin. New York: Wiley, 1988.

Peters, Alan, Sanford L. Palay, and Henry deF. Webster. *The Fine Structure of the Nervous System* (3d ed.). New York: Oxford University Press, 1991.

Plutchik, Robert, and Henry Kellerman (eds.). *Emotion: Theory, Research, and Experience, Vol. 3: Biological Foundations of Emotion.* Orlando: Academic Press, 1986.

Restak, Richard M.:

The Brain. New York: Bantam Books, 1984.

The Brain Has a Mind of Its Own. New York: Crown, 1991.

The Brain: The Last Frontier. New York: Warner Books, 1979.

The Mind. New York: Bantam Books, 1988.

Rice, James L. *Dostoevsky and the Healing Art.* Ann Arbor, Mich.: Ardis, 1985.

Rosenfield, Israel. *The Invention of Memory.* New York: Basic Books, 1988.

Sacks, Oliver W.:

Awakenings. New York: HarperCollins, 1990.

The Man Who Mistook His Wife for a Hat and Other Clinical Tales. New York: Simon & Schuster, 1985.

Silverstein, Alvin. *World of the Brain.* New York: William Morrow, 1986.

Smith, Anthony. *The Mind.* New York: The Viking Press, 1984.

Snell, Richard S., M.D. *Clinical Neuroanatomy for Medical Students* (3d ed.). Boston: Little, Brown, 1992.

Snyder, Solomon H. *Drugs and the Brain.* New York: Scientific American Books, 1986.

Springer, Sally P., and Georg Deutsch. *Left Brain, Right Brain.* New York: W. H. Freeman, 1981.

Squire, Larry. *Memory and Brain.* New York: Oxford University Press, 1987.

Thompson, Richard F.:

Introduction to Physiological Psychology. New York: Harper & Row, 1975.

The Brain. New York: W. H. Freeman, 1985.

Tortora, Gerard J., and Nicholas P. Anagnostakos. *Principles of Anatomy and Physiology* (6th ed.). New York: HarperCollins, 1990.

Vander, Arthur J., James H. Sherman, and Dorothy S. Luciano. *Human Physiology: The Mechanisms of Body Function* (5th ed.). New York: McGraw-Hill, 1990.

Wilson-Pauwels, Linda, Elizabeth J. Akesson, and Patricia A. Stewart. *Cranial Nerves.* Toronto: B. C. Decker, 1988.

Winson, Jonathan. *Brain and Psyche.* New York: Anchor/Doubleday, 1985.

Wozniak, Robert H. *Mind and Body: René Descartes to William James.* Bethesda, Md.: National Library of Medicine and Washington, D.C.: American Psychological Association, 1992.

Zeki, Semir. *Colour Vision and Functional Specialisation in the Visual Cortex* (Vol. 4, no. 2 of *Discussions in Neuroscience*). Amsterdam: Elsevier Science, 1990.

PERIODICALS

Alajouanine, T. "Dostoiewski's Epilepsy." *Brain*, June 1963.

Begley, Sharon, et al. "Mapping the Brain." *Newsweek*, Apr. 20, 1992.

Berk, Lee S., et al. "Neuroendocrine and Stress Hormone Changes During Mirthful Laughter." *The American Journal of the Medical Sciences*, Dec. 1989.

Bick, C. H. "An EEG-Mapping Study of 'Laughing': Coherence and Brain Dominances." *International Journal of Neuroscience*, 1989, Vol. 47, nos. 1-2.

Black, Donald W. "Laughter." JAMA, Dec. 7, 1984.

Blakeslee, Sandra:

"The Brain May 'See' What Eyes Cannot." *New York Times*, Jan. 15, 1991.

"Nerve Cell Rhythm May Be Key to Consciousness." *New York Times*, Oct. 27, 1992.

Bliss, T. V. P., and G. L. Collingridge. "A Synaptic Model of Memory: Long-Term Potentiation in the Hippocampus." *Nature*, Jan. 7, 1993

"The Brain Remaps Its Own Contours." *Science*, Oct. 9, 1992.

Cousins, Norman. "Anatomy of an Illness (As Perceived by the Patient)." *The New England Journal of Medicine*, Dec. 23, 1976.

Crick, Francis, and Christof Koch. "The Problem of Consciousness." *Scientific American*, Sept. 1992.

Damasio, Antonio R., and Hanna Damasio. "Brain and Language." *Scientific American*, Sept. 1992.

Derryberry, Douglas, and Don M. Tucker. "Neural Mechanisms of Emotion." *Journal of Consulting and Clinical Psychology*, June 1992.

Eichenbaum, Howard, Tim Otto, and Neal J. Cohen. "The Hippocampus—What Does It Do?" *Behavioral and Neural Biology*, Jan. 1992.

Elmer-Dewitt, Philip. "Depression: The Growing Role of Drug Therapies." *Time*, July 6, 1992.

Fischbach, Gerard D. "Mind and Brain." *Scientific American*, Sept. 1992.

Fry, William F., Jr. "The Physiologic Effects of Humor, Mirth, and Laughter." JAMA, Apr. 1, 1992.

Gazzaniga, Michael S. "Organization of the Human Brain." *Science*, Sept. 1, 1989.

Gelman, D. "Is the Mind an Illusion?" *Newsweek*, Apr. 20, 1992.

Gershon, Elliot S., and Ronald O. Rieder. "Major Disorders of Mind and Brain." *Scientific American*, Sept. 1992.

Goldman-Rakic, Patricia S. "Working Memory and the Mind." *Scientific American*, Sept. 1992.

Guérit, Jean-Michel. "Les Comas." *La Recherche*, Sept. 1990.

Haier, Richard J., et al. "Regional Glucose Metabolic Changes After Learning." *Brain Research*, 1992, Vol. 570.

Hinton, Geoffrey E. "How Neural Networks Learn from Experience." *Scientific American*, Sept. 1992.

Hoffman, Paul. "Your Mindless Brain." *Discover*, Sept. 1987.

Hubel, David H. "The Brain." *Scientific American*, Sept. 1979.

Jacobson, Robin. "Disorders of Facial Recognition, Social Behaviour and Affect after Combined Bilateral Amygdalotomy and Subcaudate Tractotomy—a Clinical and Experimental Study." *Psychological Medicine*, 1986, Vol. 16, pp. 439-450.

Kandel, Eric R., and Robert D. Hawkins. "The Biological Basis of Learning and Individuality." *Scientific American*, Sept. 1992.

Kinoshita, June. "Mapping the Mind." *New York Times Magazine*, Oct. 18, 1992.

Kolata, Gina. "Improved Scanner Watches the Brain as It Thinks." *New York Times*, July 14, 1992.

Levy, David E., et al. "Differences in Cerebral Blood Flow and Glucose Utilization in Vegetative versus Locked-in Patients." *Annals of Neurology*, Dec. 1987.

Levy, Jerre, Colwyn Trevarthen, and R. W. Sperry. "Perception of Bilateral Chimeric Figures Following Hemispheric Deconnexion." *Brain*, 1972, Vol. 95.

McAuliffe, Kathleen. "Get Smart: Controlling Chaos." *Omni*, Feb. 1990.

Mackowiak, Philip A., Steven S. Wasserman, and Myron M. Levine. "A Critical Appraisal of 98.6° F, the Upper Limit of the Normal Body Temperature, and Other Legacies of Carl Reinhold August Wunderlich." JAMA, Sept. 23/30, 1992.

Milner, Peter M. "The Mind and Donald O. Hebb." *Scientific American*, Jan. 1993.

Montgomery, Geoffrey. "The Mind in Motion." *Discover*, Mar. 1989.

Palca, Joseph. "Famous Monkeys Provide Surprising Results." *Science*, June 28, 1991.

Pennisi, E. "Neural-net Neighbors Learn from Each Other." *Science News*, Jan. 11, 1992.

"Persistent Vegetative State and the Decision to Withdraw or Withhold Life Support." JAMA, Jan. 19, 1990.

Selkoe, Dennis J. "Aging Brain, Aging Mind." *Scientific American*, Sept. 1992.

Shatz, Carla J. "The Developing Brain." *Scientific American*, Sept. 1992.

Sochurek, Howard. "Medicine's New Vision." *National Geographic*, Jan. 1987.

Squire, Larry R. "Memory and the Hippocampus: A Synthesis from Findings with Rats, Monkeys, and Humans." *Psychological Review*, Apr. 1992.

Squire, Larry R., and Stuart Zola-Morgan. "The Medial Temporal Lobe Memory System." *Science*, Sept. 20, 1991.

Stevens, Charles F. "The Neuron." *Scientific American*, Sept. 1979.

Swaab, D. F. "Brain Aging and Alzheimer's Disease, 'Wear and Tear' versus 'Use It or Lose It'." *Neurobiology of Aging*, July/Aug. 1991.

Weiss, Rick. "Shadows of Thoughts Revealed." *Science News*, Nov. 10, 1990.

"Wonder Cures from the Fringe." *U.S. News & World Report*, Sept. 23, 1991.

Zeki, Semir. "The Visual Image in Mind and Brain." *Scientific American*, Sept. 1992.

OTHER SOURCES

Bowen, D. M., and A. N. Davison. "Neurotransmitters in the Ageing Brain and Dementia." Department of Neurochemistry, Institute of Neurology, London.

"Brain Transplant." NOVA television series transcript, program #1918. Boston: WGBH Educational Foundation, Dec. 1, 1992.

INDEX

Numerals in bold indicate an illustration of the subject mentioned.

A

B

C

ACKNOWLEDGMENTS

The editors of *Mind and Brain* would like to thank these individuals for their valuable contributions:

Nancy C. Andreasen, University of Iowa, Iowa City; Anne A. Androski, The Graduate Hospital, Philadelphia; Barbara Barres, Stanford University, Stanford, Calif.; Lee S. Berk, Loma Linda University, Loma Linda, Calif.; Guido Buldrini, Rome; Robert Cohen, The Memphis Commercial Appeal, Memphis; Paul D. Coleman, University of Rochester, Rochester, N.Y.; Philippe Dacla, CNRI, Paris; Antonio R. Damasio, University of Iowa, Iowa City; Michel Ferin, Columbia University, New York; Howard L. Fields, University of California, San Francisco; Albert Fuchs, University of Washington, Seattle; Karen Gale, Georgetown University, Washington, D.C.; Charles R. Gerfen, National Institute of Mental Health, Bethesda, Md.; Alan Gevins, EEG Systems Laboratory, San Francisco; Alan Gibson, Barrow Neurological Institute, Phoenix; Richard Haier, University of California, Irvine, Calif.; Ron Harper, University of California, Los Angeles; Robert Heath, Tulane University, New Orleans; Stewart Hendry, The Johns Hopkins University, Baltimore; James Houk, Northwestern University, Evanston, Ill.; Robert L. Isaacson, State University of New York, Binghamton; Thomas M. Jessell, Columbia University, New York; Peter Jezzard, National Institutes of Health, Bethesda, Md.; Edward G. Jones, University of California, Irvine, Calif.; Lucinda Keister, National Library of Medicine, Bethesda, Md.; Mary Kritzer, Yale University, New Haven, Conn.; Irvin Kupfermann, New York State Psychiatric Institute, New York; Jan Lazarus, National Library of Medicine, Bethesda, Md.; Joseph LeDoux, New York University, New York; Thomas G. McCarter, University of Pennsylvania, Philadelphia; James McGaugh, University of California, Irvine; Wallace Mendelson, State University of New York, Stony Brook; Robert Y. Moore, University of Pittsburgh, Pittsburgh; William Pardridge, University of California, Los Angeles; Karen Pruitt, Custom Medical Stock Photo, Chicago; Marcus E. Raichle, Washington University, St. Louis; Paul E. Rapp, Medical College of Pennsylvania, Philadelphia; Allan Rechtschaffen, University of Chicago, Chicago; David A. Roberts, University of Pennsylvania, Philadelphia; Dennis Selkoe, Brigham and Women's Hospital, Boston; Ann Silverman, Columbia University, New York; Susan Spencer, Yale University, New Haven, Conn.; William Theodore, National Institutes of Health, Bethesda, Md.; Robert Turner, National Institutes of Health, Bethesda, Md.; Cornelius Vanderwolf, The University of Western Ontario, London, Ont.; Richard Wagner, National Institutes of Health, Bethesda, Md.; Joan Witkin, Columbia University, New York; Tony Yaksh, University of California, San Diego; Semir Zeki, University of London, London.

PICTURE CREDITS

The sources for the illustrations in this volume are listed below. Credits from left to right are separated by semicolons, from top to bottom by dashes.

Cover: Ray Moller, London—projected image Antonio Rosaria/The Image Bank. **7:** Art by Alfred T. Kamajian—Tim Bieber/The Image Bank—Christopher Morris/Black Star—Michael Freeman, London. **8, 9:** Walter Hodges/Westlight—Michael Freeman, London, image manipulation by Time-Life Books. **11:** CNRI/Science Photo Library/Photo Researchers. **12, 13:** Victoria Bracewell Short-Photo Illustration/Tielmans-duomo. **14, 15:** Art by Stephen R. Wagner. **16:** Howard Sochurek/Woodfin Camp and Associates. **17:** Richard J. Haier/University of California, Irvine. **18:** Dan McCoy/Rainbow—Peter Jezzard/National Institutes of Health, Bethesda, Md. **19:** Dr. Alan Gevins/EEG Systems Laboratory and SAM Technology, San Francisco. **22, 23:** National Library of Medicine (7); courtesy Columbia University, New York. **25:** Art by Alfred T. Kamajian. **26, 27:** Art by Alfred T. Kamajian, inset art by Andrew Reynolds. **28-33:** Art by Alfred T. Kamajian. **34, 35:** Tim Bieber/The Image Bank. **37:** Manny Milan/Sports Illustrated. **41:** © Guigoz/Dr. A. Privat (Petit Format) Science Source/Photo Researchers—photo by Lennart Nilsson, *The Incredible Machine*, National Geographic Society, Washington, D.C., 1986. **42, 43:** Photo by © Dr. Dennis Kunkel/PhotoTake, New York; art by Alfred T. Kamajian. **45:** Superstock—© Dr. Dennis Kunkel/PhotoTake, New York. **47:** Dr. J. M. Guerit/Catholic University of Louvain, Belgium. **49:** Art by Michael Koelsch. **50-57:** Top art by Michael Koelsch (3)—art by Edmond Alexander and Cynthia Turner of Alexander & Turner. **58, 59:** Christopher Morris/Black Star. **61:** Warren Anatomical Museum, Harvard Medical School, Boston. **62, 63:** Art by Stephen R. Wagner. **66:** Fatima Taylor; Sidney Moulds/Science Photo Library/Custom Medical Stock Photo. **69:** J. P. Laffont/Sygma. **70, 71:** Art by Stephen R. Wagner. **74, 75:** Art by Stephen R. Wagner, photo by Michael Hart/FPG. **77:** Library of Congress, *Fjodor Dostojevskij - et dikterliv*, Gyldendal Norsk Forlag A/S, Oslo, 1985; William H. Theodore, M.D. **78:** Larry R. Squire/Veteran Affairs Medical Center, San Diego, and University of California School of Medicine, San Diego—Fil Hunter. **79:** Preston Lyon/Index Stock. **80:** Nancy C. Andreasen/University of Iowa College of Medicine, Iowa City. **81:** Art by Tipy Taylor. **83:** © Dr. Dennis Kunkel/PhotoTake, New York (2), image manipulation by Time-Life Books. **84, 85:** Art by Stephen R. Wagner. **86-91:** Photos by Mark H. Rogers; art by Stephen R. Wagner. **92, 93:** Dan McCoy/Rainbow—Michael Freeman, London, image manipulation by Time-Life Books. **95:** Brian F. Alpert/Keystone. **96, 97:** Art by Matt McMullen. **100, 101:** Photo by Evan H. Sheppard—art by Matt McMullen. **102, 103:** Art by Tipy Taylor. **104, 105:** Biophoto Associates/Photo Researchers. **106:** Photo by Alan Becker/The Image Bank—art by Will Williams of Wood, Ronsaville, Harlin, Inc. **107:** Soccer art by Tipy Taylor (3)—head art by Will Williams of Wood, Ronsaville, Harlin, Inc. (2)—photo by Alan Becker/The Image Bank. **109:** Dr. Alan Gevins/EEG Systems Laboratory and SAM Technology, San Francisco. **112:** Art by Tipy Taylor. **115, 116:** Art by Will Williams of Wood, Ronsaville, Harlin, Inc. **117:** Marcus E. Raichle, M.D./Washington University School of Medicine, St. Louis. **118:** Mike Peres/Custom Medical Stock Photo, Inc. **120, 121:** Art by Will Williams of Wood, Ronsaville, Harlin, Inc.; photos by Chuck O'Rear/Westlight—art by Tipy Taylor. **125:** Paul E. Rapp. **127:** Evan H. Sheppard. **128-133:** Photos by Evan H. Sheppard—art by Stephen R. Wagner.